Cancer Drug Discovery and Development

Series Editor

Beverly A. Teicher
National Cancer Institute, Rockville, MD, USA

For further volumes:
http://www.springer.com/series/7625

Gail Lewis Phillips
Editor

Antibody-Drug Conjugates and Immunotoxins

From Pre-Clinical Development to Therapeutic Applications

Humana Press

Editor
Gail Lewis Phillips
Genentech, Inc.,
South San Francisco, CA, USA

ISBN 978-1-4614-5455-7 ISBN 978-1-4614-5456-4 (eBook)
DOI 10.1007/978-1-4614-5456-4
Springer New York Heidelberg Dordrecht London

Library of Congress Control Number: 2012948341

Printed on acid-free paper

Humana Press is a brand of Springer
Springer is part of Springer Science+Business Media (www.springer.com)

This book is dedicated to the memory of Dr. Ralph Schwall and to my mentor, colleague, and friend, Dr. Mark Sliwkowski, for their unwavering belief in the promise of antibody–drug conjugates for targeted cancer therapy.

Gail Lewis Phillips, Editor

Contents

Part I
Introduction and Development Perspectives

Chapter 1
Antibody Directed Delivery for Treatment of Cancer: Antibody Drug Conjugates and Immunotoxins

Pamela A. Trail

Introduction

A major goal in the development of cancer therapeutics is to identify agents that will effectively eradicate tumors while having minimal effects on cells of normal tissues. Unfortunately, the majority of anticancer agents developed to date have substantial side effect profiles and a narrow therapeutic index. One means to improve the selectivity and efficacy of cancer therapy is by choosing therapeutic targets with altered levels of expression on malignant versus normal cells. Following the introduction of monoclonal antibody (MAb) technology by [1], the potential to utilize the antigen-selectivity of MAbs to deliver toxic agents initiated an extensive effort to design antibody-targeted therapeutics. The clinical utility of MAb based therapeutics was substantially improved by both the chimerization and humanization of murine MAbs, both of which reduced immunogenicity and improved MAb half-life. The ability to obtain fully human MAbs from transgenic mice and by phage display has further enhanced the clinical potential of these approaches [2–4]. Monoclonal antibodies and fragments of MAbs have been used to effectively deliver radionuclides [5, 6], cytokines [7, 8], plant and bacterial toxins, [9–11], and a variety of cytotoxic drugs [12–15]. Although simple in concept, the design of effective targeting agents has required substantial investigation and modification in the selection of MAbs and their targets, the types of linkers used, and the potency of the toxic agents that are delivered. This chapter will focus on MAb-directed delivery of plant and bacterial toxins (immunotoxins) and MAb-directed delivery of cytoxic drugs (antibody drug conjugates: ADCs).

P.A. Trail (✉)
Regeneron Pharmaceuticals Inc.,777 Old Saw Mill River Road, Tarrytown, New York, NY, 10591, USA
e-mail: pamela.trail@regeneron.com

G.L. Phillips (ed.), *Antibody-Drug Conjugates and Immunotoxins: From Pre-Clinical Development to Therapeutic Applications*, Cancer Drug Discovery and Development, DOI 10.1007/978-1-4614-5456-4_1,

Targets for Immunotoxins and ADCs

In contrast to function blocking monoclonal antibodies (MAbs) and small molecules therapeutics, antibody–drug conjugates (ADCs) and immunotoxin targets do not need to be causal in tumor progression. Rather the target antigens need to be expressed on the cell surface of malignant cells, have a limited normal tissue distribution, and be internalized following antigen-specific binding of the immunotoxin or ADC. An additional consideration in the selection of both the target and the design of the targeting construct is the nature of intracellular trafficking of the antigen. Targets that are rapidly and efficiently trafficked to lysosomes are appropriate for ADCs that require lysosomal cleavage or MAb degradation for drug release but may be problematic for protein immunotoxins that would themselves be degraded.

Immunotoxin and ADC targets include cell surface antigens expressed on hematologic malignancies and epithelial tumors. For the most part, tumor-specific antigens have not been identified and as such both immunotoxins and ADCs utilize MAbs to tumor-associated antigens. These are typically antigens expressed on malignant cells with limited expression on cells of normal tissues, antigens that are expressed at much higher density on malignant versus normal cells, or antigens that are developmentally expressed. It is optimal for target antigens to be expressed homogeneously and at high density on the cell surface of malignant cells. Homogeneous antigen expression is particularly important for immunotoxins and also for those ADCs that lack bystander killing activity. Lineage specific antigens, such as CD19, that are expressed on both normal and malignant B cells but absent on progenitor cells, are attractive as targets as evidenced by the ongoing clinical evaluation of both CD19-directed immunotoxins and ADCs. Combotox, a mixture of two immunotoxins in which deglycosylated Ricin A (dgRTA) is chemically linked to MAbs to CD19 (HD37-dgRTA) and CD22 (RFB4-dgRTA) [16] is in a Phase 1 trial in relapsed/refractory B-lineage acute lymphoblastic leukemia. SAR-3419, an ADC in which an anti-CD19 MAb is linked to the maytansine analog DM4, is currently being evaluated in a Phase II trial in NHL [17]. Immunotoxin and ADC targets with disclosed targets that are currently under clinical investigation are summarized in Tables 1.1 and 1.2, respectively.

In addition to targets expressed on malignant cells, there are ongoing efforts to develop immunotoxins and ADCs to antigens expressed on the tumor vasculature. These approaches seek to exploit differences in the level of antigen expression and/or the higher proliferation rate of endothelial cells of the tumor vasculature versus those of the normal tissues. Several endothelial targets considered to meet these criteria are being evaluated in preclinical studies [18]. Endoglin (CD105) is selectively expressed on vascular and lymphatic endothelium in tumors and Ricin A-based immunotoxins of anti-CD105 MAbs have demonstrated activity and a therapeutic index in preclinical models [19, 20]. Prostate-specific antigen is expressed on prostate cancer cells and also selectively expressed on vascular endothelial cells present in malignant solid tumors but not normal vasculature [21, 22]. To date two anti-PSMA ADCs have been evaluated clinically. MLN2704 is an ADC comprised of the deimmunized anti-PSMA MAb MLN591 conjugated to the maytansinoid DM1 via

Table 1.1 Immunotoxins currently in clinical development

Designation	Target antigen	Antibody/fragment	Toxin	Construct	Developer stage[a]	Tumor indication(s)
Imtox-25 (RFT5-dgA)	CD25	Murine IgG1	Deglycosylated ricin A	Chemical	Phase II	Adult T cell leukemia/lymphoma
Combotox (HD37-dgRTA and RFB4-dgRTA)	CD19 and CD22	Murine IgG1s	Deglycosylated ricin A	Chemical	Phase I	B cell adult acute lymphoblastic leukemia/acute lymphoblastic leukemia
Hum-195/rGel	CD33	Humanized IgG1	Recombinant gelonin	Chemical	Phase I	Acute myeloid leukemia/chronic myelomonocytic leukemia
LMB-2	CD25	scFv	Pseudomonas exotoxin PE38	Recombinant	Phase II	Chronic lymphocytic leukemia/cutaneous T cell lymphoma
CAT-8015 Moxetumomab pasudotox	CD22	dsFv	Pseudomonas exotoxin PE38	Recombinant	Phase I/II	B cell non-Hodgkin lymphoma and chronic lymphocytic leukemia
SS1P	Mesothelin	dsFv	Pseudomonas exotoxin PE38	Recombinant	Phase 1	Mesothelioma
MR1-1	Epidermal growth factor receptor VIII	scFv	Pseudomonas exotoxin PE38KDEL	Recombinant	Phase I	Brain tumors

[a]Source: Clinicaltrials.gov: December 2011

Table 1.2 Antibody drug conjugates currently in clinical development[a]

ADC designations	Target antigen	Antibody	Linker	Drug class	Development stage[b]	Tumor indication(s)	Developer
Brentuximab vedotin SGN-35	CD30	Ch IgG1	Valine–citrulline	Auristatin MMAE	Approved	Hodgkin lymphoma/ALCL	Seattle Genetics
Inotuzumab ozogamicin CMC-544	CD22	Hz IgG4	Hydrazone	Calicheamicin	Phase III	non-Hodgkin lymphoma	Pfizer
Gemtuzumab ozogamicin	CD33	Hz IgG4	Hydrazone	Calicheamicin	Phase II	Relapsed AML	Pfizer
SAR3419	CD19	Hz IgG1	Hindered disulfide (SPDB)	Maytansine DM4	Phase II	non-Hodgkin lymphoma	sanofi
RG7593 DCDT2980S	CD22	Hz IgG1	Valine–citrulline	Auristatin MMAE	Phase I	Hematologic malignancies	Genentech/Roche
BT062 nBT062-SPDB-DM4	CD138	Ch IgG4	Hindered disulfide (SPDB)	Maytansine DM4	Phase I	Multiple myeloma	Biotest
Trastuzumab-emtansine T-DM1	HER2 ErbB2	Hz IgG1	Thioether (SMCC)	Maytansine DM1	Phase III	Breast cancer	Genentech/Roche
Glembatumomab vedotin CDX-011, CR011vcMMAE	Glycoprotein NMB	Hu IgG2	Valine–citrulline	Auristatin MMAE	Phase II	Breast cancer/ melanoma	Celldex Therapeutics

Lorvotuzumab mertansine IMGN901	CD56	Hz IgG1	Hindered disulfide (SPP)	Maytansine DM1	Phase I/II	Solid tumors/ multiple myeloma	Immunogen
AGS-5ME	SLC44A4	Hu IgG2	Valine–citrulline	Auristatin MMAE	Phase I	Pancreatic and prostate cancer	Astellas
SAR566658 HuDS6-DM4	CA6	Hu IgG1	Hindered disulfide (SPDB)	Maytansine DM4	Phase I	Solid tumors	Sanofi
BAY 79-4620	CA-IX	Hu IgG1	Valine–citrulline	Auristatin MMAE	Phase I	Solid tumors	Bayer
BAY 94-9343	Mesothelin	Hu IgG1	Hindered disulfide	Maytansine DM4	Phase I	Solid tumors	Bayer
SGN-75	CD70	Hz IgG1	Maleimidocaproyl	Auristatin MMAF	Phase I	Renal cell carcinoma/ non-Hodgkin lymphoma	Seattle Genetics
MDX-1203	CD70	Hu IgG1	Valine–citrulline	Duocarmycin MGBA	Phase I	Renal cell carcinoma/ non-Hodgkin lymphoma	Bristol-Myers Squibb
Anti-PSMA ADC	PSMA	Hu IgG1	Valine–citrulline	Auristatin MMAE	Phase I	Prostate cancer	Progenics
ASG-22ME	Nectin-4	Hu IgG1	Valine–citrulline	Auristatin MMAE	Phase I	Solid tumors	Astellas
hLL1-DOX	CD74	Hz IgG1	Hydrazone	Doxorubicin	Phase I	Multiple myeloma	Immunomedics

Ch chimeric; *Hz* humanized; *Hu* fully human; *MMAE* monomethyl auristatin E; *MMAF* monomethyl auristatin F; *MGBA* minor groove binding agent; *PSMA* prostate-specific membrane antigen

[a]Includes ADCs with disclosed targets currently listed on Clinicaltrials.gov

[b]Source: Clinicaltrials.gov: December 2011

a disulfide linker. The MLN2704 ADC demonstrated activity in preclinical models [23] and evidence of biologic activity (PSA reduction) in the clinic; adverse events were attributed to release of drug from the labile disulfide linker [24]. A second PSMA ADC in which an anti-PSMA MAb (IgG1) is conjugated to monomethyl auristatin E via a protease cleavable valine–citrulline linker [25, 26] is currently being evaluated in Phase 1 in patients with castration resistant metastatic prostate cancer (Table 1.2).

Immunotoxins

Immunotoxins are highly potent agents that consist of a targeting domain such as an antibody, antibody fragment, or growth factor linked to bacterial or plant-derived toxins. For the purpose of this review only antibody-based immunotoxins are discussed. The typical formats of chemically conjugated and recombinant immunotoxins are discussed below. In each case the antibody or antibody fragment is used to confer both target selectivity and facilitate internalization of the toxin into antigen-expressing cells. First-generation immunotoxins consisted of full length antibodies chemically linked to intact toxins using bi-functional cross-linking agents. The presence of the cell-binding domain of multicomponent toxins such as the bacterial exotoxins of *Corynebacterium diphtheria* and *Pseudomonas aeruginosa* as well as the plant toxin ricin resulted in "off-target" toxicities that limited their utility as therapeutics. Strategies to improved target selectivity have included eliminating or blocking the cell-binding domain of multi subunit toxins and utilizing toxins such as the plant-derived Type I ribosome inactivating proteins (RIPs) that lack a cell binding domain [11, 27]. As shown in Table 1.1, several of these chemically conjugated immunotoxins are currently in Phase I and Phase II clinical trials. In addition to chemical conjugation, immunotoxins have been produced as fusion proteins in which genes encoding the Fv region of the antibody are fused to genes encoding modified protein toxins that lack a cell-binding domain. Two formats of recombinant immunotoxins have been evaluated extensively in preclinical models, a single chain Fc (scFv) format that uses a flexible polypeptide linker between the V_H and V_L chains of the Fv [28] and a disulfide stabilized (dsFv) [9, 29]. As a result of their reduced size, recombinant immunotoxins have the potential to more rapidly penetrate solid tumors. However, rapid tumor penetration is not the sole driver of efficacy and must be balanced against the shorter half-life and lower avidity of recombinant relative to chemically linked immunotoxins prepared with full-length IgGs.

Protein Toxins used as Immunotoxins

A variety of plant and bacterial toxins have been evaluated as immunotoxins. Plant toxins can be classified into Type I and Type II RIPs. Type I and Type II RIPs induce inhibition of protein synthesis and apoptosis following immunotoxin binding, internalization, and trafficking of the toxin to the cytosol. Type I RIPs contain catalytic activity in a single chain structure and include gelonin, saporin, and bouganin [30–32]. Type II RIPs consist of a two-chain structure, with the cell-binding (B chain) subunit linked via a disulfide to an enzymatic (A chain) subunit. Type II RIPs used as immunotoxins include ricin and abrin [27, 32, 33]. Ricin has been used extensively in the construction of immunotoxins. The B chain of intact ricin can bind to most mammalian cells and efforts to improve selectivity of ricin immunotoxins have included blocking the galactose-binding sites of the B chain so that cell binding occurs primarily via the MAb or MAb fragment of the immunotoxin [34]. Ricin A-chain immunotoxins are potent and antigen selective in vitro; however, when evaluated in vivo the immunotoxins are rapidly cleared in liver and spleen as a consequence of binding to the lectin receptor on reticuloendothelial cells. Chemical deglycosylation of ricin A has resulted in reduced hepatotoxicty and improved efficacy [35–38]. Preclinical evaluation of RFT.dgA, an anti-CD25 immunotoxin in which the murine IgG1 MAb (RFT5) was conjugated to dgRTA-chain, demonstrated impressive activity in vitro and against disseminated Hodgkin lymphomas in SCID mice [39]. The RFT5.dgA immunotoxin was advanced into Phase I in patients with refractory Hodgkin lymphoma. Vascular leak syndrome (VLS) was the major dose-limiting toxicity reported. The immunotoxin was also highly immunogenic and most patients developed antibodies to the murine MAb (HAMA) and ricin components of RFT5.dgA [40]. Combotox is a mixture of two distinct dgRTA-chain immunotoxins, HD37-dgRTA and RFB4-dgTA, directed against CD19 and CD22, respectively. Both immunotoxins consist of dgRTA-chain chemically linked to their respective murine IgG1 MAbs. Combotox has shown potent activity in preclinical models [41] and as shown in Table 1.1 is currently being evaluated in Phase I studies in patients with B cell adult acute lymphoblastic leukemia or acute lymphoblastic leukemia.

The bacterial toxins Pseudomonas exotoxin A (PE), produced by *P. aeruginosa*, and diphtheria toxin (DT), produced by *C. diphtheria*, have been used extensively in the construction of immunotoxins. These A–B bacterial toxins are similar to Type II RIPs in that they consist of two distinct domains, a receptor-binding (B subunit) domain responsible for cell entry and catalytic domain (A subunit) responsible for activity. The A subunits of PE and DT contain the catalytic activity of the toxins and kill cells by ADP-ribosylation of elongation factor 2 resulting in inhibition of protein synthesis. As with Type II RIPs, the "on-target" or MAb-directed activity of PE and DT immunotoxins has been substantially improved by removal of the binding domains [9, 42, 43].

Pseudomonas exotoxin A has been extensively studied, initially as intact PE chemically conjugated to full-length IgGs and more recently as recombinant immunotoxins in which the cell-binding domain (Ia) of PE is removed and replaced with the variable domain (Fv) of monoclonal antibodies. Current efforts to further optimize PE-based therapeutics are focused on increasing therapeutic utility by decreasing immunogenicity and reducing VLS [9].

There are also ongoing efforts to utilize human proteins such as the pro-apoptotic granule-associated serine protease granzyme B [44, 45] and other endogenous human pro-apoptotic proteins [46] in the construction of immunotoxins. The use of human, rather than plant or bacterially derived proteins has the potential to reduce the immunogenicity of the toxin component of the immunotoxin and potentially further improve safety.

The immunotoxins currently being evaluated clinically (Table 1.1) include both chemical and recombinant constructs. The potency of these immunotoxins makes them desirable therapeutics, particularly for targeting cell surface antigens expressed at low density. However, the clinical utility of immunotoxins to date has been limited by the immunogenicity of the toxins used. The development of an anti-immunotoxin immune response, frequently seen as the development of neutralizing antibodies against the toxin itself, can dramatically reduce the plasma half-life of the immunotoxin and limit the number of treatment cycles a patient can receive. There are ongoing efforts to reduce the immunogenicity of toxin molecules through identification and removal of B epitopes of Pseudomonas exotoxin A [47, 48] and T epitopes of the plant toxin bouganin [49]. A combination of deletion and mutation of B cell epitopes was shown to result in a substantial reduction in the immunogenicity of an anti-CD22-PE38 immunotoxin when evaluated in mice [47, 48]. To date, VLS has been reported as the dose-limiting toxicity for the majority of immunotoxins evaluated clinically [16, 46, 50]. The targets, toxins, and characteristics of immunotoxins currently under clinical investigation, as listed in ClinicalTrials.gov as of December 2011, are shown in Table 1.1 and several of these agents are discussed in detail in later chapters.

Antibody–Drug Conjugates

Antibody–drug conjugates consist of a MAb, a linker, and a cytotoxic drug (Fig. 1.1). Each of these components should be selected in the context of the target antigen and biology of the tumor type on which the antigen is expressed. Ideally, the target antigen will be homogeneously expressed at high density on malignant cells and have limited expression on cells of normal tissues. The cytotoxic drug must be sufficiently potent to kill tumor cells at intracellular concentrations that can be achieved with MAb-mediated delivery. For the most part, ADC's are designed with linkers that liberate biologically active drug following antigen-specific internalization and trafficking to lysosomes (Fig. 1.2). Linkers with good stability and a "conditional" mechanism of drug release provide a therapeutic index to drugs that are active clinically only at doses at or beyond their maximum tolerated dose (MTD).

Early approaches to designing ADCs used murine and chimeric MAbs covalently linked to clinically approved cytotoxic drugs such as vinblastine, methotrexate, and doxorubicin. These low molecular weight drugs were already established as clinical "standards of care" and were chosen in part because their toxicity as free drugs was well understood. It was anticipated that antibody-directed delivery would improve efficacy by selectively increasing the intratumoral concentration of drug beyond what could be achieved with the free drugs. The MAbs used in early ADCs included those that were rapidly internalized following antigen-specific binding and those that

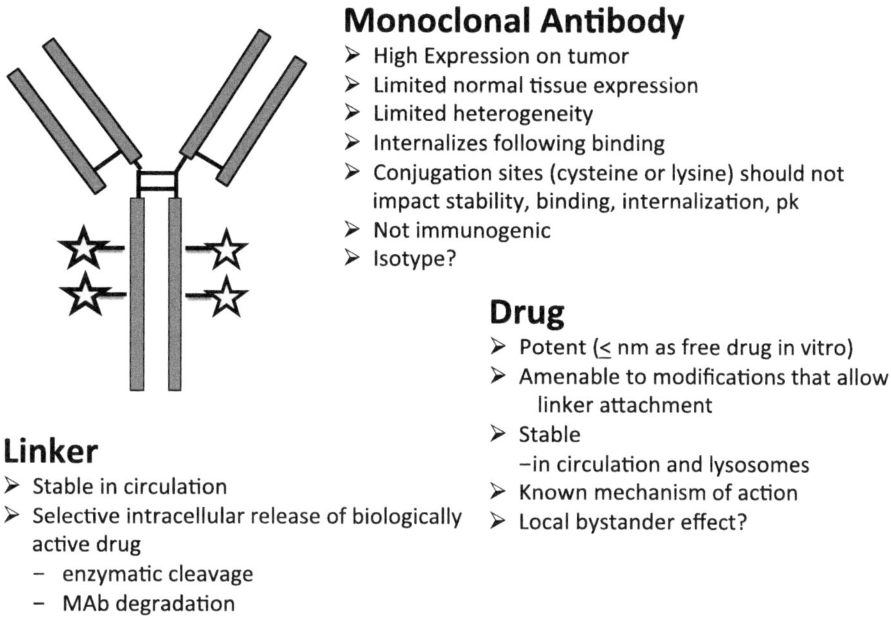

Fig. 1.1 Schematic of an ADC. An ADC consists of three components, the MAb, linker, and cytotoxic drug each of which must be optimized to design safe, potent, and effective therapeutics

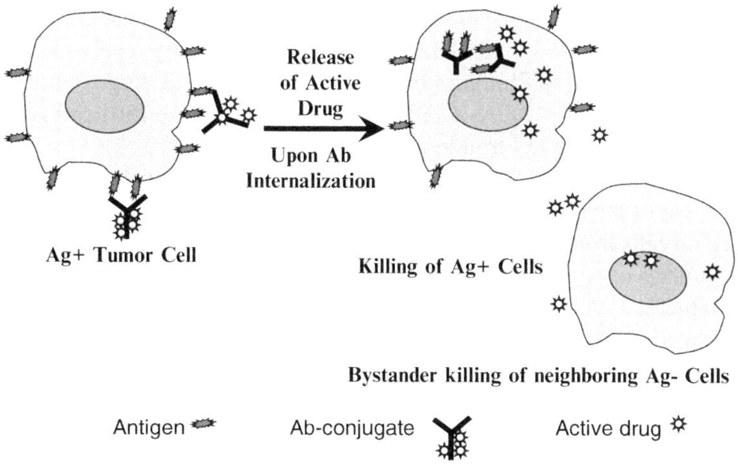

Fig. 1.2 Mechanism of ADC activity. Following tumor localization, ADCs bind to antigen-expressing cells. The ADC is internalized into endosomes/lysosomes where biologically active drug is released following enzymatic cleavage or MAb catabolism. The liberated drug enters the cytoplasm where it binds to its molecular target (typically DNA or tubulin) resulting in cell cycle arrest and apoptosis. The drug may also diffuse out of or be released from dying cells and if membrane permeable can enter cells (antigen positive or negative) in close proximity and mediate bystander killing

were not internalized to any appreciable extent. To be effective, the noninternalizing ADCs needed to be stable in the circulation and yet selectively release biologically active drug following tumor localization. These ADCs were designed with peptidyl linkers that could be cleaved by enzymes such as cathepsins and matrix metalloproteinases expressed by tumor cells or linkers that would release drug by hydrolysis at the slightly acidic pH observed in many solid tumors. For the most part, noninternalizing ADCs did not show significant antigen-specific activity in vitro or in vivo [51, 52]. The use of MAbs that rapidly internalize has enabled the design of conditional linkers that efficiently release biologically active drug following internalization and trafficking to the endosomal/lysosomal compartments of antigen expressing cells (Fig. 1.2). The optimal characteristics of the MAb, linker, and drug are shown in Fig. 1.1 and will be discussed individually below.

Characteristics of Targets and MAbs used in ADCs

To date, the use of ADCs as therapeutics has focused almost exclusively on the treatment of cancer. There are at least 25 ADCs in various stages of clinical development and those for which the target has been disclosed are included in Table 1.2. Of the 18 ADCs listed in Table 1.2, 6 ADCs are being evaluated in hematologic malignancies, 10 in various solid tumors, and 2 ADCs that bind CD70 are being evaluated in both non-Hodgkin Lymphoma (NHL) and renal cell carcinoma. The majority of ADCs in clinical development utilize humanized or fully human MAbs. An exception is brentuximab vedotin (SGN-35) an ADC that utilizes a chimeric IgG1 anti-CD30 MAb [53, 54]. Brentuximab vedotin recently received accelerated approved for treatment of Hodgkin lymphoma and anaplastic large cell lymphoma [55]. BT062, an anti-CD138 ADC also uses a chimeric MAb [56] and is currently being evaluated in a Phase I trial in multiple myeloma.

As the majority of target antigens are tumor selective rather than tumor specific, it is important to select MAbs that cross-react with the corresponding target antigen expressed on cells from normal nonhuman primates. This enables preclinical toxicology assessments of "on-target" toxicities that may result from binding of the ADC to antigen expressed on cells of normal tissues. Preclinical pharmacology studies are also facilitated by MAbs that cross-react with rodent species as this allows for an understanding of efficacy in the background of normal tissue expression.

Although there is a general agreement that effective ADC conjugation strategies should not reduce affinity relative to that of the unconjugated MAb, there are limited data available that can be used to define the optimal, or even the minimal, affinity that is required for an effective ADC. Rather than MAb affinity being the sole driver of ADC efficacy it is likely that affinity, internalization rate, intracellular trafficking, and selectivity of a given MAb in composite that will define an efficacious and safe ADC.

The selection of the isotype of the MAb is another important consideration in ADC design as it will influence whether the ADC has the potential to kill cells via immune-mediated effector functions such as antibody-dependent cellular cytotoxicity (ADCC) and/or complement dependent cytotoxicity (CDC) in addition to killing mediated by the cytotoxic drug. IgG1 MAbs have the potential to mediate CDC, via binding the complement component C1q, and ADCC, via binding to Fcγ receptors expressed on various effector cells whereas IgG2 and IgG4 MAbs are inefficient in these effector functions [57]. Whether the ADCC and/or CDC activity of a given IgG1 MAb is retained following attachment of the linker/drug is likely to be influenced by both the sequence of the particular MAb, the site of drug conjugation, the drug load, and the drug itself. Notably, Trastuzumab-DM1, an anti-HER2 ADC currently in Phase III, has been shown to retain in vitro ADCC activity [58]. It is frequently assumed that retaining effector functions may contribute to the antitumor activity of ADCs. However, the relative contribution of the effector function of IgG1 versus IgG2 and IgG4 ADCs to the potency, selectivity, and off-target toxicity of the respective ADCs is not clear and difficult to model in preclinical studies in rodents. At present, the majority of ADCs in clinical development (13/18) are IgG; however, both IgG2 (2/18) and IgG4 (3/18) ADCs are being evaluated. The relative safety and tolerability of ADCs that differ only in isotype could be addressed by studies in nonhuman primates, assuming appropriate species cross-reactivity. However, a comprehensive comparison of the safety profile of ADCs that differ only in isotype has not been published to date.

Drugs and Linkers Used in ADCs

To be effective, an ADC must achieve an intracellular concentration of biologically active drug that is sufficient to result in cell death. The copy number and heterogeneity of antigen expression must be considered in the selection of drug and linker. This is particularly important for antigens with heterogeneous expression where ADCs with bystander activity may be desirable. Ideally, the stability of the linker will exploit the long circulating half-life of the MAb and release biologically active drug following antigen-mediated internalization of the ADC. Linkers currently used in ADCs can be broadly classified as cleavable linkers that release drug by hydrolysis or enzymatic cleavage following internalization and noncleavable linkers, in which the drug is released by degradation of the MAb in lysosomes following antigen-specific internalization. In addition to the mechanism of drug release, the site of conjugation, the potency of the drug, and the average number of drug molecules per antibody molecule need to be considered in the selection of the linker.

Early approaches to ADC design incorporated cytotoxic drugs such as methotrexate [59–61], vinblastine [62, 63], and doxorubicin [12, 64–66] that displayed clinical activity and an exploitable therapeutic index as free drugs. In general these ADCs demonstrated antigen-specific activity in vitro and in vivo but required high dose levels to achieve substantial antitumor activity. One approach to increasing the potency of these ADCs was to increase the quantity of drug delivered per MAb. In the case of doxorubicin conjugates, increasing the drug:MAb ratio over a range of 1–25 molecules of drug/MAb was achieved through direct conjugation [67], the use of branched linkers [68, 69], or through polymeric carriers [70]. In general, as long as the method of conjugation did not result in a loss of MAb affinity, the in vitro potency of these ADCs increased as the drug:MAb ratio increased.

The importance of drug potency to the therapeutic efficacy of ADCs was shown in the clinical evaluation of an ADC termed BR96-DOX (BMS-182248), a chimeric IgG1 anti-Lewis^y MAb conjugated to doxorubicin via an acid-labile hydrazone linker. The BR96-DOX conjugate was rapidly internalized following antigen-specific binding and doxorubicin was released in the acidic environment of endosomes/lysosomes. The BR96-DOX conjugate, at an average drug:MAb of 8, produced cures of established human tumors in immune deficient mice and rats and curative activity was seen for both doxorubicin sensitive and insensitive tumors [12, 65]. However, the dose levels required were high (>100 mg/kg) likely reflecting the low potency of doxorubicin and the suboptimal half-life of the hydrazone linker. The BR96-DOX conjugate was evaluated in Phase I trials in patients with solid tumors confirmed to express the Lewis^y antigen by immunohistochemistry. The observed toxicities were primarily gastrointestinal and resulted from binding of the BR96 MAb to Lewis^y antigen expressed in the gastrointestinal tract. The results of this Phase I trial were disappointing, with objective responses seen in only 2 of 66 patients treated every 3 weeks with various dose levels of BR96-DOX. Tumor biopsies were obtained from patients with accessible lesions 48 h after infusion of the ADC. Localization of the BR96 MAb was shown by immunohistochemistry and importantly, intranuclear deposition of doxorubicin was also seen by confocal microscopy demonstrating tumor localization of both the MAb and drug components of the ADC [71]. The demonstrated tumor localization of the ADC and minimal clinical activity observed indicate the limitations of using a low potency drug such as doxorubicin for MAb-targeted delivery and the limitations of linkers that do not adequately exploit the half life of the MAb.

A major advance in ADC optimization resulted from incorporating highly potent cytotoxics such as calicheamicin, maytansinoids, auristatins, and duocarmycins into ADCs. These cytotoxics are 100–1,000-fold more potent than the drugs used in first-generation ADCs. For the most part these cytotoxics failed clinically as free drugs as they were very toxic and lacked a therapeutic index. Delivery in the form of an ADC provides a means to clinically exploit the potency of these agents while minimizing their systemic toxicities. As shown in Table 1.2, ADCs that utilize each of these drug classes are currently under clinical evaluation. Of these 18 ADCs, the majority utilize drugs that function as tubulin inhibitors (6/18 maytansines and 8/18 auristatins) and 4 utilize drugs that target DNA (2/18 calicheamicin, 1/18 duocarmycin, and 1/18 doxorubicin).

The calicheamicins bind to the minor groove of DNA resulting in double strand breaks in DNA and cell death at subpicomolar concentrations. Calicheamicin conjugates utilizing a hydrazone linker (Fig. 1.3) were very potent, producing durable, antigen-specific activity in preclinical models at doses of ~100 μg/kg [13]. Gemtuzumab ozogamicin, is an ADC in which calicheamicin is conjugated to a humanized anti-CD33 (IgG4) MAb via an acid-labile hydrazone linker. The average drug:MAb ratio is 3–4; however, the distribution of drug in the ADC is skewed in

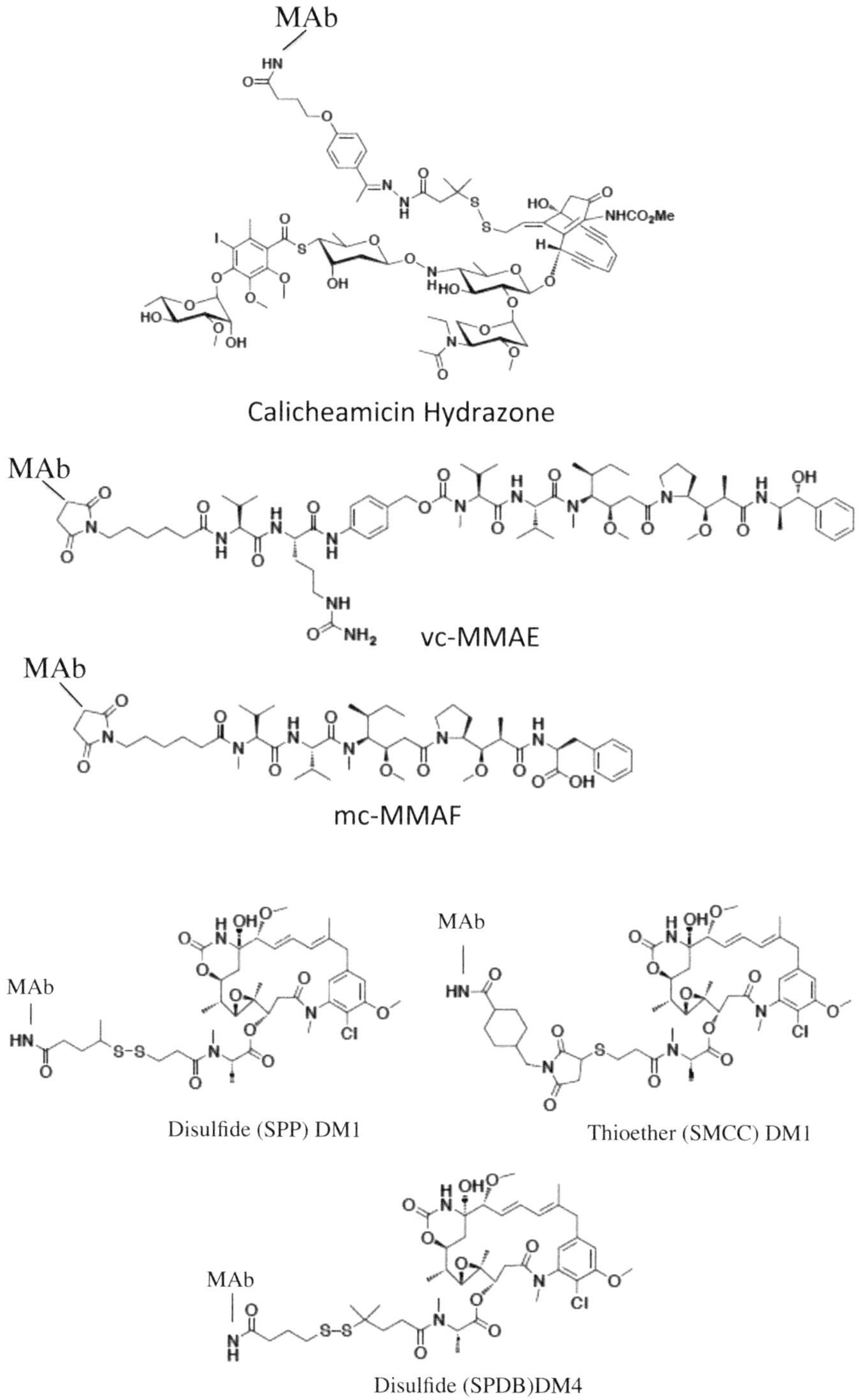

Fig. 1.3 Drugs and linkers used in ADCs under clinical development

that approximately half of the MAb has 4–6 mol of calicheamicin per mole of MAb and the remaining half of the MAb is not conjugated to calicheamicin. Gemtuzumab ozogamicin received accelerated approval by the FDA in 2000 for treatment of CD33 positive acute myeloid leukemia in first relapse in patients over 60 years of age [72]. Accelerated approval was granted based on the results of three single arm open-label Phase II studies in which 227 patients were treated with Gemtuzumab ozogamicin (9 mg/m^2) and 26% achieved remission [73]. The drug was voluntarily withdrawn from the market in 2010 due to concerns about the relative therapeutic benefit seen in post marketing studies [74]. As shown in Table 1.2, there are ongoing Phase II and III studies of gemtuzumab ozogamicin in additional clinical settings. A second calicheamicin ADC termed inotuzumab ozogamicin (CMC-544) that consists of an IgG4 anti-CD22 MAb conjugated to the same calicheamicin analog via a hydrazone linker is now in Phase III studies in NHL. The ADC demonstrated potent activity in preclinical models [75]. A Phase I study of inotuzumab ozogamicin was completed in relapsed or refractory CD22 expressing B cell NHL and demonstrated evidence of clinical activity of the ADC. At the MTD (1.8 mg/m^2 every 4 weeks) 15% of patients with diffuse large B-cell lymphoma ($n=26$) and 68% of patients with follicular lymphoma ($n=22$) achieved an objective response. The major grade 3/4 toxicity was thrombocytopenia [76]. This likely reflects "off-target" toxicity of the ADC as a consequence of nonspecific release of drug from hydrolysis of the hydrazone linker and suggests that improvements in linker stability are required to fully exploit the potency of calicheamicin-based ADCs.

The auristatins [15, 77, 78] and maytansinoids [79–81] are two classes of highly potent (pM-nM IC50s) tubulin inhibitors being developed as ADCs (Fig. 1.3). The auristatins MMAE and MMAF are fully synthetic analogs of the marine natural product dolastatin [15]. The maytansines DM1 and DM4 are benzoansamacrolides derived semi-synthetically from ansamitocin [80]. The auristatins and maytansinoids are structurally distinct; however, they both bind to tubulin at the same site as the vinca alkaloids and inhibit tubulin polymerization resulting in G2/M arrest and cell death [15, 80, 81].

Auristatin-based ADCs comprise 45% (8/18) of the ADCs with disclosed targets currently in clinical development and the majority of these use a cleavable valine–citrulline (vc) dipeptide linker (Table 1.2). The dipeptide linker is stable in circulation and is cleaved by lysosomal enzymes, including cathepsin B, following antigen-specific internalization [82]. The auristatin derivative MMAE is conjugated to MAbs via a valine–citrulline dipeptide-based linker attached to solvent accessible thiols present in MAb cysteines [83]. Biologically active MMAE is released from the ADC following antigen-specific internalization, and importantly, due to the membrane permeability of MMAE, the released drug is able to kill cells that are in close proximity, including those that lack CD30 expression [84]. The ability of a targeted drug, released in an antigen-specific manner to mediate bystander killing, is an important selection criteria for those ADCs directed to antigens that are heterogeneously expressed in tumors. The most advanced of the vc-MMAE ADCs is brentuximab vedotin (SGN-35), an anti-CD30 vc-MMAE ADC with an average drug:MAb ratio of 4, that recently received accelerated approval for treatment of Hodgkin lymphoma and anaplastic large cell lymphoma [55].

In addition to the cleavable vc-MMAE ADCs, noncleavable maleimidocaproyl (mc) linked conjugates of the auristatin analog MMAF are being pursued [85, 86]. As with vc-MMAE-based ADCs the mc linkers are attached to solvent accessible thiols present in MAb cysteines. Conjugates of MMAF demonstrate potent activity in vitro and in vivo [77, 85, 86]. The intracellular release of biologically active drug is believed to be a consequence of MAb degradation in lysosomes. In contrast to MMAE, the MMAF analog is cell impermeable and as such does not display significant bystander killing activity. An MMAF-based ADC termed SGN-75 and directed against CD70 [86] is currently in Phase 1 evaluation in NHL and renal cell carcinoma (Table 1.2).

Maytansine-based ADCs represent 33% (6/18) of currently active clinical programs (Table 1.2). There are two maytansine analogs, DM1 and DM4, being used in ADCs currently under clinical evaluation. These derivatives differ in steric hindrance around the disulfide bridge (Fig. 1.3) with the DM4 derivative demonstrating improved linker stability relative to disulfide-linked derivatives of DM1 [79, 87]. In each case, maytansine linkers are conjugated through amino groups of MAb lysine residues. The most advanced of the maytansine-based ADCs is trastuzumab emtansine (T-DM1), currently in Phase III clinical trials for treatment of HER2-positive metastatic breast cancer. This ADC will be discussed in detail later in this book and as such is only described briefly here. T-DM1 consists of the clinically approved MAb trastuzumab (humanized IgG1) conjugated to DM1 via a noncleavable thioether (SMCC) linker. It is anticipated that drug release from the ADC occurs as a result of degradation of the MAb in lysosomes. T-DM1 has an average of 3.5 molecules of DM1/MAb. In preclinical studies, T-DM1 demonstrated potent antigen-specific activity in vitro, was more efficacious and was better tolerated than ADCs prepared with derivatives of DM1 with various degrees of steric hindrance around the disulfide. Importantly, the pharmacokinetics demonstrated impressive stability of the T-DM1 with the concentration of the ADC equivalent to 70% of the antibody at 7 days [87]. T-DM1 demonstrated significant biologic activity in a Phase 1 trial in patients with advanced HER2-positive breast cancer. Clinical benefit was seen in 73% of the 15 patients treated at the MTD, 3.6 mg/kg every 3 weeks and 44% of 9 patients with measurable disease achieved an objective response [88]. The dose-limiting toxicity of T-DM1 was transient thrombocytopenia. Phase II studies were performed in patients with HER2-positive metastatic breast cancer that had previously progressed following treatment with Trastuzumab and chemotherapy. T-DM1 administered every 3 weeks at a dose of 3.6 mg/kg demonstrated impressive biologic activity [89].

Maytansine-based ADCs prepared with cleavable linkers are also being evaluated clinically (Table 1.2). The most advanced of these is SAR3419, an ADC that consists of a humanized (IgG1 MAb) conjugated to DM4 using a cleavable hindered disulfide linker. The ADC releases biologically active DM4 following antigen-specific internalization and intracellular cleavage of the disulfide linker [17]. The preclinical and clinical development of SAR3419 will be discussed in detail later in this book.

Optimization of ADCs

Major advances in the efficacy and safety of ADCs have resulted from incorporating highly potent drugs and utilizing linkers with stability sufficient to better exploit the half-life of the MAb component of the ADC. However, the choice of appropriate targets remains a critical challenge to ADC design as the target must be selectively expressed on tumor relative to normal tissues and also be expressed at sufficient copy number on the majority of malignant cells. Characteristics of the ADC target such as copy number, heterogeneity and specificity of expression, internalization rate, and intracellular trafficking can be used to define the selection of an ADC linker (cleavable or noncleavable) and the characteristics of the drug released (cell permeable or impermeable). There are currently 18 ADCs, directed to 16 distinct cell surface targets, under clinical investigation. Evolving clinical data from these ADCs will provide critical insight into the design of next generation ADCs.

References

1. Kohler G, Milstein C (1975) Continuous cultures of fused cells secreting antibody of predefined specificity. Nature 256:495–497
2. Carter PJ (2006) Potent antibody therapeutics by design. Nat Rev Immunol 6:343–357
3. Jakobovits A (1998) The long-awaited magic bullets: therapeutic human monoclonal antibodies from transgenic mice. Expert Opin Investig Drugs 7:607–614
4. Lonberg N (2005) Human antibodies from transgenic animals. Nat Biotechnol 23:1117–1125
5. Goldenberg DM, Sharkey RM (2010) Radioactive antibodies: a historical review of selective targeting and treatment of cancer. Hosp Pract (Minneap) 38:82–93
6. Steiner M, Neri D (2011) Antibody-radionuclide conjugates for cancer therapy: historical considerations and new trends. Clin Cancer Res 17:6406–6416
7. Frey K, Zivanovic A, Schwager K, Neri D (2011) Antibody-based targeting of interferon-alpha to the tumor neovasculature: a critical evaluation. Integr Biol (Camb) 3:468–478
8. Halin C, Niesner U, Villani ME, Zardi L, Neri D (2002) Tumor-targeting properties of antibody-vascular endothelial growth factor fusion proteins. Int J Cancer 102:109–116
9. Weldon JE, Pastan I (2011) A guide to taming a toxin—recombinant immunotoxins constructed from Pseudomonas exotoxin A for the treatment of cancer. FEBS J 278:4683–4700
10. Lorberboum-Galski H (2011) Human toxin-based recombinant immunotoxins/chimeric proteins as a drug delivery system for targeted treatment of human diseases. Expert Opin Drug Deliv 8:605–621
11. Choudhary S, Mathew M, Verma RS (2011) Therapeutic potential of anticancer immunotoxins. Drug Discov Today 16:495–503
12. Trail PA, Willner D, Lasch SJ, Henderson AJ, Hofstead S, Casazza AM et al (1993) Cure of xenografted human carcinomas by BR96-doxorubicin immunoconjugates. Science 261:212–215
13. Hinman LM, Hamann PR, Wallace R, Menendez AT, Durr FE, Upeslacis J (1993) Preparation and characterization of monoclonal antibody conjugates of the calicheamicins: a novel and potent family of antitumor antibiotics. Cancer Res 53:3336–3342
14. Liu C, Chari RV (1997) The development of antibody delivery systems to target cancer with highly potent maytansinoids. Expert Opin Investig Drugs 6:169–172
15. Doronina SO, Toki BE, Torgov MY, Mendelsohn BA, Cerveny CG, Chace DF et al (2003) Development of potent monoclonal antibody auristatin conjugates for cancer therapy. Nat Biotechnol 21:778–784

16. Schindler J, Gajavelli S, Ravandi F, Shen Y, Parekh S, Braunchweig I et al (2011) A phase I study of a combination of anti-CD19 and anti-CD22 immunotoxins (Combotox) in adult patients with refractory B-lineage acute lymphoblastic leukaemia. Br J Haematol 154:471–476
17. Blanc V, Bousseau A, Caron A, Carrez C, Lutz RJ, Lambert JM (2011) SAR3419: an anti-CD19-maytansinoid immunoconjugate for the treatment of B-cell malignancies. Clin Cancer Res 17:6448–6458
18. Gerber HP, Senter PD, Grewal IS (2009) Antibody drug-conjugates targeting the tumor vasculature: current and future developments. MAbs 1:247–253
19. Seon BK, Matsuno F, Haruta Y, Kondo M, Barcos M (1997) Long-lasting complete inhibition of human solid tumors in SCID mice by targeting endothelial cells of tumor vasculature with antihuman endoglin immunotoxin. Clin Cancer Res 3:1031–1044
20. Burrows FJ, Derbyshire EJ, Tazzari PL, Amlot P, Gazdar AF, King SW et al (1995) Up-regulation of endoglin on vascular endothelial cells in human solid tumors: implications for diagnosis and therapy. Clin Cancer Res 1:1623–1634
21. Baccala A, Sercia L, Li J, Heston W, Zhou M (2007) Expression of prostate-specific membrane antigen in tumor-associated neovasculature of renal neoplasms. Urology 70:385–390
22. Haffner MC, Kronberger IE, Ross JS, Sheehan CE, Zitt M, Muhlmann G et al (2009) Prostate-specific membrane antigen expression in the neovasculature of gastric and colorectal cancers. Hum Pathol 40:1754–1761
23. Henry MD, Wen S, Silva MD, Chandra S, Milton M, Worland PJ (2004) A prostate-specific membrane antigen-targeted monoclonal antibody-chemotherapeutic conjugate designed for the treatment of prostate cancer. Cancer Res 64:7995–8001
24. Galsky MD, Eisenberger M, Moore-Cooper S, Kelly WK, Slovin SF, DeLaCruz A et al (2008) Phase I trial of the prostate-specific membrane antigen-directed immunoconjugate MLN2704 in patients with progressive metastatic castration-resistant prostate cancer. J Clin Oncol 26:2147–2154
25. Ma D, Hopf CE, Malewicz AD, Donovan GP, Senter PD, Goeckeler WF et al (2006) Potent antitumor activity of an auristatin-conjugated, fully human monoclonal antibody to prostate-specific membrane antigen. Clin Cancer Res 12:2591–2596
26. Wang X, Ma D, Olson WC, Heston WD (2011) In vitro and in vivo responses of advanced prostate tumors to PSMA ADC, an auristatin-conjugated antibody to prostate-specific membrane antigen. Mol Cancer Ther 10:1728–1739
27. Vitetta ES, Thorpe PE (1991) Immunotoxins containing ricin or its A chain. Semin Cell Biol 2:47–58
28. Chaudhary VK, Queen C, Junghans RP, Waldmann TA, FitzGerald DJ, Pastan I (1989) A recombinant immunotoxin consisting of two antibody variable domains fused to Pseudomonas exotoxin. Nature 339:394–397
29. Brinkmann U, Reiter Y, Jung SH, Lee B, Pastan I (1993) A recombinant immunotoxin containing a disulfide-stabilized Fv fragment. Proc Natl Acad Sci USA 90:7538–7542
30. Bolognesi A, Polito L, Tazzari PL, Lemoli RM, Lubelli C, Fogli M et al (2000) In vitro anti-tumour activity of anti-CD80 and anti-CD86 immunotoxins containing type 1 ribosome-inactivating proteins. Br J Haematol 110:351–361
31. Rosenblum M (2004) Immunotoxins and toxin constructs in the treatment of leukemia and lymphoma. Adv Pharmacol 51:209–228
32. Stirpe F (2004) Ribosome-inactivating proteins. Toxicon 44:371–383
33. Kreitman RJ, Pastan I (2006) Immunotoxins in the treatment of hematologic malignancies. Curr Drug Targets 7:1301–1311
34. Lambert JM, Goldmacher VS, Collinson AR, Nadler LM, Blattler WA (1991) An immunotoxin prepared with blocked ricin: a natural plant toxin adapted for therapeutic use. Cancer Res 51:6236–6242
35. Thorpe PE, Wallace PM, Knowles PP, Relf MG, Brown AN, Watson GJ et al (1988) Improved antitumor effects of immunotoxins prepared with deglycosylated ricin A-chain and hindered disulfide linkages. Cancer Res 48:6396–6403

36. Ghetie V, Vitetta ES (2001) Chemical construction of immunotoxins. Mol Biotechnol 18:251–268
37. Ghetie V, Vitetta E (1994) Immunotoxins in the therapy of cancer: from bench to clinic. Pharmacol Ther 63:209–234
38. Blakey DC, Watson GJ, Knowles PP, Thorpe PE (1987) Effect of chemical deglycosylation of ricin A chain on the in vivo fate and cytotoxic activity of an immunotoxin composed of ricin A chain and anti-Thy 1.1 antibody. Cancer Res 47:947–952
39. Winkler U, Gottstein C, Schon G, Kapp U, Wolf J, Hansmann ML et al (1994) Successful treatment of disseminated human Hodgkin's disease in SCID mice with deglycosylated ricin A-chain immunotoxins. Blood 83:466–475
40. Schnell R, Borchmann P, Staak JO, Schindler J, Ghetie V, Vitetta ES et al (2003) Clinical evaluation of ricin A-chain immunotoxins in patients with Hodgkin's lymphoma. Ann Oncol 14:729–736
41. Herrera L, Yarbrough S, Ghetie V, Aquino DB, Vitetta ES (2003) Treatment of SCID/human B cell precursor ALL with anti-CD19 and anti-CD22 immunotoxins. Leukemia 17:334–338
42. Shapira A, Benhar I (2010) Toxin-based therapeutic approaches. Toxins (Basel) 2:2519–2583
43. Dosio F, Brusa P, Cattel L (2011) Immunotoxins and anticancer drug conjugate assemblies: the role of the linkage between components. Toxins (Basel) 3:848–883
44. Rosenblum MG, Barth S (2009) Development of novel, highly cytotoxic fusion constructs containing granzyme B: unique mechanisms and functions. Curr Pharm Des 15:2676–2692
45. Liu Y, Cheung LH, Hittelman WN, Rosenblum MG (2003) Targeted delivery of human pro-apoptotic enzymes to tumor cells: in vitro studies describing a novel class of recombinant highly cytotoxic agents. Mol Cancer Ther 2:1341–1350
46. Mathew M, Verma RS (2009) Humanized immunotoxins: a new generation of immunotoxins for targeted cancer therapy. Cancer Sci 100:1359–1365
47. Onda M, Beers R, Xiang L, Nagata S, Wang QC, Pastan I (2008) An immunotoxin with greatly reduced immunogenicity by identification and removal of B cell epitopes. Proc Natl Acad Sci USA 105:11311–11316
48. Pastan I, Onda M, Weldon J, Fitzgerald D, Kreitman R (2011) Immunotoxins with decreased immunogenicity and improved activity. Leuk Lymphoma 52(Suppl 2):87–90
49. Cizeau J, Grenkow DM, Brown JG, Entwistle J, MacDonald GC (2009) Engineering and biological characterization of VB6-845, an anti-EpCAM immunotoxin containing a T-cell epitope-depleted variant of the plant toxin bouganin. J Immunother 32:574–584
50. Kreitman RJ, Hassan R, Fitzgerald DJ, Pastan I (2009) Phase I trial of continuous infusion anti-mesothelin recombinant immunotoxin SS1P. Clin Cancer Res 15:5274–5279
51. Dubowchik GM, Walker MA (1999) Receptor-mediated and enzyme-dependent targeting of cytotoxic anticancer drugs. Pharmacol Ther 83:67–123
52. Trail PA, Bianchi AB (1999) Monoclonal antibody drug conjugates in the treatment of cancer. Curr Opin Immunol 11:584–588
53. Younes A, Bartlett NL, Leonard JP, Kennedy DA, Lynch CM, Sievers EL et al (2010) Brentuximab vedotin (SGN-35) for relapsed CD30-positive lymphomas. N Engl J Med 363:1812–1821
54. Katz J, Janik JE, Younes A (2011) Brentuximab Vedotin (SGN-35). Clin Cancer Res 17:6428–6436
55. DeFrancesco L (2011) Seattle Genetics rare cancer drug sails through accelerated approval. Nat Biotechnol 29:851–852
56. Ikeda H, Hideshima T, Fulciniti M, Lutz RJ, Yasui H, Okawa Y et al (2009) The monoclonal antibody nBT062 conjugated to cytotoxic Maytansinoids has selective cytotoxicity against CD138-positive multiple myeloma cells in vitro and in vivo. Clin Cancer Res 15:4028–4037
57. Jiang XR, Song A, Bergelson S, Arroll T, Parekh B, May K et al (2011) Advances in the assessment and control of the effector functions of therapeutic antibodies. Nat Rev Drug Discov 10:101–111
58. Junttila TT, Li G, Parsons K, Phillips GL, Sliwkowski MX (2011) Trastuzumab-DM1 (T-DM1) retains all the mechanisms of action of trastuzumab and efficiently inhibits growth of lapatinib insensitive breast cancer. Breast Cancer Res Treat 128:347–356

59. Smyth MJ, Pietersz GA, McKenzie IF (1987) The mode of action of methotrexate-monoclonal antibody conjugates. Immunol Cell Biol 65(Pt 2):189–200
60. Ghose T, Ferrone S, Blair AH, Kralovec Y, Temponi M, Singh M et al (1991) Regression of human melanoma xenografts in nude mice injected with methotrexate linked to monoclonal antibody 225.28 to human high molecular weight-melanoma associated antigen. Cancer Immunol Immunother 34:90–96
61. Elias DJ, Kline LE, Robbins BA, Johnson HC Jr, Pekny K, Benz M et al (1994) Monoclonal antibody KS1/4-methotrexate immunoconjugate studies in non-small cell lung carcinoma. Am J Respir Crit Care Med 150:1114–1122
62. Schrappe M, Bumol TF, Apelgren LD, Briggs SL, Koppel GA, Markowitz DD et al (1992) Long-term growth suppression of human glioma xenografts by chemoimmunoconjugates of 4-desacetylvinblastine-3-carboxyhydrazide and monoclonal antibody 9.2.27. Cancer Res 52:3838–3844
63. Petersen BH, DeHerdt SV, Schneck DW, Bumol TF (1991) The human immune response to KS1/4-desacetylvinblastine (LY256787) and KS1/4-desacetylvinblastine hydrazide (LY203728) in single and multiple dose clinical studies. Cancer Res 51:2286–2290
64. Yang HM, Reisfeld RA (1988) Doxorubicin conjugated with a monoclonal antibody directed to a human melanoma-associated proteoglycan suppresses the growth of established tumor xenografts in nude mice. Proc Natl Acad Sci USA 85:1189–1193
65. Trail PA, King HD, Dubowchik GM (2003) Monoclonal antibody drug immunoconjugates for targeted treatment of cancer. Cancer Immunol Immunother 52:328–337
66. Shih LB, Goldenberg DM, Xuan H, Lu HW, Mattes MJ, Hall TC (1994) Internalization of an intact doxorubicin immunoconjugate. Cancer Immunol Immunother 38:92–98
67. Trail PA, Willner D, Lasch SJ, Henderson AJ, Greenfield RS, King D et al (1992) Antigen-specific activity of carcinoma-reactive BR64-doxorubicin conjugates evaluated in vitro and in human tumor xenograft models. Cancer Res 52:5693–5700
68. King HD, Yurgaitis D, Willner D, Firestone RA, Yang MB, Lasch SJ et al (1999) Monoclonal antibody conjugates of doxorubicin prepared with branched linkers: a novel method for increasing the potency of doxorubicin immunoconjugates. Bioconjug Chem 10:279–288
69. King HD, Dubowchik GM, Mastalerz H, Willner D, Hofstead SJ, Firestone RA et al (2002) Monoclonal antibody conjugates of doxorubicin prepared with branched peptide linkers: inhibition of aggregation by methoxytriethyleneglycol chains. J Med Chem 45: 4336–4343
70. Shih LB, Goldenberg DM, Xuan H, Lu H, Sharkey RM, Hall TC (1991) Anthracycline immunoconjugates prepared by a site-specific linkage via an amino-dextran intermediate carrier. Cancer Res 51:4192–4198
71. Saleh MN, LoBuglio AF, Trail PA (1998) Immunoconjugate therapy of solid tumors: studies with BR96-doxorubicin. In: Grossbard ML (ed) Monoclonal antibody-based therapy of cancer, Ith edn. Marcel Dekker, Inc., New York, pp 397–416
72. Bross PF, Beitz J, Chen G, Chen XH, Duffy E, Kieffer L et al (2001) Approval summary: gemtuzumab ozogamicin in relapsed acute myeloid leukemia. Clin Cancer Res 7:1490–1496
73. Larson RA, Sievers EL, Stadtmauer EA, Lowenberg B, Estey EH, Dombret H et al (2005) Final report of the efficacy and safety of gemtuzumab ozogamicin (Mylotarg) in patients with CD33-positive acute myeloid leukemia in first recurrence. Cancer 104:1442–1452
74. Jurcic JG (2012) What happened to anti-CD33 therapy for acute myeloid leukemia? Curr Hematol Malig Rep 7:65–73
75. DiJoseph JF, Dougher MM, Evans DY, Zhou BB, Damle NK (2011) Preclinical anti-tumor activity of antibody-targeted chemotherapy with CMC-544 (inotuzumab ozogamicin), a CD22-specific immunoconjugate of calicheamicin, compared with non-targeted combination chemotherapy with CVP or CHOP. Cancer Chemother Pharmacol 67:741–749
76. Advani A, Coiffier B, Czuczman MS, Dreyling M, Foran J, Gine E et al (2010) Safety, pharmacokinetics, and preliminary clinical activity of inotuzumab ozogamicin, a novel immunoconjugate for the treatment of B-cell non-Hodgkin's lymphoma: results of a phase I study. J Clin Oncol 28:2085–2093

77. Doronina SO, Mendelsohn BA, Bovee TD, Cerveny CG, Alley SC, Meyer DL et al (2006) Enhanced activity of monomethylauristatin F through monoclonal antibody delivery: effects of linker technology on efficacy and toxicity. Bioconjug Chem 17:114–124
78. Francisco JA, Cerveny CG, Meyer DL, Mixan BJ, Klussman K, Chace DF et al (2003) cAC10-vcMMAE, an anti-CD30-monomethyl auristatin E conjugate with potent and selective antitumor activity. Blood 102:1458–1465
79. Widdison WC, Wilhelm SD, Cavanagh EE, Whiteman KR, Leece BA, Kovtun Y et al (2006) Semisynthetic maytansine analogues for the targeted treatment of cancer. J Med Chem 49:4392–4408
80. Oroudjev E, Lopus M, Wilson L, Audette C, Provenzano C, Erickson H et al (2010) Maytansinoid-antibody conjugates induce mitotic arrest by suppressing microtubule dynamic instability. Mol Cancer Ther 9:2700–2713
81. Chari RV, Martell BA, Gross JL, Cook SB, Shah SA, Blattler WA et al (1992) Immunoconjugates containing novel maytansinoids: promising anticancer drugs. Cancer Res 52:127–131
82. Dubowchik GM, Firestone RA, Padilla L, Willner D, Hofstead SJ, Mosure K et al (2002) Cathepsin B-labile dipeptide linkers for lysosomal release of doxorubicin from internalizing immunoconjugates: model studies of enzymatic drug release and antigen-specific in vitro anticancer activity. Bioconjug Chem 13:855–869
83. Doronina SO, Bovee TD, Meyer DW, Miyamoto JB, Anderson ME, Morris-Tilden CA et al (2008) Novel peptide linkers for highly potent antibody-auristatin conjugate. Bioconjug Chem 19:1960–1963
84. Okeley NM, Miyamoto JB, Zhang X, Sanderson RJ, Benjamin DR, Sievers EL et al (2010) Intracellular activation of SGN-35, a potent anti-CD30 antibody-drug conjugate. Clin Cancer Res 16:888–897
85. Jackson D, Gooya J, Mao S, Kinneer K, Xu L, Camara M et al (2008) A human antibody-drug conjugate targeting EphA2 inhibits tumor growth in vivo. Cancer Res 68:9367–9374
86. Oflazoglu E, Stone IJ, Gordon K, Wood CG, Repasky EA, Grewal IS et al (2008) Potent anticarcinoma activity of the humanized anti-CD70 antibody h1F6 conjugated to the tubulin inhibitor auristatin via an uncleavable linker. Clin Cancer Res 14:6171–6180
87. Lewis Phillips GD, Li G, Dugger DL, Crocker LM, Parsons KL, Mai E et al (2008) Targeting HER2-positive breast cancer with trastuzumab-DM1 an antibody-cytotoxic drug conjugate. Cancer Res 68:9280–9290
88. Krop IE, Beeram M, Modi S, Jones SF, Holden SN, Yu W et al (2010) Phase I study of trastuzumab-DM1, an HER2 antibody-drug conjugate, given every 3 weeks to patients with HER2-positive metastatic breast cancer. J Clin Oncol 28:2698–2704
89. Burris HA 3rd, Rugo HS, Vukelja SJ, Vogel CL, Borson RA, Limentani S et al (2011) Phase II study of the antibody drug conjugate trastuzumab-DM1 for the treatment of human epidermal growth factor receptor 2 (HER2)-positive breast cancer after prior HER2-directed therapy. J Clin Oncol 29:398–405

Chapter 2
Antibody–Drug Conjugate Development

Aakanksha Khandelwal, Haleh Saber, Marjorie A. Shapiro, and Hong Zhao

Introduction

Antibody–drug conjugate (ADC) development started about three decades ago with the hypothesis that toxins conjugated to antibodies would enhance antitumor activity and reduce toxicity by delivering toxins to specific tumor sites. Since then, the field has evolved to include potent small molecule drugs (SMD) and radiolabeled drugs conjugated to antibodies targeting both solid tumors and hematologic malignancies. Improved ADC technology has paved the way for increased drug delivery to the target tumors and decreased normal tissue exposure to cytotoxic agents. Radioimmunoconjugates (RICs) present a different set of challenges leading to unique development pathways. Several factors need to be taken into consideration when developing RICs, such as decay of radioactivity, potentially higher exposure to normal tissue caused by lower specificity, and dehalogenation leading to a loss of signal. This chapter focuses on antibodies conjugated to SMDs.

Administration of unconjugated SMDs that have a narrow therapeutic window often leads to serious adverse events in patients, which limits their use in achieving maximal effectiveness. Increasing the dose of these agents is not a viable option because of the lack of specificity and resulting toxicity. However, targeting these agents to a particular marker on a cancer cell can reduce the toxic side effects and potentially increases efficacy. There are several steps involved in the mechanism of

---

Disclaimer. The views expressed in this chapter are those of the authors and do not necessarily reflect the views of the United States Food and Drug Administration (FDA).

A. Khandelwal (✉) • H. Saber • M.A. Shapiro • H. Zhao
Food and Drug Administration (formerly), Silver Spring, MD 20993, USA
e-mail: aakanksha.khandelwal@hotmail.com

G.L. Phillips (ed.), *Antibody-Drug Conjugates and Immunotoxins: From Pre-Clinical Development to Therapeutic Applications*, Cancer Drug Discovery and Development,
DOI 10.1007/978-1-4614-5456-4_2,

ADC activity: circulation, antigen binding, internalization, drug release, and eventual drug action. When in circulation, the activity of the ADC is heavily dependent on the stability of the linkage. An unstable linker could lead to premature release of the payload (either a SMD or a toxin), before reaching the site of action. Additionally, the antibody component of the ADC should retain a high affinity for its target; this affinity should ideally remain unhindered by the linker and payload. Furthermore, internalization of the payload can be challenging given the limited number of antigen targets on the cell surface. Upon internalization, the antibody must release the payload and allow the payload to exert its mechanism of action [1]. While the various mechanisms involved in ADC action are important, so are the various components that comprise the ADC product: the SMD, linker, and monoclonal antibody (mAb).

Several challenges present themselves in ADC development, and multiple considerations need to be taken. Ideally, the ADC should have a potent cytotoxic agent with a proven mechanism of action, a mAb with high affinity and selectivity for the target, and a linker with suitable stability to deliver the ADC to the site of action and also labile after getting inside of the tumor cell. Some ADCs have a mAb that possesses its own therapeutic activity whereas others have a mAb whose only function is targeting and delivering SMDs or toxins. Trastuzumab emtansine (T-DM1), for example, is trastuzumab conjugated to DM1, a maytansine derivative. In this case, trastuzumab, the mAb, targets HER-2 and possesses ADCC (antibody-dependent cellular cytotoxicity) activity among other intracellular activities [2, 3]. The SMD component, DM1, acts as a microtubule disrupting agent to inhibit cell division [4]. However, it is not necessary for a mAb in the ADC to have therapeutic activity. In the case of inotuzumab ozogamicin (CMC-544), a conjugate of G544 and calicheamicin connected by an acetyl butyrate linker, the anti-CD22 mAb, G544, does not possess any antitumor activity of its own [5]. The lack of activity of the mAb does not preclude inotuzumab ozogamicin from having anticancer activity in patients with relapsed or refractory CD22-positive B-cell non-Hodgkin's lymphoma [6]. Brentuximab vedotin (Adcetris or SGN-35), a newly approved ADC for CD30-postivie Hodgkin lymphoma and systemic anaplastic large cell lymphoma, also utilizes a mAb (cAC10), which according to Younes and colleagues does not possess antitumor activity of its own [7].

This chapter aims to cover the nonclinical and clinical pharmacology aspects of ADC development. The chemistry, manufacturing, and controls information is not discussed in this chapter but can be found in a public document entitled, "*Points to Consider in the Manufacture and Testing of Monoclonal Antibody Products for Human Use*" [8]. The overall clinical development program of an ADC from an efficacy and safety standpoint is similar to that of any other agent depending on the indication. Since most ADCs in development are for oncology indications, the clinical trial design would have to take into consideration the complexities involved in treating a cancer patient population.

Nonclinical Development

Most ADCs in development are intended to treat cancer in patients with serious and life-threatening conditions. Therefore, the discussion on nonclinical studies will focus on experience to date in oncology ADC development and the relevance of the principles described in the *International Conference on Harmonization (ICH) Guidance S9, Nonclinical Evaluation for Anticancer Pharmaceuticals* [9]. Therapeutic radioisotope- and toxin-conjugated products are not discussed as there is little experience with their safety assessment or the safety assessment requires considerations in addition to those encountered in traditional drug development. It should be noted that these products are also excluded from the ICH S9 guideline. For the purpose of this discussion, the term conjugate refers to the ADC. Nonclinical approaches described in this section are based on the experience gained with ADCs currently in development, but other approaches not described below may also be applicable.

As for any pharmaceutical agent, nonclinical evaluations to support first-in-human studies are conducted to identify the pharmacologic properties of the product, to understand the toxicity profile of the product and guide adequate monitoring in patients, and to establish a safe-starting dose in humans.

Prior to first-in-human studies, preliminary characterization of the mechanism of action of the conjugate is conducted. For a conjugate, in addition to evaluating the anticancer activity of the product, it is generally necessary to conduct appropriate pharmacology studies to select relevant species for toxicology studies, unless such data are already available, for example, when a previously approved antibody is being linked to a SMD.

Most conjugates thus far in development for treatment of cancer contain a cytotoxic agent as a SMD. These SMDs are genotoxic and target rapidly dividing cells (e.g., crypt cells and bone marrow) in general toxicology studies; they usually interact directly with the DNA or components of DNA synthesis or cell division. In a conjugate, the SMD is covalently attached to the antibody via a linker. The linker is intended to provide a stable product in the plasma and result in efficient release of the drug inside the cell. The antibody is used to direct the SMD to a specific epitope on the target cell; this is followed by internalization and release of the SMD inside the cell. The proposed advantage of developing a conjugate is to direct high concentrations of the SMD to the site of action, usually the tumor site (via tumor-specific or overexpressed antigens). Hypothetically, the targeted binding will reduce systemic exposure to the free SMD and reduce off-target adverse effects. In order to achieve this goal, the conjugate is expected to be stable in the plasma. As discussed in ICH S9, plasma stability of the conjugate in the test species and in humans is assessed to assure stable products and to guide in interpretation of study results when differences in plasma stability exist in test species compared to humans.

The primary goal of toxicology studies is to assess the potential for toxicity associated with the conjugate, the compound to which patients are exposed in clinical trials. As described in ICH S9, a more limited evaluation could be done on the safety of the free SMD if such data do not already exist. The rationale for an assessment of toxicity associated with free SMD is the intended or unintended dissociation of the conjugate in the biologic system or the presence of unconjugated drug in the dosing solution; experience to date with conjugates in development shows that toxicities of conjugates are mainly related to the SMD moiety. Toxicities of the linker are assumed to have been evaluated in toxicology studies conducted with the conjugate. In addition, as stated above, toxicities related to the SMD have been shown to be the primary cause of nonclinical and clinical toxicities. Therefore, it has not been generally necessary to assess the safety profile of the linker alone in general toxicology studies. This approach will be reevaluated in the future if non-toxic SMDs will be conjugated to the antibody or the nature of linkers evolves. The state of the current science of linkers and conjugation methods has been recently reviewed by Alley and colleagues [10].

To support the first-in-human study of most anticancer drugs, general toxicology studies in two relevant species (rodent and non-rodent) with an appropriate dose–response evaluation are usually conducted. A similar pathway has been used for many ADCs. Criteria used for the selection of a pharmacologically relevant species for an antibody may be used to select the relevant species for toxicology studies of the conjugate [11]. In some cases, only a single species with the intended target of the conjugate was available. In this case, to support first-in-human clinical trials of the ADC, a study of the conjugate in a second species was deemed not necessary. In another example, a study in a second species with the conjugate was conducted and provided useful information even in the absence of the epitope (described below).

If the antibody does not bind to its target in species that are typically used for toxicology studies (e.g., mouse, rat, monkey), a toxicology study of the conjugate could be still conducted in one species with appropriate dose–response. The rationale for conducting this study in the absence of antibody-target binding is the experience with conjugates to date, demonstrating that dose-limiting toxicities in nonclinical studies have been primarily due to toxicities associated with the cytotoxic agent. Hence, the study conducted with the conjugate has provided useful information on the toxicities associated with the SMD. Characterization of toxicities associated with the free SMD could possibly be done through reference to available data for a well-characterized substance, through inclusion of an arm of the free SMD in toxicology study(ies), or by conducting a separate toxicology study with the free SMD. Studies that do not specifically comply with good laboratory practice (GLP) regulations have sometimes been conducted with the free SMD to characterize drug-related toxicities, although in some cases these studies predate the GLP regulations. However, the studies were judged to be of sufficient quality to adequately describe the toxicities of the SMD. Pivotal studies, for example, toxicology studies conducted with the conjugate and used to set the first-in-human starting dose, are usually GLP-compliant (see 21CFR58).

Per ICH S9, "an assessment of the pharmaceutical's effect on vital organ functions (including cardiovascular, respiratory, and central nervous systems) should be available before the initiation of clinical studies; such parameters could be included in general toxicology studies. Detailed clinical observations following dosing and appropriate electrocardiographic measurements in non-rodents are generally considered sufficient." When the SMD moiety is known to cause cardiovascular toxicities, ECG monitoring in non-rodents may not be necessary as the conjugate may be considered a cardiovascular toxicant and appropriate clinical monitoring is expected. As stated in ICH S9, stand-alone safety pharmacology studies are generally not needed for drugs intended for patients with advanced disease. If the sponsor chooses to conduct stand-alone studies to assess a specific concern, it is important to consider the appropriateness of the model, for example, the hERG assay is generally not considered useful for large molecules such as a conjugate but may be more appropriate for the free SMD.

An assessment of the immune response to the conjugate may be useful in the interpretation of study results. Samples may be stored and analyzed retrospectively as needed. When the SMD is a cytotoxic agent, a class of products known to cause bone marrow suppression, immunogenicity may be reduced as doses of the conjugate are increased in animals.

As toxicities of the conjugates investigated to date arise mainly from the SMD moiety, a toxicokinetic evaluation to assess the levels of conjugate and the free SMD in studies conducted with the conjugate are expected, as discussed in ICH S9. These studies provide useful information in interpreting the study results.

Examples of different clinical schedules and the nonclinical studies to support clinical development are provided in ICH S9. For initial IND (Investigational New Drug) submissions, the commonly used clinical schedules of dosing for conjugates have been once every 3 weeks, once every 2 weeks, or once per week. In general, the schedule and route of administration in pivotal toxicology studies are expected to simulate the proposed clinical protocol, taking into account the available pharmacokinetic and pharmacodynamic data. A more frequent dosing schedule in animals could be considered in certain conditions, for example, if formation of anti-product antibodies (APAs) results in reduced half-life of and exposure to the conjugate. Single-dose toxicology studies have been successful in defining toxicities of the conjugate and in selecting a clinical starting dose when dosing in patients was once every 3–4 weeks in the initial clinical trial.

The clinical starting dose for conjugates has been set as per existing practice for SMDs. When a rodent study was deemed relevant, 1/10th the STD_{10} (severely toxic dose in 10% of animals) was used to select the starting dose in patients. When a non-rodent study was considered more relevant, the human starting dose was set at 1/6th the HNSTD (highest non-severely toxic dose). The animal-to-human dose extrapolation based on body weight (mg/kg) has been considered appropriate for large molecules such as a conjugate. Because a conversion based on the body surface area (mg/m^2) results in a smaller starting dose, this approach has been accepted when proposed by the sponsors. Other approaches used include a starting dose based on the no observed adverse effects level (NOAEL). When proposed by the sponsor and based on adequate scientific justification, a human starting dose based on pharmacodynamic and/or pharmacokinetic data was also accepted. Other approaches may be equally acceptable. These different approaches used to date are being evaluated as experience is gained with this product class.

Long-term toxicology studies of the conjugate are generally conducted in two appropriate species. When a second relevant species (e.g., containing the target of the antibody) was not identified, a study in the second species has not always been deemed necessary. However, this study, when conducted, did provide useful information on toxicities associated with the SMD. There might be other circumstances for which the long-term study in the second species may not be considered essential, for example, when short-term toxicology studies and clinical data indicate that toxicities of the conjugate are due to the SMD moiety and toxicities of the SMD have been characterized in long-term studies. Justification for conducting the chronic study in one species is expected. As discussed in ICH S9, for conjugates (and other pharmaceuticals) developed to treat cancer in patients with serious and life-threatening conditions, the duration of chronic study(ies) may be limited to 3 months or 3–4 cycles, and these studies are expected to be submitted prior to Phase 3 clinical development.

Genotoxicity studies are performed to support a marketing application [9, 12]. When the free SMD was a well-characterized molecule and known to be positive in genetic toxicology studies, additional studies to characterize genotoxicity of the conjugate have not been needed; the conjugate was considered genotoxic. If the genotoxicity potential of the conjugate or the SMD is unknown, the in vitro genotoxicity studies may be conducted with the free SMD. For the approved ADC, Adcetris, the genetic toxicology studies were conducted with the SMD. Per ICH S9, if the in vitro assays for a drug intended to treat patients with life-threatening cancer are positive, an in vivo assay might not be warranted.

Per ICH S9, embryofetal toxicity studies of anticancer pharmaceuticals should be available when the marketing application is submitted. When the free SMD is a well-characterized molecule and is clearly toxic to embryo and/or fetus (e.g., SMD is teratogenic or causes embryofetal lethality), an additional embryofetal toxicity study with the conjugate may not be essential. Moreover, in accordance with ICH S9, these studies may not be essential for conjugates containing cytotoxic SMDs when the SMD is genotoxic and toxicities associated with the cytotoxic SMD are observed in general toxicity studies, showing toxicities primarily in rapidly diving cells (e.g., bone marrow and crypt cells).

Clinical Pharmacology

The field of ADCs has taken leaps since gemtuzumab ozogamicin (Mylotarg); the first ADC was approved in 2000 under the Accelerated Approval pathway [13]. Advances in linker and assay technology have allowed the field to progress over the past decade. Moreover, lessons learned from the approval, use, and eventual market withdrawal of Mylotarg in 2010 have led the development of novel ADCs. In the ADC of gemtuzumab ozogamicin, for example, approximately 50% of the antibodies are not linked to the calicheamicin derivative [13]. Improved conjugation methods and linkers providing greater stability have since been produced [1].

The selected antigen is among a number of factors that can affect the clinical pharmacology profile of the ADC. Certain antigens allow faster internalization of the ADC compared to the naked mAb [14], while others do not affect the rate of internalization [15]. Upon internalization, the ADC undergoes receptor-mediated endocytosis, in which the antigen and antibody are localized in clathrin-coated pits [10]. This rate of internalization affects the half-life of the ADC and the kinetics of the SMD. The linker technology used plays a critical role in the activity and potency of the ADC. The stability of the drug linker in circulation is essential to providing a long half-life for the ADC. SMDs directly linked to mAbs and ADCs with protease-cleavable linkers have generally been shown to be more stable in circulation than disulfide and hydrazone linkers [16–18]. However, as linker technology continues to evolve, more stable and favorable linkers will be developed.

Analytes

Characterization of the clinical pharmacology profile of an ADC is essential during product development. Earlier in the development of ADCs, researchers strove to determine the levels of each component in the investigational ADC, including the conjugate, total SMD, free SMD, total antibody, and free antibody. However, as the field has evolved and more insight has been gained on the analytical challenges in ADC development, it has been determined that measuring all of these components may not be feasible and essential for characterization of the disposition of the ADC. Now, the most important and useful parameters stem from three key measurements in systemic circulation: intact conjugate, total antibody [19], and free (unbound) SMD. Measurement of these three components is important because the intact conjugate plays the role of proving the concept that the entity not only is in fact acting as a conjugate but also is stable in circulation; plasma levels of total antibody and unbound SMD give information as to what is happening to the conjugate once in circulation. For example, high levels of free SMD would raise both efficacy and safety concerns because high SMD concentrations would indicate less drug available at the target site for exerting efficacy, and a higher systemic exposures could lead to greater toxicity. Low levels of total antibody relative to unbound SMD would hint premature release of the payload. A measure of these three components would be expected to provide concentration–time profiles to adequately characterize the single- and multiple-dose pharmacokinetics (PK) of the ADC.

To optimally design an ADC, it is critical to understand the distribution and exposure of the ADC in the body and in various tissues. Ideally, the distribution and accumulation of the three key components would be determined in both target and nontarget tissues in addition to that in circulation. This data would support the hypothesis that the

ADC provides preferential tumor targeting and exposure compared to nontarget containing tissues. The free SMD should have a very low plasma concentration to minimize toxicity due to its systemic exposure. Theoretically, total antibody concentrations should be higher than ADC concentrations, which is also what has been observed in the clinical studies [6, 20]. In the case of T-DM1, total trastuzumab has serum concentrations 10,000–100,000-fold higher than DM1, and T-DM1 (conjugate) has serum concentrations 1,000–10,000-fold higher than DM1 [20]. This data demonstrates the degree to which the levels of the different components in circulation vary.

It is critical to determine the levels of SMD early on in nonclinical and clinical testing to ensure that there is little free SMD in circulation. A large amount of SMD in circulation in comparison to the ADC and total antibody indicates premature release of the SMD from the ADC. The levels of SMD in circulation and at the target site would also guide further clinical pharmacology development of the ADC. For example, characterization of the levels of SMD at the target site and in circulation may explain the onset of certain clinical adverse events. It is of note that although assays are designed to measure free SMD, most liquid chromatography linked to mass spectrometry (LC–MS) assays limited by the sample extraction technique are unable to differentiate between complete free SMD, SMD bound to linker, and SMD bound to plasma proteins such as albumin or alpha acid glycoprotein. The extent of plasma protein binding of the SMD can be assessed in a separate assay and is often useful in characterizing the disposition of the SMD.

In addition to those listed above, there may be other entities in circulation resulting from the ADC, such as catabolites of the mAb or metabolites of the SMD. The metabolism of the SMD should be initially characterized in vitro, before conjugation with the mAb. Early characterization of the individual components of the ADC, the antibody, the SMD, and the linker may dictate the further studies that need to be conducted.

Assay Development

The complexity of the ADC and its various by-products poses a number of challenges in developing assay methodologies for both the mAb and SMD. In certain instances, the same assay may be used for more than one component. For example, an assay that can determine total antibody may also be able to differentiate between the conjugate and unconjugated forms of the antibody. A separate assay would be needed to measure the drug-to-antibody ratio or drug load of the ADC and how this changes over time. Total and free SMD would have to be assessed by a different extraction procedure. Thorough characterization of the antibody and the SMD individually prior to analyzing the ADC would be beneficial in help predicting the time course of the individual components in circulation. Prior determination of metabolites of the SMD would also help plan the number and scope of further assays that would need to be developed for the characterization of the SMD component of the ADC.

Different ELISA (enzyme-linked immunosorbent assay) methods have been used to quantify the conjugate and the total antibody and may differ in format (sandwich versus bridging), while LC–MS has generally been used to quantify free SMD. Levels of linker-SMD may also be present in circulation although it is not expected to be in large amount. Similar to the free SMD, the linker–SMD complex can be identified by LC–MS or other chromatography and spectrometry methods; however, as mentioned above, the complex cannot be differentiated between specific and nonspecific protein binding. It is useful to identify the amount of SMD that is bound to plasma proteins in the early development stage since this helps to predict the extent of SMD reaching the site of action. In theory, the amount of linker–SMD transfer from the ADC to plasma proteins should be low; however, the potential for this transfer still exists. An assay developed to determine the level of this transfer will help ensure that the transferred SMD only accounts for a small percent of the circulating conjugated SMD.

The importance of sensitive bioanalytical methods cannot be overstressed. An article by DeSilva et al. covers recommendations for bioanalytical method development and validation that can be applied to assays for ADCs [21]. Further information can be obtained from the FDA Guidance on bioanalytical assays [22].

Drug-to-Antibody Ratio

The DAR (drug-to-antibody ratio), or the number of SMDs per antibody, affects the levels of SMD in circulation. The DAR has been shown to have an impact on the PK of the ADC. In general, the more loaded the antibody with SMD, the more the PK of the ADC behaves like a SMD; the less the SMD loading, the PK of the ADC behaves more like the naked antibody. This has been demonstrated by changes in the clearance of the ADC with changes of the DAR. As the DAR increases, the ADC clears faster from the body and the half-life is shorter. ADCs with a DAR of 2–4 have been shown to have a more favorable PK profile (longer half-life, slower rate of clearance, and greater efficacy) than more heavily loaded conjugates [23, 24]. However, reducing the DAR can also reduce conjugate yield and increase heterogeneity in the average number of payload per antibody. For example, attempting to achieve a DAR of 2 has been difficult since a large amount of antibody remains unconjugated. The effect of conjugate site and stoichiometry on safety and efficacy of ADCs is not clear and is the subject of continuing research.

It is important to point out that the DAR only refers to the average payload per antibody. Each antibody can have several different sites of conjugation, but even with improving methods, it remains difficult to control where each SMD is conjugated. This leaves a high level of heterogeneity in the conjugates. Moreover, the ADC product contains a distribution of payload as well as some unconjugated antibody.

Immunogenicity

ADCs represent a classical hapten-carrier antigen, where the hapten (SMD) is not immunogenic on its own, but when conjugated to a carrier protein (mAb), animals can mount a heterogenous immune response to the hapten, including Ig class-switched, high-affinity antibodies [25–28].

While most studies of hapten-carrier antigens used a foreign protein as a carrier, a few demonstrated anti-hapten immune responses when autologous proteins were used as the carrier [29, 30]. Most therapeutic mAbs currently in development, including ADCs, use chimeric, humanized, or human mAbs, all of which can be immunogenic [31]. Therefore, the immunogenic potential of both the SMD and mAb should be studied during clinical development.

Immunogenicity testing for ADCs is similar to that for a mAb. While in recent years, immunogenicity has not resulted in serious adverse events as seen with the development of neutralizing antibodies against erythropoietin [32], the development of immunogenicity can still result in a decrease in efficacy and/or a change in PK [33, 34]. Even some chimeric and humanized antibodies have shown high rates of immunogenicity, similar to mouse monoclonal antibodies [35].

Assay methods for immunogenicity testing have included ELISA and ECL (Electrochemiluminescence) for detection of APAs. A tiered approach has been often utilized in nonclinical and clinical studies where samples are first screened for APAs and those samples that test positive are further evaluated to determine the APA titer. APA positive samples are subsequently evaluated for the ability to neutralize the activity of the ADC. The FDA's draft guidance for industry on immunogenicity describes the multitiered approach and considerations for assay development in further detail [36].

The immunogenicity of ADCs can be complex because it may be difficult to determine if the immune response is towards the mAb portion or the linker portion of the ADC. In the case of gemtuzumab ozogamicin, two patients developed antibody titers against the calicheamicin/calicheamicin-linker portion of the ADC, while no patients developed an antibody response to the mAb portion of the ADC. Thus, it is important to determine if the APAs that develop are to the linker or to the mAb portion of the ADC.

Metabolism and Elimination

Metabolism studies are not generally performed for biologic products such as mAbs because these products are proteins that are degraded into amino acids that are then recycled into other proteins. In the case of the ADCs, the SMD portion of the conjugate is evaluated for its ability to be metabolized by the liver or gut mucosa. Major metabolites are expected to be further evaluated for their pharmacologic activity and PK.

There are a number of factors that contribute to the elimination of mAbs including binding to FcRn, binding to target antigen, antigen density, binding to Fcγ receptors as part of the antibody–antigen immune complex, nonspecific proteolysis, and the ability of the antibody to reach the site of disease [34]. Elimination studies of the SMD should be conducted, and amount of SMD excreted in urine and feces should be measured. Although a mass balance study of the SMD has limitations because free SMD behaves differently than conjugated SMD, this study would provide insight on the need and extent of possible organ impairment studies. In certain cases, population PK analysis may be used to evaluate the effect of organ impairment on the PK of the SMD, which is discussed in subsequent sections.

Drug Interaction

Drug interaction studies constitute an integral part of the clinical pharmacology development of SMDs. Generally, a SMD is initially screened in vitro to determine whether it is a substrate, inhibitor, or inducer of cytochrome P-450 isozymes (CYPs). Whether or not the SMD is a substrate or inhibitor of phase 2 enzymes, P-glycoprotein, and other transporters is also assessed. These studies help determine the need for in vivo drug–drug interaction studies.

In the case of ADCs, these in vitro studies are only conducted for the SMD portion of the conjugate. The antibody portion of the ADC is not metabolized by CYPs or other drug metabolizing enzymes. Thus, a mAb is unlikely to have an effect on these enzymes in terms of inhibition or induction unless the mAb is a cytokine modulator.

Pharmacokinetic Comparability

Manufacturing changes during the development of an ADC can present several challenges in demonstrating comparability between the pre- and post-change products. One approach in PK comparability assessment has been to determine the AUC and C_{max} of each key component that is characterized in the clinical pharmacology studies of the ADC. This generally includes the conjugate, total antibody, and free SMD. Similar to PK comparability evaluation for other therapeutic biologics, the point estimate of the geometric mean ratio with the 90% confidence interval for AUC and C_{max} falling between 80% and 125% has been used to assess the PK comparability between the pre- and post-change products [37]. Examining the intrasubject and intersubject variability of the PK parameters would provide additional information regarding the PK comparability between the pre- and post-change products.

Organ Impairment

Since ADCs behave more like therapeutic proteins than SMDs, the need for hepatic or renal impairment studies for ADCs is similar as for therapeutic proteins. Further information on renal impairment studies for therapeutic proteins can be found in the draft guidance for industry entitled, "*Pharmacokinetics in Patients with Impaired Renal Function — Study Design, Data Analysis, and Impact on Dosing and Labeling*" [38]. A recent review of data revealed that therapeutic proteins larger than 69 kDa are unlikely to be cleared in the kidneys via glomerular filtration. Thus, a dedicated renal impairment study may not be needed for this class of therapeutics. In the case of ADCs, a dedicated renal impairment study may be needed if the free SMD has substantial systemic exposure and renal elimination. The mass balance data generated for the SMD will determine the need for a dedicated renal or hepatic impairment study for the SMD. The effect of renal impairment as well as hepatic impairment on the PK of the ADCs can also be assessed through population PK analyses for both the SMD and the ADC. Additionally, certain safety concerns may necessitate organ impairment studies for the ADC; however, this is not generally the case and would be specific to the product of concern.

Exposure-Response

The exposure-response analysis is a very useful approach in exploring the relationships between the systemic exposure of the ADC and the clinical responses including efficacy and safety and may determine the attribution of each component of the ADC to the clinical responses. Comparing the exposure of the SMD and the conjugate in terms of efficacy and safety would provide an insight of what is occurring in the biological system.

Population PK analyses can be performed to assess the clinical pharmacology of ADCs in various population subgroups. This approach has been used to evaluate the effect of various intrinsic factors including, but not limited to, age, weight, gender, and race on the PK of the ADCs. Population PK analysis is extremely useful for analyzing sparse PK data collected from larger clinical studies in which intensive PK sampling may not be feasible [39, 40].

ECG Evaluation

The effect of the ADC on ventricular repolarization as measured by the QT/QTc interval needs to be determined during development. While ECG monitoring has been sufficient in the past for therapeutic mAbs given their low likelihood for ion channel interactions, this may not be the case for ADCs [41]. Because ADCs have the propensity to release SMD into circulation prior to reaching the target and in certain instances, the levels of SMD in circulation may be high enough to enter the hERG channel leading to the potential for QT/QTc prolongation, an adequate ECG monitoring may be needed. ECG monitoring in early clinical studies may provide safety signals as to whether further rigorous evaluation is needed. At a minimum, 12-lead ECG monitoring is generally recommended to be taken at baseline, at the time of the maximum plasma concentration of the drug, during steady state, and during the follow-up visit in early and late clinical studies for an assessment of safety. However, a well-designed and adequately conducted QT study with ability to detect small QTc changes can often eliminate the need for ECG monitoring in multiple clinical trials for cancer indications. There are several factors to be considered when designing a QT study such as blood sampling times for PK or immunogenicity, doses being tested, comorbidities, co-medications, and control arm to name a few [42–44].

Discussion

Clinical research in ADC development is increasing steadily with the FDA seeing a number of pre-IND and IND submissions for new ADCs. On August 19, 2011, the FDA approved brentuximab vedotin (Adcetris), currently the only ADC on the market. This recent approval and a greater understanding of the science behind ADC development pave the way for future development in this growing field.

As the development of ADCs continues, the science behind it is expected to evolve and grow. Safety evaluation of ADCs is a dynamic process. As more experience is gained with this class of products and technology advances to produce conjugates containing non-cytotoxic drugs, or containing different types of linkers and antibodies (e.g., antibody with double antigen-binding domain), current approaches will be reevaluated. In addition, nonclinical studies described above are for products indicated for patients with advanced cancers. Consulting appropriate guidances and discussing with appropriate FDA divisions are encouraged when the indication sought is for a non-life-threatening condition.

Clinical pharmacology of ADCs poses several challenges and nuances. The experience gained and lessons learned from the SMD development may not always apply to ADCs [45, 46]. Assay design is an important component of the development plan where poorly designed assays may indicate the need to reanalyze samples or repeat clinical and nonclinical studies. A recent report on assay development showed that the quantitation (level of detection) of a specific mAb in serum may be different depending on the bioanalytical method used [34].

As with all therapeutic drug development, the benefit must be weighed against the risk to patients. Approval decisions will not only be made based on the efficacy of an ADC but also the safety profile of the ADC that presents to patients. Not all studies are required for each ADC under development, and the nonclinical and clinical pharmacology programs should be tailored to the ADC under development. The FDA continues to be open to discussion with industry regarding the science and rationale behind recommended studies.

References

1. Ducry L, Stump B (2010) Antibody-drug conjugates: linking cytotoxic payloads to monoclonal antibodies. Bioconjug Chem 21(1):5–13
2. Barok M et al (2011) Trastuzumab-DM1 causes tumor growth inhibition by mitotic catastrophe in trastuzumab-resistant breast cancer cells in vivo. Breast Cancer Res 13(2):R46
3. Barok M et al (2007) Trastuzumab causes antibody-dependent cellular cytotoxicity-mediated growth inhibition of submacroscopic JIMT-1 breast cancer xenografts despite intrinsic drug resistance. Mol Cancer Ther 6(7):2065–2072
4. Remillard S et al (1975) Antimitotic activity of the potent tumor inhibitor maytansine. Science 189(4207):1002–1005
5. DiJoseph JF et al (2004) Antibody-targeted chemotherapy with CMC-544: a CD22-targeted immunoconjugate of calicheamicin for the treatment of B-lymphoid malignancies. Blood 103(5):1807–1814
6. Advani A et al (2010) Safety, pharmacokinetics, and preliminary clinical activity of inotuzumab ozogamicin, a novel immunoconjugate for the treatment of B-cell non-Hodgkin's lymphoma: results of a phase I study. J Clin Oncol 28(12):2085–2093
7. Younes A et al (2010) Brentuximab vedotin (SGN-35) for relapsed CD30-positive lymphomas. N Engl J Med 363(19):1812–1821
8. FDA (1997) Points to Consider in the Manufacture and Testing of Monoclonal Antibody Products for Human Use, CBER, Editor: Rockville; weblink last assessed January 3, 2012: http://www.fda.gov/downloads/BiologicsBloodVaccines/GuidanceComplianceRegulatoryInformation/OtherRecommendationsforManufacturers/UCM153182.pdf
9. FDA (2010) Guidance for Industry: ICH S9 Nonclinical Evaluation for Anticancer Pharmaceuticals. Weblink last assessed January 3, 2012: http://www.fda.gov/downloads/Drugs/GuidanceComplianceRegulatoryInformation/Guidances/ucm085389.pdf
10. Alley SC, Okeley NM, Senter PD (2010) Antibody-drug conjugates: targeted drug delivery for cancer. Curr Opin Chem Biol 14(4):529–537
11. FDA (1997) Guidance for Industry: ICH S6 Preclinical Safety Evaluation of Biotechnology-Derived Pharmaceuticals. Weblink last assessed January 3, 2012: http://www.fda.gov/downloads/regulatoryinformation/guidances/ucm129171.pdf
12. FDA (1996) Guideline for Industry: ICH S2A Specific Aspects of Regulatory Genotoxicity Tests for Pharmaceuticals. Weblink last assessed January 3, 2012: http://www.fda.gov/downloads/Drugs/GuidanceComplianceRegulatoryInformation/Guidances/ucm074925.pdf
13. Bross PF et al (2001) Approval summary: gemtuzumab ozogamicin in relapsed acute myeloid leukemia. Clin Cancer Res 7(6):1490–1496
14. Law CL et al (2004) Efficient elimination of B-lineage lymphomas by anti-CD20-auristatin conjugates. Clin Cancer Res 10(23):7842–7851
15. Sutherland MS et al (2006) Lysosomal trafficking and cysteine protease metabolism confer target-specific cytotoxicity by peptide-linked anti-CD30-auristatin conjugates. J Biol Chem 281(15):10540–10547
16. Alley SC et al (2008) Contribution of linker stability to the activities of anticancer immunoconjugates. Bioconjug Chem 19(3):759–765
17. Lewis Phillips GD (2008) Targeting HER2-positive breast cancer with trastuzumab-DM1, an antibody-cytotoxic drug conjugate. Cancer Res 68(22):9280–9290

18. Sanderson RJ et al (2005) In vivo drug-linker stability of an anti-CD30 dipeptide-linked auristatin immunoconjugate. Clin Cancer Res 11(2 Pt 1):843–852
19. Kuang B, King L, Wang HF (2010) Therapeutic monoclonal antibody concentration monitoring: free or total? Bioanalysis 2(6):1125–1140
20. Krop IE et al (2010) Phase I study of trastuzumab-DM1, an HER2 antibody-drug conjugate, given every 3 weeks to patients with HER2-positive metastatic breast cancer. J Clin Oncol 28(16):2698–2704
21. DeSilva B et al (2003) Recommendations for the bioanalytical method validation of ligand-binding assays to support pharmacokinetic assessments of macromolecules. Pharm Res 20(11):1885–1900
22. FDA (2001) Guidance for Industry: Bioanalytical Method Validation. Weblink last assessed January 3, 2012: http://www.fda.gov/downloads/Drugs/GuidanceComplianceRegulatoryInformation/Guidances/ucm070107.pdf
23. Hamblett KJ et al (2004) Effects of drug loading on the antitumor activity of a monoclonal antibody drug conjugate. Clin Cancer Res 10(20):7063–7070
24. McDonagh CF et al (2006) Engineered antibody-drug conjugates with defined sites and stoichiometries of drug attachment. Protein Eng Des Sel 19(7):299–307
25. Imanishi T, Makela O (1974) Inheritance of antibody specificity. I. Anti-(4-hydroxy-3-nitrophenyl)acetyl of the mouse primary response. J Exp Med 140(6):1498–1510
26. Imanishi T, Makela O (1974) Inheritance of fine-specificity in mouse anti-hapten antibodies. Ann Immunol (Paris) 125C(1–2):199–200
27. Bothwell AL et al (1981) Heavy chain variable region contribution to the NPb family of antibodies: somatic mutation evident in a gamma 2a variable region. Cell 24(3):625–637
28. Berek C, Griffiths GM, Milstein C (1985) Molecular events during maturation of the immune response to oxazolone. Nature 316(6027):412–418
29. Paul WE, Siskind GW (1970) Hapten specificity of cellular immune responses as compared with the specificity of serum anti-hapten antibody. Immunology 18(6):921–930
30. Yamashita U, Kitagawa M (1974) Induction of anti-hapten antibody response by hapten-isologous carrier conjugate. I. Development of hapten-reactive helper cells by hapten-isologous carrier. Cell Immunol 14(2):182–192
31. Harding FA et al (2010) The immunogenicity of humanized and fully human antibodies: residual immunogenicity resides in the CDR regions. MAbs 2(3):256–265
32. McKoy JM et al (2008) Epoetin-associated pure red cell aplasia: past, present, and future considerations. Transfusion 48(8):1754–1762
33. Buttel IC et al (2011) Taking immunogenicity assessment of therapeutic proteins to the next level. Biologicals 39(2):100–109
34. Swann PG, Shapiro MA (2011) Regulatory considerations for development of bioanalytical assays for biotechnology products. Bioanalysis 3(6):597–603
35. Getts DR et al (2010) Have we overestimated the benefit of human(ized) antibodies? MAbs 2(6):682–694
36. FDA (2009) Guidance for Industry: Assay Development for Immunogenicity Testing of Therapeutic Proteins. Weblink last assessed January 3, 2012: http://www.fda.gov/downloads/Drugs/GuidanceComplianceRegulatoryInformation/Guidances/UCM192750.pdf
37. FDA (2005) Guidance for Industry: Q5E Comparability of Biotechnological/Biological Products Subject to Changes in Their Manufacturing Process, CDER/CBER. Weblink last assessed January 3, 2012: http://www.fda.gov/downloads/RegulatoryInformation/Guidances/ucm128076.pdf
38. FDA (2010) Draft Guidance for Industry: Pharmacokinetics in Patients with Impaired Renal Function—Study Design, Data Analysis, and Impact on Dosing and Labeling. 2010; weblink last assessed January 3, 2012: http://www.fda.gov/downloads/Drugs/GuidanceComplianceRegulatoryInformation/Guidances/UCM204959.pdf
39. FDA (2003) Guidance for Industry: Exposure-Response Relationships—Study Design, Data Analysis, and Regulatory Applications. Weblink last assessed January 3, 2012: http://www.

fda.gov/downloads/Drugs/GuidanceComplianceRegulatoryInformation/Guidances/ucm072109.pdf
40. FDA (1999) Guidance for Industry: Population Pharmacokinetics. Weblink last assessed January3,2012:http://www.fda.gov/downloads/ScienceResearch/SpecialTopics/WomensHealthResearch/UCM133184.pdf
41. Rodriguez I et al (2010) Electrocardiographic assessment for therapeutic proteins—scientific discussion. Am Heart J 160(4):627–634
42. Curigliano G et al (2008) Drug-induced QTc interval prolongation: a proposal towards an efficient and safe anticancer drug development. Eur J Cancer 44(4):494–500
43. Rock EP et al (2009) Assessing proarrhythmic potential of drugs when optimal studies are infeasible. Am Heart J 157(5):827–836, 836.e1
44. Sarapa N, Britto MR (2008) Challenges of characterizing proarrhythmic risk due to QTc prolongation induced by nonadjuvant anticancer agents. Expert Opin Drug Saf 7(3):305–318
45. Lalonde RL, Honig P (2008) Clinical pharmacology in the era of biotherapeutics. Clin Pharmacol Ther 84(5):533–536
46. Mould DR, Green B (2010) Pharmacokinetics and pharmacodynamics of monoclonal antibodies: concepts and lessons for drug development. BioDrugs 24(1):23–39

Part II
Development of Antibody-Drug Conjugates

Chapter 3
Assay Methodologies and Challenges

Katherine R. Kozak and Helga Raab

Abbreviations

ADC	Antibody–drug conjugate
ADCC	Antibody-dependent cell-mediated cytotoxicity
CDC	Complement-dependent cytotoxicity
DAR	Drug-to-antibody ratio
ELISA	Enzyme-linked immunosorbent assay
HIC	Hydrophobic interaction chromatography
MALDI	Matrix-assisted laser desorption/ionization
MS	Mass spectrometry
RP-HPLC	Reversed-phase high-pressure liquid chromatography
TOF	Time of flight

Challenges Associated with Analytical Characterization of ADCs

The development of safe and efficacious antibody–drug conjugates (ADCs) requires their accurate characterization throughout all phases of the discovery, optimization, and development life cycle. This process includes straightforward in vitro characterization, such as measurements of purity, aggregation, and stability, and more

K.R. Kozak (✉)
Department of Biochemical and Cellular Pharmacology, Genentech, Inc., MS#98, 1 DNA Way, South San Francisco, CA 94080, USA
e-mail: kkozak@gene.com

H. Raab
Department of Protein Chemistry, Genentech, Inc., MS#63, 1 DNA Way, South San Francisco, CA 94080, USA
e-mail: raab.helga@gene.com

G.L. Phillips (ed.), *Antibody-Drug Conjugates and Immunotoxins: From Pre-Clinical Development to Therapeutic Applications*, Cancer Drug Discovery and Development, DOI 10.1007/978-1-4614-5456-4_3,

complex measurements of drug load, drug distribution, cytotoxicity, internalization, and binding to antigen or Fc gamma receptor (FcγR). Assessment of biological efficacy and preclinical safety in vivo requires the deployment of a panel of bioanalytical assays to quantitate total antibody (conjugated and unconjugated), conjugated antibody, free drug, and immunogenicity in plasma samples from a variety of animals used in preclinical studies. The sum of these data allows thorough assessments of ADC plasma stability, pharmacokinetics, safety, and efficacy.

The current analytical methods used to characterize ADCs evolved from assay methods and technologies previously implemented to investigate either small molecule cytotoxic compounds or therapeutic antibodies. The complete analytical profiling of ADCs requires methods geared to evaluating their multicomponent properties such as the average number of drugs on the antibody (drug-to-antibody ratio or DAR) and location of drug on the antibody (drug distribution). The drug heterogeneity of ADC's is one of the challenging characteristics that requires additional evaluation and method development compared to an unconjugated antibody. Depending on the conjugation method, ADCs can be a mixture of different antibodies with different drug loads where the number of drugs on each antibody molecule can vary. The variation in this DAR generally results in antibodies with 0–8 drugs, depending on the conjugation chemistry and the final targeted average DAR. Because the number of drugs per antibody can influence the antigen binding, potency, clearance, and possibly the bio-distribution and toxicity of the ADC, it is necessary to measure precisely the different circulating ADC DAR species. A second challenging characteristic of ADCs is the fact that the conjugation chemistry can result in positional heterogeneity. Thus, the antibodies with similar DAR may differ significantly as a result of different positions of the small molecules on the antibody. When the primary sites used for protein-directed conjugation are the lysine amino groups or the sulfhydryl groups of the interchain cysteine residues on the ADC molecule, this can yield a heterogeneous mixture with respect to the distribution of cytotoxic drug species. These unique characteristics of drug loading and distribution heterogeneity of ADCs represent unique analytical challenges because the different subpopulations for a given ADC could have different biological properties.

In addition to the increased level of ADC complexity due to drug load and position on the antibody, covalent conjugation of drug to antibodies can affect ADC stability, solubility [1–3], and binding [4]. Thus, depending on the characteristics of the drug, the linker, and the conjugation site, analytical methods that can be applied to the parent antibody may not always be applicable to the ADC or may yield misleading information. The challenge for the researcher is to build upon the methods used for analyzing the parent small molecule drug and unconjugated antibody to devise new, unique assays that are appropriate for the specific conjugation process and heterogeneity of the ADC's in question. In this respect, some methods have been more challenging than others to optimize for analyzing ADCs.

ADC Analytical Methods and Applications

There are a variety of assay methods that have been used to analyze ADCs, many of which have recently been captured in comprehensive reviews [5, 6]. Wakankar et al. [5] published a thorough review of analytical methods for physicochemical characterization of ADCs, while Stephan et al. [6] discussed analytical and bioanalytical assays and their challenges. Summaries of some of the more challenging methods and assays used to characterize ADCs are highlighted in this chapter (Table 3.1).

Chromatography

Chromatographic separation of ADCs and their enzymatic digests can provide important information such as the number and location of conjugation sites, amount of free drug, and average DAR. Chromatography is also a useful tool to purify DAR fractions used for assay characterization. Chromatographic methods based on hydrophobicity (reversed-phase high-pressure liquid chromatography—RP-HPLC, hydrophobic interaction chromatography—HIC), charge (ion-exchange chromatography), and size (size-exclusion chromatography) have all been used to help characterize ADCs. Reversed-phase high-pressure liquid chromatography (RP-HPLC) has been used to separate and quantify intact ADCs and their light and heavy chain fragments with different drug loads for characterization of ADCs, DAR fractions, and free drug content. This column separation uses alkyl chains bonded covalently to the support surface and a nonpolar stationary phase at high column temperatures (60–80°C) for high resolution of intact antibody. For example, RP-HPLC has been used to determine the location of drug attachment to the anti-CD30 antibody heavy and light chains [7, 8] and to determine DAR of conjugates containing auristatin drugs [9–12]. This method has also been used to determine free drug levels in various ADCs [7, 9, 13–16]. For instance, RP-HPLC in combination with mass spectrometry (MS) has been used to monitor the free drug species released in plasma [15] and in cultured tumor cell lines [17]. RP-HPLC polymer columns such as PLRP-S (Agilent, Santa Clara, CA, USA) with porous, hydrophobic, nonbonded stationary phases are routinely used to analyze intact ADCs or ADC fragments. However, heat and the use of denaturing mobile phases (containing organic solvents such as acetonitrile and acid modifiers) are usually necessary for resolution and recovery of the protein molecules from the column. These conditions do not preserve the native structure of the ADCs.

HIC is another chromatographic separation technique, which has been used to analyze ADCs. However, this technique can also be used to purify intact ADCs as it can have mild binding and elution conditions. Like RP-HPLC, HIC relies on the change in hydrophobicity imparted by conjugating one or more hydrophobic linker-drug moieties to an antibody. Successful resolution of DAR species depends on the

Table 3.1 Utility and challenges of ADC technologies

Technology	Utility	Challenges
Chromatography	Determine number of conjugation sites Determine location of conjugation sites Measure amount of free drug Purify DAR fractions Determine DAR average	Conjugation through lysine residues more difficult to resolve due to greater heterogeneity Conjugation with a hydrophobic drug can alter the solubility of an antibody Conjugation may induce aggregation which can alter column retention time and peak tailing
Immunoassays	Measure ADC binding to target Quantitate ADC conjugate, antibody, and drug Determine stability of linker and drug Measure FcγR binding Evaluate immunogenicity	DAR of sample may not match DAR of standard Conjugation can alter binding of ADC to capture and/or detection reagent Assay format can impact signal Antidrug antibodies used as capture may not measure all ADCs of different drug loads equally Antidrug antibodies used as detection may not provide signals proportional to drug load
Mass spectrometry	Characterize ADC DAR Analyze free drug & metabolites Characterize DAR fractions Evaluate linker stability	ADCs may not ionize equally Hydrolytically labile linkers may be affected by acidic conditions resulting in erroneous DAR assignments Conjugation at interchain disulfide bonds can cause antibody subunit dissociation Loss of drug may be induced by ionization energy
Spectrophotometry	Detect impurities Determine average DAR Measure ADC concentrations	Drug and antibody must have different wavelength spectra Extinction coefficient or λ_{max} of drug may change once bound or is in different buffer
Cell-based viability	Evaluate potency of ADC Measure ADCC and CDC	Assay incubation of more than 12 h can cause cell death Drug may be released before reaching the incubation time required to measure cell killing

hydrophobic nature of both the antibody and the linker-drug used. There are a variety of stationary phases available (phenyl, butyl, hexyl) with different hydrophobicity and selectivity characteristics. High salt aqueous mobile phases are generally used to bind the protein followed by elution with decreasing salt gradients. These mild binding and elution conditions typically maintain the native structure of the conjugated antibodies and allow the antibody to remain intact during analysis, even if the interchain disulfide bond is reduced during the conjugation process. ADC species purified by preparative HIC retain their cytotoxic activities and have been used to (i) determine the effects of drug loading on efficacy and toxicity in vitro and in vivo [10], (ii) evaluate ADC stability in plasma from treated animals [18], (iii) evaluate conjugation methodology [7], (iv) characterize the distribution of drug-linked species and determine the average DAR [12], and (v) investigate the impact of assay format on the detection of different DAR species [4].

Other forms of chromatography such as ion-exchange chromatography have been used to estimate the heterogeneity [19] and drug distribution of ADCs (e.g., Mylotarg™, [20]), while size-exclusion chromatography has been used to (i) characterize ADCs for protein fractionation, aggregation or contaminant removal, and degradation during storage in liquid formulations [21], (ii) to analyze the drug distribution [22], and (iii) to study the thermal stability [23].

There are a variety of challenges associated with analyzing ADCs using chromatography. With RP-HPLC, conjugates produced using linkage through lysine residues are not easily resolved due to their high degree of heterogeneity, and thus, this method generally yields only enriched fractions of lysine conjugates for assay characterization [4]. In contrast, HIC purification of cysteine conjugates can readily yield specific DAR fractions; however, conjugation with a particularly hydrophobic drug can alter the solubility of an antibody [1] or can lead to increased column retention time and peak tailing [9]. Addition of an organic modifier, such as acetonitrile or 25% propylene glycol, to the mobile phase has been used successfully to improve chromatographic performance [2, 14]; this may be by altering aggregated states of the drug in solution.

Immunoassays

Immunoassays are the most common methods used to characterize ADCs. These assays can be used to measure the ADC binding to target protein; quantitation of ADC, antibody, and drug; stability of the linker and the drug; FcγR binding; and immunogenicity. These measurements are important for understanding the efficacy, pharmacokinetics, and safety of ADCs. Enzyme-linked immunosorbent assays (ELISAs) have commonly been used to evaluate ADC concentrations and antigen binding.

Specific Total Antibody ELISA

Total antibody ELISAs are commonly used to measure the concentration of ADCs with a DAR higher (conjugated) or equal to 0 (unconjugated). These assays usually rely on the antibody target antigen or anti-idiotypic antibody as coat material to capture the antibody on a plate, and the binding of the ADC to the antigen-coated wells is then detected using a species-specific anti-immunoglobulin secondary antibody coupled to an enzyme [4, 24]. When an antigen or an anti-idiotypic antibody is used in an ELISA, the assay is referred to as a specific ELISA. For example, specific ELISAs using an antigen as capture have been used to quantitate ricin A chain-conjugated anti-human α-fetoprotein [13, 24], anti-CD33-calicheamicin ADC [25], Trastuzumab-DM1[26],anti-MUC16-vc-MMAE[12],andanti-GPNMB-vc-MMAE [27, 28]. Anti-idiotypic antibodies have also been utilized as capture to quantify ADC total antibody for anti-CD30 cAC10 vc-MMAE [10], anti-PSMA-DM1 [29], anti-CD30-vc-MMAE [8, 18, 30], anti-CD70-vc-MMAF [31], and anti-Steap1 MC-vc-PAB-MMAE [32].

Generic Total Antibody ELISA

In the absence of antigen or anti-idiotypic antibody, generic ELISAs (using anti-human IgG or anti-Fc for both capture and detection) have been implemented to quantitate ADCs in preclinical PK studies. For example, in a generic total antibody ELISA used to measure huC242-DM1 in mouse plasma (cantuzumab mertansine, [33]), the capture reagent was an antibody that recognizes all human IgG (hence the term generic) rather than an antigen that is specifically recognized by the variable region of the ADC.

Semi-homogeneous ELISA

We have shown that semi-homogeneous ELISAs, where both the capture and detection antibodies are allowed to form a complex with the ADC prior to immobilization on a plate, provide a significant advantage for characterizing ADCs with different drug loads. This assay format can bridge a biotinylated antigen, anti-idiotypic antibody, or anti-human IgG antibody with the ADC in the sample and an anti-human Fc or IgG-HRP detection antibody. The complex formed during a preincubation step can then be captured on either streptavidin- or neutrAvidin-coated plates and washed prior to detection. To select the optimal assay reagents and format for quantitating an ADC, it is recommended to first characterize ELISAs using purified or enriched ADC DAR fractions. These ELISAs yield comparable concentration results for antibodies with different drug loads whereas concentration data from sequential ELISAs can vary depending on the ADC DAR (unpublished). Thus, the semi-homogeneous ELISA, with its reduced washing, offers advantages, especially when it is necessary to quantify a mixture of DARs generated during the conjugation process.

Competitive ELISA

Competitive ELISAs have also been used to help characterize ADCs. For a competition ELISA, the higher the sample concentration (ADC or free drug), the weaker the eventual signal. In general, a capture molecule (target antigen or antidrug antibody) is coated onto a plate in order to bind a fixed amount of labeled-detection reagent (ADC or free drug). Standards or samples containing ADC or free drug (competitor) are titrated and preincubated with the fixed labeled-detection reagent. The mixture is then added to the pre-coated wells, washed, and detected. There are few examples of using competitive ELISAs to quantitate total antibody [34], as compared to using competitive assays to measure free drug [18, 25, 28, 29, 33–36]. Tolcher et al. [34] reported the use of an anti-idiotypic antibody in a competition ELISA measuring anti-MUC1-DM1 in human plasma from a phase I clinical study. In this study, the assay lower limit of detection was 1.56 μg/ml, indicating that this method was significantly less sensitive than other quantification methods. Competition ELISAs have more frequently been used to measure free drug. For example, this assay has been implemented to detect free maytansinoid in various samples [33–35] and to quantify calicheamicin derivatives [25]. The competition ELISA is particularly useful in measuring the average drug quantity conjugated to an antibody by quantifying free drug after induced release. For example, Sanderson et al. [18] determined the total amount of MMAE bound to circulating cAC10-vc-MMAE, by incubating plasma samples with cathepsin B and then detecting the drug in a competition ELISA.

Conjugated Antibody ELISA

Although preexisting ELISA formats have been useful to characterize ADCs by measuring total antibody concentration and free drug, measurement of the conjugated ADC has required specific assay development. One such assay, the conjugated antibody ELISA, measures only antibody with drug attached (DAR greater than or equal to 1) and does not measure unconjugated antibody. This is done by capturing the drug portion of the ADC using an antidrug antibody in combination with an extracellular domain or anti-idiotypic antibody (specific conjugated antibody ELISA) or in combination with an anti-human IgG antibody (generic conjugated antibody ELISA). Quantification of drug-loaded antibody is particularly useful for understanding exposure, drug pharmacokinetics, and pharmacodynamics in in vivo efficacy studies. Measurement of the percent conjugation (relative amount of conjugated antibody compared to total antibody) can be used as a general indicator of linker stability [37], which is useful in evaluating linker stability in plasma either in vitro or ex vivo. For instance, Sung et al. [38] determined linker stability in a human anti-CD70 antibody conjugated to a prodrug containing DNA alkylating cytotoxic drug A using a specific total and conjugated antibody assay. For conjugated antibody assay quantitation, many investigators have used antidrug-specific antibodies as capture reagents, while others have used antidrug antibodies as detection reagents (Table 3.2).

Table 3.2 Antidrug antibodies used in conjugated Ab ELISAs

Target	Antidrug antibody	Antidrug antibody used as capture	Antidrug antibody used as detection
Anti-CanAg-DM1	Anti-DM1	[33, 35]	[34]
Anti-B7-H4-DM1	Anti-DM1	[39]	
Anti-HER2 T-DM1	Anti-DM1	[26]	
Anti-CD22 MCC-DM1	Anti-DM1	[4]	[4]
Anti-CD25-ricin A-chain	Anti-Ricin	[40, 41]	
Anti-CD30-vc-MMAE	Anti-MMAE	[18]	[18]
Anti-MUC16-vc-MMAE ch3A5	Anti-MMAE		[12]
Anti-GPNMB-vc-MMAE	Anti-MMAE	[28]	
Anti-Steap1-vc-MMAE	Anti-MMAE	[32]	
Anti-CD22-MC-MMAF	Anti-MMAF	[4]	[4]
Anti-CD70-MC-MMAF	Anti-MMAF		[31]
Anti-CD22-calicheamicin	Anti-calicheamicin		[42]
Anti-CD22-calicheamicin	Anti-calicheamicin	[36]	

Immunoassay Challenges

A challenge with using immunoassays to characterize ADCs has been that as drug is released from the ADC in circulation, the resulting changes in DAR may lead to ADCs that are different from the ADC used as assay standard. Another challenge is that drug conjugation to the antibody has the potential to alter binding of ADC to its capture and/or detection reagent. This is generally not observed with assays where only one binding site is required for measurement (e.g., SPR, FACS). For example, different total antibody ELISA formats and reagents have been shown to impact the binding of ADCs. The extent of this impact depends on which linker and drug is conjugated to the antibody (e.g., MCC-DM1, MC-MMAF, vc-MMAE). Stephan et al. [4] demonstrated the impact drug load has on the ADC quantification with ELISAs, by comparing the quantification of ADCs in different assay formats, utilizing enriched fractions of anti-CD22-MCC-DM1 (average DAR of 0, 1, 3.1, 4.2, 6.5 and 8.5) and purified DAR fractions of anti-CD22-MC-MMAF (DAR0, 2, 4, 6 and 8). In this way, the authors evaluated the negative impact of increasing DM1 load on the antigen-binding activity of the ADC. Because the influence of drug load on the total antibody assay can be assessed using DAR fractions, it is best to evaluate the recovery of these fractions in different assay formats. A challenge specific to conjugated antibody ELISAs is that when using antidrug antibodies as capture, they may not measure all ADCs of different drug loads equally, while assays using antidrug antibodies as detection may not provide detection signals proportional to the number of drug molecules [4,12,18]. In general, ELISAs using antidrug as coating antibody tend to be less sensitive to differences in drug load ([39]; Phillips et al. 2008; [4]), compared to the ELISAs using antidrug antibodies as detection [4, 18]. Thus, the extent of drug impact binding is dependent upon the antibody reagents used, emphasizing the value of characterizing assays with enriched or purified DAR fractions.

Mass Spectrometry

MS has been utilized to evaluate linker stability, analyze free drug and metabolites, characterize DAR fractions, and more recently to determine the relative ratios of ADCs with different DARs. The MS principle consists of ionizing molecules to generate charged species or molecular fragments and measuring their mass-to-charge ratios. Specific MS methods used to characterize ADCs include electrospray ionization MS (ESI-MS), coupled to time-of-flight (TOF) [43, 44] or triple quadrupole mass detectors [45]. Used in combination with HIC and RP-HPLC, MS (LC–MS) or MS/MS (LC–MS/MS) has been used to (i) analyze the structural or compositional characteristics of huN901-SPP-DM1 [46] and C242-DM4 [22], (ii) evaluate linker stability of 1F6-C4v2-bac-MMAF [31], (iii) analyze the number of drugs conjugated per antibody to Thio-trastuzumab-MC-vc-PAB-MMAE and -MPEO-DM1 [12, 47], (iv) investigate the impact of assay formats on the detection of anti-CD22-MC-MMAF [4], (v) elucidate the exact position of a coumarin linker conjugation [48], and (vi) determine the relative ratios of ADCs with different DARs [43, 49]. The latter authors developed a method to immuno-affinity purify ADCs using antigen-coated beads, followed by reversed-phase chromatographic separation and analysis by electrospray quadrupole TOF MS. Using this approach, the relative percentage of ADCs with different DARs was determined. The characterization of plasma trastuzumab-MCC-DM1 was performed by capturing the ADC using a target receptor extracellular domain or an antidrug mouse monoclonal antibody immobilized onto a membrane or a bead-based support. The immobilized ADC was then washed and eluted and analyzed by LC–MS. This method also successfully identified antibody species whose mass was consistent with drug loss from engineered site-specific ADCs [43, 44]. Finally, concentrations of free drug released from the ADCs in samples from in vivo plasma or plasma stability studies can be measured using LC–MS/MS, as is common practice for small molecule therapeutics [9, 15, 32]. Aliquots of cAC10-vc-MMAE incubated in human, mouse, or dog plasma were analyzed by LC–MS/MS for the release of free MMAE [15].

Matrix-assisted laser desorption/ionization (MALDI) is a soft ionization technique allowing analysis of biomolecules, which tend to fragment when ionized. When combined with UV (UV MALDI-TOF MS), MALDI has also been used to characterize ADCs. For example, MALDI has been used to compare unconjugated antibody with ADCs conjugated through lysine residues to calicheamicin, methotrexate, or mitoxantrone [3, 50] and lysine-linked conjugates prepared using activated paclitaxel [51]. Infrared combined with MALDI (IR/MALDI) has been used to analyze calicheamicin conjugates [52]. Finally, MALDI-TOF MS has been used to measure levels of DOTA and DM1 on PSMA antibody conjugates [53] and to measure levels of drug conjugation of anti-B7-H4 to DM1 [39].

One of the challenges of MS is that it assumes that all species, whether of high or low drug load, ionize the same as the unconjugated species. Thus, the integration of the deconvoluted mass spectrum used to estimate the DAR assumes equivalent recovery and ionization of all species. This may not always be the case since drug conjugation to positively charged amines leads to changes in both charge and hydrophobicity. Therefore, it is important to evaluate that all antibody speciesionize similarly during method development. Additionally, hydrolytically labile linkers (such as those containing a hydrazone) can be affected by the acidic LC/MS conditions or by acidic matrices frequently used for MALDI analysis, resulting in erroneous DAR assignments. MS-based approaches used to analyze ADC DAR ratios face another challenge. Although MS-based approaches can be readily implemented for lysine residue conjugations where intact disulfides are present and the antibody chains do not dissociate in the presence of the denaturing conditions used to effect chromatography and ionization, it is more challenging for characterization of ADCs conjugated via maleimide linkage to cysteine residues (unless the cysteine residues are engineered outside the internal disulfide bonds). Conjugation of drugs to the interchain disulfide bonds leaves the antibody held together with mostly noncovalent bonds, which inevitably dissociate under the conditions used for optimal resolution and ionization. It has been recently shown that, if analysis occurs in the absence of organic solvent and acidic ion-pairing reagents, this softer ionization may allow the heavy and light chain of the ADC to remain together [54].

Ultraviolet–Visible Spectrophotometry

Ultraviolet–visible spectrophotometry (UV/Vis) has been used historically to analyze ADCs, in order to detect impurities and determine average DAR and ADC concentrations. Using the measured absorbances of the ADC and the extinction coefficients of the monoclonal antibody at its A_{max} of ~280 nm and the drug at its A_{max}, the individual concentrations of monoclonal antibody and drug can be calculated. Examples of this include the characterization of the vinca alkaloid conjugate 4-desacetylvinblastine [14], maytansinoid DM1 [55], doxorubicin [56], calicheamicin analogues [57], and dipeptide-linked auristatins such as MC-vc-MMAE [10]. Hamblett et al. [10] confirmed the quantification of a different drug-loaded ADC by comparing the results obtained using UV analysis described above with those obtained with chromatographic (HIC) methods. This method requires that the UV/Vis spectra of the drug and of the unconjugated antibody have different λ_{max} values [10, 14, 55–57]. Another challenge is that the extinction coefficient or λ_{max} of the drug may change once bound or in a different buffer. Siegel et al. [50] demonstrated some of these differences when using UV by comparing UV/Vis to UV-MALDI MS.

Cell-Based Viability Assays: Anti-proliferation and Cytotoxicity

Cell-based viability assays can be used to measure the in vitro anti-proliferative efficacy and cytotoxicity of ADCs. ADC potency studies are typically conducted by comparing the anti-proliferative activity of the ADC with that of the unconjugated antibody, using paired or distinct cell lines that do or do not express the ADC surface antigen. Frequently, a nonrelevant drug-conjugated antibody may be used as a negative control. In practice, mammalian cells expressing a target protein are exposed to the ADC for a period of about 6 h to 5 days, and cell viability is assessed during this time period or at a specific end point. A variety of methods for evaluating cell viability have been used, including cell counting [55], dye exclusion [24], dye reduction [58], and incorporation of radiolabeled precursors [59, 60]. Colorimetric approaches [61] that use dyes such as Alamar Blue [62], Vybrant™, and UptiBlue™ or to monitor cellular metabolic activity [8, 17, 63] are also extensively used. CellTiter-Glo™, another indicator of metabolically active cells that indirectly monitors ATP levels, is frequently used to measure the cellular anti-proliferative activity of ADCs ([12, 64, 65–67]).

In addition to understanding the efficacy of an ADC, the mechanism of action is also important. ADC-induced target cell killing can also be mediated via antibody-dependent cell-mediated cytotoxicity or ADCC. ADCC is a cell-mediated reaction in which nonspecific cytotoxic cells that express Fc receptors recognize bound antibody on a target cell leading to their lysis. Because certain ADC conjugation techniques involve limited reduction of intra- or interchain disulfide bonds by treatment with reducing agents, the potential for the ADC to bind to Fc receptors and trigger ADCC may be altered and thus needs to be evaluated. An example of ADC conjugation reducing Fc binding has been shown by [68], where amine coupling at high load ratios had a significant effect on binding to the Fc domain. A typical ADCC assay consists of treating a target cell line, which may have been pre-labeled and is expressing the surface-exposed antigen of interest, with the ADC. After washing, effector cells expressing Fc receptors are coincubated with the ADC-treated target cells. Target cell lysis is subsequently quantitated by measuring the release of intracellular label or enzyme using a scintillation counter, fluorometer, or spectrophotometry. ADC, unconjugated antibody, and an ADCC positive control are generally evaluated during assessment of ADCC. In addition, the ADC should also be tested without the addition of effector cells to ensure that there is no killing by the ADC within the duration of the assay. ADCC assays have been used to investigate the mechanism of action of ADC-induced cell death [69, 70]. For example, DiJoseph et al. [69] utilized CD22 expressing Ramos B-lymphoma cells as target cells and peripheral blood mononuclear cells as effector cells in the presence of an anti-CD22 antibody covalently linked to calicheamicin. These authors treated the Ramos cells with anti-CD22 calicheamicin conjugate for 4 h at 37°C, and then, the release of LDH in the cell-free culture medium was assessed using a Cytotox-1 homogeneous membrane integrity assay. The negative controls included Ramos cells alone, PBMCs alone, a mixture of Ramos cells and PBMCs in the absence of antibodies, Ramos cells and antibodies without PBMCs, and PBMCs and antibodies without Ramos cells. Maximum release of LDH was derived from cells treated with the lysis buffer. They found the ADC not to have effector function, thus attributing potency to efficient internalization and subsequent intracellular delivery.

Another cell-killing mechanism is complement-dependent cytotoxicity (CDC) in which complement-dependent cell lysis occurs as a result of binding of antibody to the cell surface and subsequent activation of the complement pathway. CDC assays can assess whether a molecule ADC causes lysis of target cells in the presence of complement can be assessed using complement for either normal human serum or rabbit serum [69, 71, 72]. DiJoseph et al. [69] treated Ramos cells with anti-CD22 antibody covalently linked to calicheamicin for 4 h at 37°C with or without mouse blood serum as a source of murine complement. CDC assays, in the context of in vivo efficacy studies, provide critical data for the characterization of the ADC.

The potent anti-proliferative or cytotoxicity activity of many ADCs can pose a challenge for measuring antigen binding in a cellular context, because any binding assessment that may require an incubation of more than 12 h can cause cell death. Cell-based assays with short incubation times such as cell-binding assays (30 min to several hours) or even CDC assays are less impacted by this issue, although even these assays are performed using the unconjugated antibody as control along with the ADC. However, evaluating certain ADC-induced cell killing can be more difficult. Thus, these assays require careful optimization of the time course of cell growth. The challenge of monitoring the timing cell growth can be minimized by applying real-time cell-based technologies such as Incucyte™ (Essen BioScience, Ann Arbor, MI) or xCELLegence™ (Roche, Indianapolis, IN, USA). Both of these technologies allow faster optimization of the best end point of assays measuring potency or anti-proliferation. Another challenge with anti-proliferation assays is that the drug portion of the ADC could be released before reaching the incubation time required to measure cell killing. For example, Sharkey et al. [58] showed that despite differences in antigen expression, Emab–SN-38 and Vmab–SN-38 had similar potencies as the non-binding Lmab–SN-38 anti-anti-CEACAM5 conjugate in a MTS dye assay. This was likely due to dissociation of SN-38 during the 4-day assay. Annexin V staining after a 1-day exposure also failed to find differences between untreated and treated cells. Because these conjugates require a 48-h exposure before early signs of apoptosis could be seen, it was concluded that in vitro testing would not be able to discriminate the potency, and therefore, the authors resorted to in vivo studies [58].

Conclusion

Although there have been efforts made to minimize ADC heterogeneity using reduction/oxidation strategies [7] and protein engineering of antibodies where serine residues replace interchain cysteines [8], or cysteine residues are engineered at sites selected for drug conjugation [12, 73], due to the complex structural nature of ADCs, appropriate ADC characterization is required. Preexisting and novel bioanalytical strategies have been required to support the characterization of a growing collection of novel ADCs that have emerged from drug discovery pipelines. In this review, we have attempted to emphasize some of the particular challenges of some of the current methods used to characterize these ADCs. Although we continue to overcome analytical challenges of our current tools used to characterize ADCs, development of new assay technologies for implementing bioanalytical methods will allow for better understanding of ADCs in vivo.

Acknowledgements We thank Cris Lewis, Hicham Alaoui, and Ola Saad for their useful comments on the manuscript.

References

1. King HD, Dubowchik GM, Mastalerz H et al (2002) Monoclonal antibody conjugates of doxorubicin prepared with branched peptide linkers: inhibition of aggregation by methoxytriethyleneglycol chains. J Med Chem 45:4336–4343
2. Hollander I, Kunz A, Hamann PR (2008) Selection of reaction additives used in the preparation of monomeric antibody-calicheamicin conjugates. Bioconjugate Chem 19:358–361
3. Quiles S, Raisch KP, Sanford LL et al (2010) Synthesis and preliminary biological evaluation of high-drug-load paclitaxel-antibody conjugates for tumor-targeted chemotherapy. J Med Chem 53:586–594
4. Stephan JP, Chan P, Lee C et al (2008) Anti-CD22-MCC-DM1 and MC-MMAF conjugates: impact of assay format on pharmacokinetic parameters determination. Bioconjugate Chem 19:1673–1683
5. Wakankar A, Chen Y, Gokarn Y et al (2011) Analytical methods for physicochemical characterization of antibody drug conjugates. Landes Biosci 3(2):161–172
6. Stephan JP, Kozak KR, Wong WL (2011) Challenges in developing bioanalytical assays for characterization of antibody-drug conjugates. Bioanalysis 3(6):677–700
7. Sun MM, Beam KS, Cerveny CG et al (2005) Reduction-alkylation strategies for the modification of specific monoclonal antibody disulfides. Bioconjugate Chem 16:1282–1290
8. McDonagh CF, Turcott E, Westendorf L et al (2006) Engineered antibody-drug conjugates with defined sites and stoichiometries of drug attachment. Protein Eng Des Sel 19:299–307
9. Doronina SO, Toki BE, Torgov MY et al (2003) Development of potent monoclonal antibody auristatin conjugates for cancer therapy. Nat Biotechnol 21:778–784
10. Hamblett KJ, Senter PD, Chace DF et al (2004) Effects of drug loading on the anti-tumor activity of a monoclonal antibody drug conjugate. Clin Cancer Res 10:7063–7070
11. Erickson HK, Park PU, Widdison WC et al (2006) Antibody-maytansinoid conjugates are activated in targeted cancer cells by lysosomal degradation and linker-dependent intracellular processing. Cancer Res 66:4426–4433
12. Junutula JR, Raab H, Clark S et al (2008) Site-specific conjugation of a cytotoxic drug to an antibody improves the therapeutic index. Nat Biotech 26:925–932
13. Hurwitz E, Levy R, Maron R et al (1975) The covalent binding of daunomycin and adriamycin to antibodies, with retention of both drug and antibody activities. Cancer Res 35:1175–1181
14. Laguzza BC, Nichols CL, Briggs SL et al (1989) New antitumor monoclonal antibody-vinca conjugates LY203725 and related compounds: design, preparation, and representative in vivo activity. J Med Chem 32:548–555
15. Francisco JA, Cerveny CG, Meyer DL et al (2003) cAC10-Val-CitMMAE, an anti-CD30-monomethyl auristatin E conjugate with potent and selective anti-tumor activity. Blood 102:1458–1465

16. Fleming MS, Zhang W, Lambert JM et al (2005) A reversed-phase high-performance liquid chromatography method for analysis of monoclonal antibody-maytansinoid immunoconjugates. Anal Biochem 340:272–278
17. Doronina SO, Mendelsohn BA, Bovee TD et al (2006) Enhance activity of monomethylauristatin F through monoclonal antibody delivery: effect of linker technology on efficacy and toxicity. Bioconjugate Chem 17:114–124
18. Sanderson RJ, Hering MA, James SF et al (2005) In vivo drug-linker stability of anti-CD30 dipeptide-linked auristatin immunoconjugate. Clin Cancer Res 11:843–852
19. Maeda E, Urakami K, Shimura K et al (2010) Charge heterogeneity of a therapeutic monoclonal antibody conjugated with a cytotoxic antitumor antibiotic, calicheamicin. J Chromatogr A 1217:7164–7171
20. Kunz A (2004) Calicheamycin derivative carrier conjugates, United States patent application publication pub. no. US 2004/0192900 A1
21. Cordoba AJ, Shyong BJ, Breen D et al (2005) Non-enzymatic hinge region fragmentation of antibodies in solution. J Chromatogr B Analyt Technol Biomed Life Sci 818:115–121
22. Lazar AC, Wang L, Blattler WA et al (2005) Analysis of the composition of immunoconjugates using size-exclusion chromatography coupled to mass spectrometry. Rapid Commun Mass Spectrom 19:1806–1814
23. Wakankar A, Feeney MB, Rivera J et al (2010) Physicochemical stability of the antibody-drug conjugate trastuzumab-DM1: changes due to modification and conjugation processes. Bioconjugate Chem 21(9):1588–1595
24. Tsukazaki K, Hayman EG, Rusolahti E (1985) Effects of ricin A chain conjugates of monoclonal antibodies to human a-fetoprotein and placental alkaline phosphatase on antigen-producing tumor cells in culture. Cancer Res 45:1834–1838
25. Dowell JA, Korth-Bradley J, Liu H et al (2001) Pharmacokinetics of gemtuzumab ozogamicin, an antibody-targeted chemotherapy agent for the treatment of patients with acute myeloid leukemia in first relapse. J Clin Pharmacol 41:1206–1214
26. Phillips GDL, Li G, Dugger DL et al (2008) Targeting HER2-positive breast cancer with trastuzumab-DM1, an antibody-cytotoxic drug conjugate. Cancer Res 68:9280–9290
27. Pollack VA, Alvarez E, Tse KF et al (2007) Treatment parameters modulating regression of human melanoma xenografts by an antibody-drug conjugate (CR011-vcMMAE) targeting GPNMB. Cancer Chemother Pharmacol 60:423–435
28. Sznol M, Hamid O, Hwu P et al (2009) Pharmacokinetics of CR011-vcMMAE, an antibody-drug conjugate, in a phase I study of patients with advanced melanoma. Poster 2009 ASCO annual meeting. J Clin Oncol 27:15s (suppl; abstr 9063)
29. Henry MD, Wen S, Silva MD et al (2004) A Prostate-specific membrane antigen-targeted monoclonal antibody-chemotherapeutic conjugate designed for the treatment of prostate cancer. Cancer Res 64:7995–8001
30. McDonagh CF, Kim KM, Turcott E et al (2008) Engineered anti-CD70 antibody-drug conjugate with increased therapeutic index. Mol Cancer Ther 7:2913–2931
31. Alley SC, Benjamin DR, Jeffrey SC et al (2008) Contribution of linker stability to the activities of anticancer immunoconjugates. Bioconjugate Chem 19:759–765
32. Boswell CA, Mundo EE, Zhang C et al (2011) Impact of drug conjugation on pharmacokinetics and tissue distribution of anti-STEAP1 antibody-drug conjugates in rats. Bioconjugate Chem 22:1994–2004
33. Xie H, Audette C, Hoffee M et al (2004) Pharmacokinetics and biodistribution of the anti-tumor immunoconjugate, cantuzumab mertansine (huC242-DM1), and its two components in mice. J Pharmacol Exp Ther 308:1073–1082
34. Tolcher AW, Ochoa L, Hammond LA et al (2003) Cantuzumab mertansine, a maytansinoid immunoconjugate directed to the CanAg antigen: a phase I, pharmacokinetic, and biologic correlative study. J Clin Oncol 21:211–222
35. Kovtun YV, Audette CA, Ye Y et al (2006) Antibody-drug conjugates designed to eradicate tumors with homogeneous and heterogeneous expression of the target antigen. Cancer Res 66: 3214–3221

36. Advani A, Coiffier B, Czuczman MS et al (2010) Safety, pharmacokinetics, and preliminary clinical activity of inotuzumab ozogamicin, a novel immunoconjugate for the treatment of B-cell Non-Hodgkin's Lymphoma: results of a phase I study. J Clin Oncol 28:2085–2093
37. Ferraiolo BL, Mohler MA (1994) Analytical methods for biotechnology products. In: Welling PG, Balant LP (eds) Pharmacokinetics of drugs, vol 110, Handbook of experimental pharmacology. Springer-Verlag, Berlin, New York
38. Sung J, Derwin D, Vemuri K et al (2010) In vitro plasma stability of human anti-CD70 antibody drug conjugate, MDX-1203. USA Association of American Cancer Research Abstract #2587
39. Hsieh FY, Tengstrand E, Li LY et al (2008) Toxicological protein biomarker analysis—an investigative one-week single dose intravenous infusion toxicity and toxicokinetic study in cynomolgus monkeys using an antibody–cytotoxic conjugate against ovarian. Pharm Res 25(6):1309–1317
40. Engert A, Diehl V, Schnell R et al (1997) A phase-I study of an anti-CD25 Ricin A-chain immunotoxin (RFT5-SMPT-dgA) in patients with refractory Hodgkin's lymphoma. Blood 89(2):403–410
41. Schnell R, Vitetta E, Schindler JB et al (2000) Treatment of refractory Hodgkin's lymphoma patients with an anti-CD25 ricin A-chain immunotoxin. Leukemia 14:129–135
42. Dijoseph JF, Armellino DC, Boghaert ER et al (2004) Antibody-targeted chemotherapy with CMC-544: a CD22-targeted immunoconjugate of calicheamicin for treatment of B-lymphoid malignancies. Blood 103:1807–1814
43. Xu K, Liu L, Saad OM et al (2011) Characterization of intact antibody-drug conjugates from plasma/serum in vivo by affinity capture capillary liquid chromatography-mass spectrometry. Anal Biochem 412(1):56–66
44. Shen B-Q, Xu K, Liu L et al (2012) Conjugation site modulates the in vivo stability and therapeutic activity of antibody-drug conjugates. Nat Biotechnol 30(2):184–189
45. Zhang Z, Pan H, Chen X (2009) Mass spectrometry for structural characterization of therapeutic antibodies. Mass Spectrom Rev 28:147–176
46. Wang L, Amphlett G, Blattler WA et al (2005) Structural characterization of the maytansinoid-monoclonal antibody immunoconjugate, huN901-DM1, by mass spectrometry. Protein Sci 14:2436–2446
47. Junutula JR, Flagella KM, Graham RA et al (2010) Engineered thio-trastuzumab-DM1 conjugate with an improved therapeutic index to target human epidermal growth factor receptor 2-positive breast cancer. Clin Cancer Res 16:4769–4778
48. Chih H-W, Gikanga B, Tang Y et al (2011) Identification of amino acid responsible for the release of free drug from an antibody-drug conjugate utilizing lysine-succinimidyl ester chemistry. J Pharm Sci 100(7):2518–2525
49. Xu K, Saad O, Baudys J et al (2007) Bioanalytical strategies for antibody drug conjugate (ADC) biopharmaceutical development: characterization of trastuzumab-MCC-DM1 in plasma by affinity mass spectrometry. AAPS National Biotechnology Conference. J Am Soc Mass Spec 18(5):S11–S15
50. Siegel MM, Hollander IJ, Hamann PR et al (1991) Matrix-assisted UV-laser desorption/ionization mass spectrometric analysis of monoclonal antibodies for the determination of carbohydrate, conjugated chelator, and conjugated drug content. Anal Chem 63:2470–81
51. Safavy A, Bonner JA, Waksal HW et al (2003) Synthesis and biological evaluation of paclitaxel-C225 conjugate as a model for targeted drug delivery. Bioconjugate Chem 14:302–310
52. Siegel MM, Tabei K, Kunz A et al (1997) Calicheamicin derivatives conjugated to monoclonal antibodies: determination of loading values and distributions by infrared and UV matrix-assisted laser desorption/ionization mass spectrometry and electrospray ionization mass spectrometry. Anal Chem 69:2716–2726
53. Lu SX, Takach EJ, Solomon M et al (2005) Mass spectral analyses of labile DOTA-NHS and heterogeneity determination of DOTA or DM1 conjugated anti-PSMA antibody for prostate cancer therapy. J Pharm Sci 94(4):788–797
54. Valliere-Douglass JF, McFee WA, Salas-Solano O (2012) Native intact mass determination of antibodies conjugated with monomethyl auristatin E and F at interchain cysteine residues. Anal Chem 84:2843–2849

55. Chari RV, Martell BA, Gross JL et al (1992) Immunoconjugates containing novel maytansinoids: promising anticancer drugs. Cancer Res 52:127–131
56. Willner D, Trail PA, Hofstead SJ et al (1993) (6-Maleimidocaproyl)hydrazone of doxorubicin—a new derivative for the preparation of immunoconjugates of doxorubicin. Bioconjugate Chem 4:521–527
57. Hinman LM, Hamann PR, Wallace R et al (1993) Preparation and characterization of monoclonal antibody conjugates of the calicheamicins: a novel and potent family of antitumor antibiotics. Cancer Res 53:3336–3342
58. Sharkey RM, Govindan SV, Cardillo TM et al (2012) Epratuzumab-SN-38: a new antibody-drug conjugate for the therapy of hematologic malignancies. Mol Cancer Ther 11:224–234
59. Lambert JM, Senter PD, Yay-Young A et al (1985) Purified immunotoxins that are reactive with human lymphoid cells. J Biol Chem 260:12035–12041
60. Tai YT, Li XF, Catley L et al (2005) Immunomodulatory drug lenalidomide (CC-5013, IMiD3) augments anti-CD40 SGN-40-induced cytotoxicity in human multiple myeloma: clinical implications. Cancer Res 65:11712–11720
61. DiJoseph JF, Dougher MM, Kalyandrug LB et al (2006) Antitumor efficacy of a combination of CMC-544 (inotuzumab ozogamicin), a CD22-targeted cytotoxic immunoconjugate of calicheamicin, and rituximab against non-Hodgkin's B-cell lymphoma. Clin Cancer Res 12(1):242–249
62. Petrul HM, Schatz CA, Kopitz CC et al (2012) Therapeutic mechanism and efficacy of the antibody-drug conjugate BAY 79-4620 targeting human carbonic anhydrase 9. Molecular Cancer Ther 11:340–349
63. Kim KM, McDonagh CF, Westendorf L et al (2008) Anti-CD30 diabody-drug conjugates with potent anti-tumor activity. Mol Cancer Ther 7:2486–2497
64. Ingle G, Chan P, Elliott JM et al (2007) High CD21 expression inhibits internalization of anti-CD19 antibodies and cytotoxicity of an anti-CD19-drug conjugate. British J Haematol 140:46–58
65. Dornan D, Bennett F, Chen Y et al (2009) Therapeutic potential of an anti-CD79b antibody-drug conjugate, anti-CD79b-vc-MMAE, for the treatment of non-Hodgkin lymphoma. Blood 114(13):2721–2729
66. Ryan MC, Kostner H, Gordon KA et al (2010) Targeting pancreatic and ovarian carcinomas using the auristatin-based anti-CD70 antibody–drug conjugate SGN-75. British J Cancer 103:676–684
67. Erickson HK, Widdison WC, Mayo MF et al (2010) Tumor delivery and in vivo processing of disulfide-linked and thioether-linked antibody-maytansinoid conjugates. Bioconjugate Chem 21:84–92
68. Acchione M, Kwon H, Jochheim CM et al (2012) Impact of linker and conjugation chemistry on antigen binding, Fc receptor binding and thermal stability of model antibody-drug conjugates. mAbs 4(3):362–372
69. DiJoseph JF, Dougher MM, Armellino DC et al (2007) CD20-specific antibody-targeted chemotherapy of non-Hodgkin's B-cell lymphoma using calicheamicin-conjugated rituximab. Cancer Immunol Immunother 56:1107–1117
70. McEarchern JA, Smith LM, McDonagh CF et al (2008) Preclinical characterization of SGN-70, a humanized antibody directed against CD70. Clin Cancer Res 14(23):7763–7772
71. Gazzano-Santoro H, Ralph P, Ryskamp TC et al (1997) A non-radioactive complement-dependent cytotoxicity assay for anti-CD20 monoclonal antibody. J Immunol Methods 202:163–171
72. Ferrone S, Cooper NR, Pellegrino MA et al (1971) The lymphocytotoxic reaction: the mechanism of rabbit complement action. J Immunol 107:939–947
73. Junutula JR, Bhakta S, Raab H et al (2008) Rapid identification of reactive cysteine residues for site-specific labeling of antibody-Fabs. J Immunol Methods 332:41–52

Chapter 4
Clinical Pharmacology Strategies in the Development of Antibody–Drug Conjugates

Sandhya Girish and Manish Gupta

History of ADCs

Antibody–drug conjugates (ADCs) are monoclonal antibodies (mAbs) linked with cytotoxic agents through a linker. They are designed to selectively deliver the cytotoxic agent to tumor cells via tumor-specific and/or overexpressed cell surface antigens. Targeted delivery of the cytotoxic drugs to tumors means that ADCs have the potential to harness and improve their antitumor effects while minimizing the impact on normal tissues.

The concept of ADC as a platform for targeted delivery of cytotoxic agents has been around for over 25 years (Fig. 4.1). Four products have been launched in the past 10 years. The first ADC approved was in 2000, Mylotarg®, with calicheamicin as the cytotoxic agent and a hydrazone linker. The antibody in Mylotarg® targets CD33 antigen that is expressed in malignant plasma cells of myeloid lineage and was approved for treating Acute Myeloid Leukemia. It is linked to the cytotoxic agent calicheamicin via the acid-labile hydrazone "AcBut" linker. Approximately 50% of the mAb is loaded with 4–6 calicheamicin per molecule in Mylotarg® and the rest is unconjugated. However, in 2010, this ADC was withdrawn from the market because of product safety and lack of efficacy concerns [1].

Bexxar® (2003) [2] and Zevalin® (2002) [3], both approved for treating Non-Hodgkin's lymphoma (NHL), contain radiolabeled antibodies, I131 and Y90, respectively and target CD20 antigen. These approved radioimmunoconjugates can be viewed as a separate class of ADCs as they pose challenges that are unique to their class. Due to the nature of their radioactivity (type of radioactive energy,

S. Girish (✉) • M. Gupta
Senior Scientist/ Group Leader Antibody Drug Conjugates, Clinical Pharmacology,
gRED Genentech Inc., 1 DNA Way, Bristol Myers Squib, South San Francisco, CA 94080, USA
e-mail: sandhyag@gene.com; Manish.Gupta2@bms.com

G.L. Phillips (ed.), *Antibody-Drug Conjugates and Immunotoxins: From Pre-Clinical Development to Therapeutic Applications*, Cancer Drug Discovery and Development,
DOI 10.1007/978-1-4614-5456-4_4,

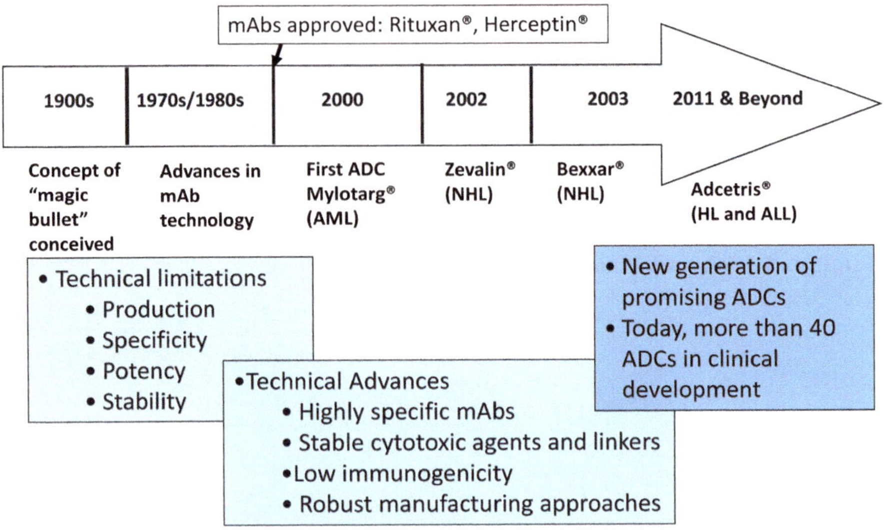

Fig. 4.1 The history of ADCs. *AML* acute myeloid leukemia, *NHL* non-Hodgkin's lymphoma, *HL* Hodgkin's lymphoma, *ALL* anaplastic large cell lymphoma

radioactive decay) and poor internalization at target site, accumulation of radioactivity in normal tissues is common. Further, loss of radiolabel due to dehalogenation and metabolism in systemic circulation is also likely. In the past decade advances in mAb and conjugation technology have produced a new generation of ADCs with more desirable attributes. More recently Adcetris®, a CD30-directed ADC was approved [4]. Based on response rate this ADC was approved for the treatment of patients with Hodgkin's lymphoma (HL) after failure of autologous stem cell transplant (ASCT) or after failure of at least two prior multiagent chemotherapy regimens in patients who are not ASCT candidates. It was also approved for the treatment of patients with systemic anaplastic large cell lymphoma (ALL) after failure of at least one prior multiagent chemotherapy regimen.

There are over 40 ADCs in various stages of clinical development, Phase I through III. Each of these ADCs has different target, linker, and/or cytotoxic agent characteristics that make them distinct from one another. Trastuzumab emtansine (T-DM1) belongs to the newer generation of ADCs and is in late stage clinical development for treating solid tumors. Several confirmatory, randomized, international, multicenter, Phase III trials (EMILIA, MARIANNE) are underway for T-DM1 for treating HER2-positive cancers [5]. Another ADC in late stage development is Inotuzumab ozogamicin (CMC-544) for treating NHL. In this case, the cytotoxic agent from the class of calicheamicins similar to Mylotarg® is linked to a humanized mAb (for CD22). It is undergoing several clinical trials for treating NHL and acute lymphoblastic leukemia.

From a clinical pharmacology perspective, the biggest challenge is to identify the component that is most likely to contribute to the safety and efficacy of the product. Because ADCs contain both small and large molecules (biologic) as components,

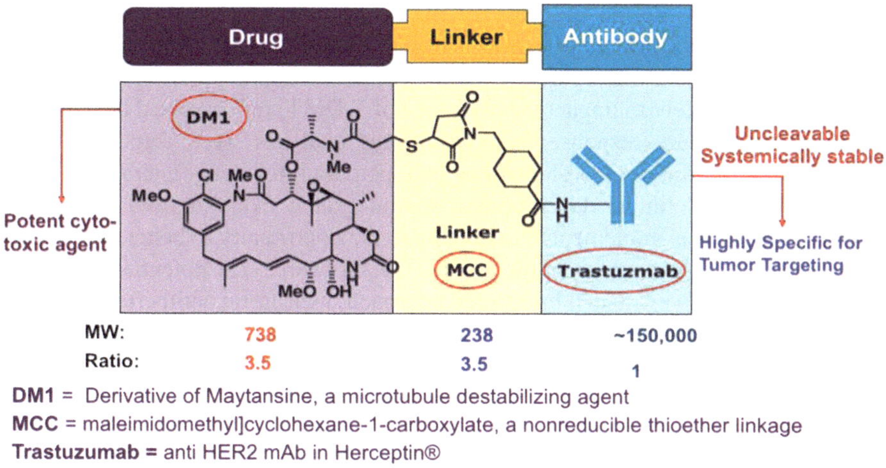

Fig. 4.2 Trastuzumab emtansine structure and complexity

it is unclear whether a small or large molecule drug development paradigm is appropriate and given the recent advances in technologies there is limited relevance of approved ADCs like radioimmunoconjugates and Mylotarg®, primarily due to differences in linker-cytoxic agent stability for the newer ADCs compared to earlier ones. Further, the historical precedence is limited and not entirely applicable towards the new generation of ADCs. Lack of specific guidance around global development of ADCs is also limiting. There are also increased regulatory expectations around establishing exposure–safety and exposure–efficacy relationships for a new molecular entity now than a decade ago.

Therefore, designing a customized clinical pharmacology strategy incorporating relevant aspects of small molecule and large molecule drug development strategies to address safety and efficacy (patient and regulatory needs) is probably the best approach. Given the in-depth clinical pharmacology experience gained with T-DM1, currently in development for treating metastatic breast cancer (MBC), strategies applied are highlighted and discussed in this chapter. The recent approval of Adcetris® also sheds some light on the clinical pharmacology of ADCs [4, 6].

T-DM1 is an ADC that contains DM1 linked to the humanized anti-HER2 IgG1, trastuzumab, primarily through antibody lysine residues using the heterobifunctional reagent, succinimidyl trans-4-[maleimidylmethyl]cyclohexane-1-carboxylate (SMCC) (Fig. 4.2).

Clinical Pharmacology Testing Strategy

The clinical pharmacology of T-DM1 incorporates elements of small molecule and mAb (large molecule) development strategies. Given the structural complexity, multiple analytes were measured across Phase I and Phase II clinical pharmacology studies to characterize the pharmacokinetics (PK) of T-DM1, including, but not limited to the primary analyte T-DM1 (conjugate) and other analytes such as total trastuzumab (TT) and the cytotoxic agent DM1. Demographic and pathophysiologic covariates likely to impact the clearance of T-DM1 were assessed using population PK. Exposure–response (safety/efficacy) analyses were conducted. The potential for QT interval prolongation and potential for drug interaction were assessed early in clinical development. An integrated modeling and simulation (M&S) strategy was implemented to maximize the opportunity to better understand pharmacokinetic/pharmacodynamic (PK/PD) relationships. The potential for immunogenicity was also evaluated by a tiered approach, measuring antitherapeutic antibody (ATA) responses to all the molecular components of the ADC.

Bioanalytical Strategy

Developing assays to characterize the PK and PD of ADCs is challenging as the ADCs are heterogenous mixtures and have different DM1 drug-to-antibody ratio (DAR) species ranging from DAR 1 to 8, with an average of approximately 3.5 DM1 moieties for most ADCs. The abundance of DAR species in systemic circulation changes with time and it is not always feasible to measure the changing DAR species in serum samples.

Specifically, T-DM1 has the molecular characteristics of both a large molecule biologic and a small molecule drug. T-DM1 is composed of trastuzumab with 1–8 DM1 molecules linked via MCC ((maleimidomethyl)cyclohexane-1-carboxylate, a nonreducible thioether linkage), primarily to lysine residues. The DAR approximates a Poisson distribution with an average DAR of ~3.5.

Thus two key technologies, enzyme linked immunosorbent assay (ELISA) and liquid chromatography tandem mass spectrometry (LC–MS/MS), typical for large and small molecule quantification were used for T-DM1 bioanalysis. Validated PK assays were used to measure T-DM1 (conjugate), TT (trastuzumab conjugated as well as unconjugated), and DM1. Exploratory LC–MS/MS assays were developed to measure some catabolites like MCC–DM1 and Lysine–MCC–DM1 in plasma samples.

The T-DM1 PK ELISA was designed to measure the drug conjugate containing one or more covalently bound DM1 (1–8) molecule. The TT PK ELISA measured T-DM1, with variable DAR (in the ADC conjugate) plus unconjugated trastuzumab (with no bound DM1). The DM1 PK through LC–MS/MS assayed DM1 and any disulfide-bound forms of released DM1 (e.g., dimers, glutathione, cysteine, and albumin adducts). It did not measure DM1 linked to trastuzumab via MCC–DM1. As DM1 contains a free sulfhydryl, DM1 released from T-DM1 is likely to dimerize or react with other thiol-containing molecules in plasma. Therefore, to avoid an under quantification of released DM1, plasma samples were treated with a reducing agent to release disulfide-bound DM1. The free thiol was then blocked with N-ethylmaleimide (NEM) to prevent any further reactions. The LC–MS/MS assay quantified DM1–NEM. The assay approach measured all disulfide-bound forms of DM1.

Immunogenicity assessment of T-DM1 required a strategy and a method that enabled measurement of ATA responses to the molecular components of the ADC. A tiered approach was used to detect and characterize any ATA response to T-DM1 using robust validated bridging immunoassay methods designed to detect all ATAs in the presence of circulating T-DM1.

Characterization of Clinical PK

During the development of T-DM1, data from multiple Phase I, II, and III single-agent and combination studies were used to investigate the clinical pharmacology of this molecule (Table 4.1; Fig. 4.3). Given that the intended use for the drug is to treat patients with breast cancer, no studies were conducted in healthy volunteers. Also since T-DM1 includes an antibody and is administered via the intravenous route, traditional studies with human biomaterial to assess permeability or to assess metabolic pathways were not conducted.

The Phase I, first-in-human study (TDM3569g) was a dose escalation trial assessing the safety, tolerability, and PK of single-agent T-DM1 administered by IV infusion, on both a q3w- and weekly (qw)-dosing regimen, to HER2 positive MBC patients who had previously received a trastuzumab-containing regimen [7, 8]. Doses ranging from 0.3 to 4.8 mg/kg were administered in the q3w regimen. In the remaining studies (TDM4258g, TDM4374g, and TDM4688g), T-DM1 was administered as a 30–90-min IV infusion at 3.6 mg/kg on a q3w dosing regimen, the recommended dosing regimen for Phase II studies [7–12]. In the Phase I trial, an extensive PK sampling program was used to characterize T-DM1 disposition, whereas in the Phase II trials, peak and trough data were collected with frequent sampling in later cycles (Cycles 1 and, at steady state, Cycle 3 or 4). Standard non-compartmental methods were used in individual studies to determine relevant PK parameters.

PK data from the Phase I dose escalation study was primarily used to characterize T-DM1 PK, assess dose dependence, determine single and repeat dose kinetics of different schedules (weekly and q3w), and help determine an optimal dose and regimen for Phase II/III studies. Data from Phase II studies were used to further characterize the PK of T-DM1 (and other analytes) in a larger population. Population PK was done to assess the interindividual variability (IIV) and to determine if any specific dose adjustments might be necessary. Also, relevant pathophysiological covariates likely to impact T-DM1 clearance were determined using a population PK model (POP PK). Additionally, Phase II data were also used to explore exposure–safety (platelet, liver enzymes) and exposure–efficacy (tumor size, response rate) relationships.

Clinical PK data from the above-mentioned studies were adequately described by a linear two-compartment model with first-order elimination from the central

Table 4.1 Summary of study designs and pharmacokinetic (PK) sampling schedules for four single-agent Phase I/II studies of T-DM1

Study[a]	No. of enrolled patients	Prior therapies required for eligibility	T-DM1 doses and regimens	PK sampling
TDM3569g, phase I	q3w: $n=24$	Trastuzumab	q3w: 0.3, 0.6,1.2, 2.4, 3.6, and 4.8 mg/kg	Intensive sampling in cycle 1; peak/trough PK sampling in subsequent cycles; NCA of PK data
TDM4258g, phase II	112	≥1 HER2-directed therapy and ≥1 chemotherapy for MBC	3.6 mg/kg q3w	Frequent sampling in cycles 1 and 4 for NCA of PK data; peak/trough PK sampling in subsequent cycles
TDM4374g, phase II	110	Trastuzumab, lapatinib, capecitabine, a taxane, an anthracycline; ≥2 HER2-directed therapies for MBC	3.6 mg/kg q3w	Frequent sampling in cycles 1 and 4 for NCA of PK; peak/trough PK sampling in subsequent cycles
TDM4688g, phase II	51	Trastuzumab	T-DM1 at up to 3.6 mg/kg q3w for 1 year[b]	Frequent sampling in cycles 1 and 3 for NCA of PK data; QTc assessment pre- and post-T-DM1 dosing

HER2 human epidermal growth factor receptor 2; *MBC* metastatic breast cancer; *NCA* noncompartmental analysis; *PK* pharmacokinetic; *q3w* every 3 weeks; *QTc* corrected QT; *T-DM1* trastuzumab emtansine

In all studies, the analytes measured were T-DM1, total trastuzumab, and DM1; incidence of antitherapeutic antibodies to T-DM1 was also examined

[a]A population PK analysis was conducted using T-DM1 PK data for all studies except TDM4688g

[b]The earliest a patient could begin treatment with T-DM1 in combination with pertuzumab was cycle 4, day 1, after all PK samples for single-agent T-DM1 had been obtained in cycle 3. Pertuzumab dose: 840-mg loading dose, followed by 420 mg q3w for 1 year

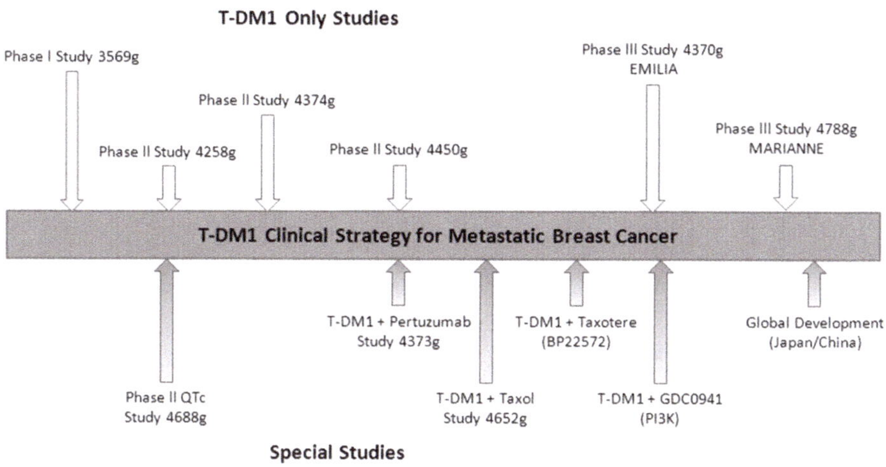

Fig. 4.3 Additional clinical studies with T-DM1 that have a clinical pharmacology strategy

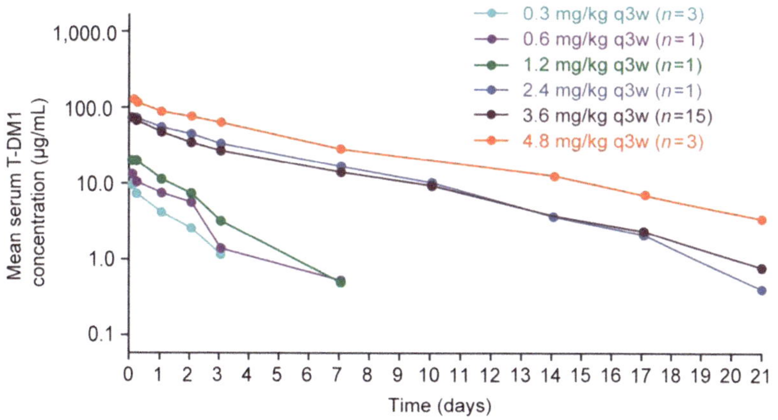

Fig. 4.4 Pharmacokinetics profiles

compartment. In the Phase I study TDM3569g, following T-DM1 administration in a q3w schedule, a trend toward faster T-DM1 clearance was observed at T-DM1 doses of ≤1.2 mg/kg. In doses ranging from 2.4 to 4.8 mg/kg q3w, T-DM1 exhibited linear PK (Fig. 4.4). This supports the dual mechanism of clearance for T-DM1, similar to other mAbs—target (HER2) antigen-specific and nonspecific (in part by Fc mediated) mechanisms.

At the maximally tolerated 3.6 mg/kg q3w dose, T-DM1 disposition is characterized by mean clearance values ranging from 7 to 13 mL/day/kg, a volume of distribution limited to the plasma volume, and a terminal half life of approximately 4 days.

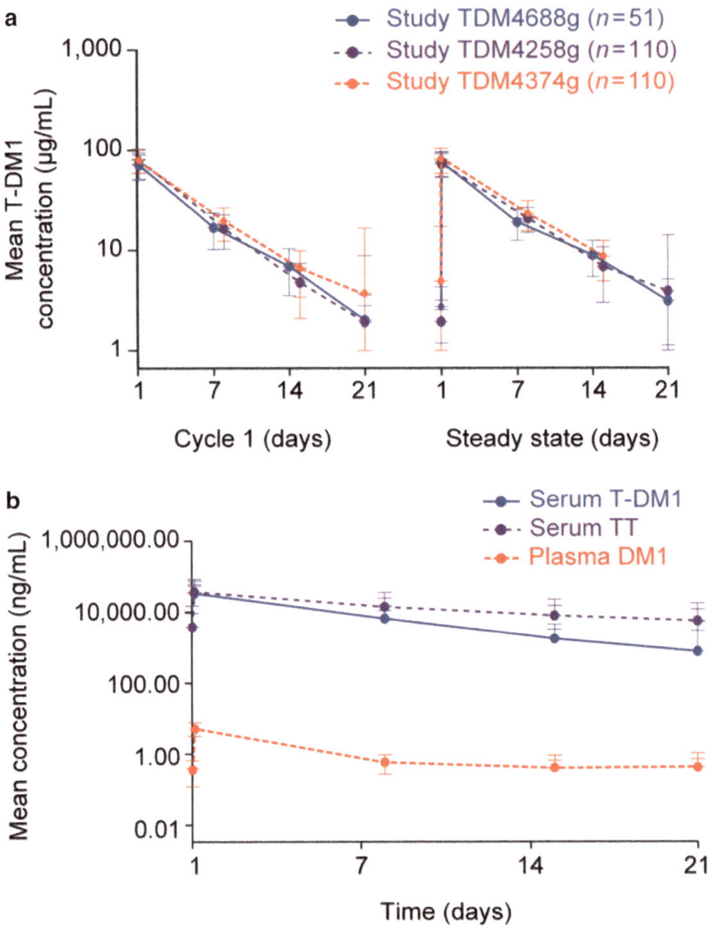

Fig. 4.5 Steady state levels

Although a higher cumulative dose could be safely administered to patients with a weekly schedule (7.2 mg/kg in a 21-day cycle; 2.4 mg/kg qw × 3 weeks), a q3w regimen was considered best suited for late stage clinical studies in consideration of patient convenience and similar clinical benefit rates/antitumor activity across both schedules.

Consistent PK was observed across 3 Phase II studies as shown in Fig. 4.5. The half-life of T-DM1 ranged from 3.1 to 4.5 days and the clearance in the linear range was 7.3–12.7 mL/day/kg. The half-life of TT averaged ~10 days and clearance was 4.21 mL/day/kg. Modest accumulation was observed for this analyte. The half-life of T-DM1 was shorter than that of TT. The shorter half-life and faster clearance for T-DM1 can be attributed to the combined clearance mechanisms of deconjugation and proteolytic degradation. The systemic exposure to DM1 was consistently low with mean maximum levels not exceeding 6 ng/mL.

Integrated Modeling and Simulation (M&S) Strategy

An integrated M&S strategy was conceived and applied early in clinical development of T-DM1 to leverage all available clinical data to establish PK/PD relationships. POP PK modeling using conjugate T-DM1 concentrations as an analyte of interest was developed to assess the effects of demographic and pathophysiologic covariates on the PK of T-DM1 in order to better understand clinical factors that might affect exposure in individual patients [12]. Additionally, in an attempt to streamline the number of analytes being collected and analyzed during clinical development, integrated models with multiple analytes of T-DM1 were developed [13–15].

Semi-mechanistic and empirical models were developed to explain exposure–safety (alanine aminotransferase (ALT), aspartate aminotransferase (AST), platelets) and exposure–efficacy (objective response rate (ORR), tumor size) relationships [16, 17]. Additionally, population approaches were used to assess potential for drug interactions for T-DM1 in combination with taxanes (docetaxel and paclitaxel) and pertuzumab [13, 18, 19].

Population PK (POP PK)

As the mechanism of action of T-DM1 requires both trastuzumab and DM1, a POP PK model was developed using T-DM1 (conjugate) concentrations [20]. T-DM1 PK was best described by a linear two-compartment model. Population estimates (IIV) for pharmacokinetic parameters were clearance, 0.7 L/day (21.0%); central compartment volume (V_c), 3.33 L (13.2%); peripheral compartment volume (V_p), 0.89 L (50.4%); and intercompartmental clearance, 0.78 L/day. A number of demographic, body size-specific, and pathophysiological covariates were tested to determine if they might have an impact on T-DM1 PK. The interindividual variability (IIV) in T-DM1 pharmacokinetic parameters from the base model (18–48%) before inclusion of any covariates was similar to the IIV observed for other mAbs like trastuzumab, pertuzumab, and bevacizumab. Body weight, albumin, tumor burden, and AST levels were identified as statistically significant covariates accounting for IIV in T-DM1 PK, with body weight having a greater effect on IIV of clearance and V_c than other covariates. The IIV of clearance was reduced from 26.4 to 21% (decrease of 36.7%) after adding these covariates. The interindividual variability for central volume was reduced from 18.3 to 13.2% (decrease of 47.9%) after adding body weight as a covariate for V_c. Baseline trastuzumab TmAb (from prior trastuzumab treatment), specific to this MBC patient population, and HER2 shed antigen (HER2ECD) were found to have no effect on T-DM1 CL.

Independently, other models were developed using all available T-DM1 and TT data. Lu et al. developed an empirical integrated POP PK model that simultaneously fitted T-DM1 and TT PK data [13]. This model provided quantitative estimates of deconjugation and proteolytic degradation rates of T-DM1 and assisted in understanding the kinetics of conversion from T-DM1 to unconjugated trastuzumab. The model provided a hypothesis for the observed differences in clearance between T-DM1 and TT. As T-DM1 CL is comprised of both degradation and deconjugation processes, its faster clearance than trastuzumab was partly explained. Chudasama et al. and Bender et al. have also developed semi-mechanistic POP PK models based on PK data in cynomolgous monkeys and patients to provide additional insight into the kinetics of each deconjugation step of T-DM1 from high DAR moieties to low DAR moieties [14, 15]. Such integrated models may be useful in predicting PK profile for T-DM1 and other analytes and can potentially eliminate the necessity of dense PK sampling for multiple analytes in future clinical trials.

Exposure–Response Models/Relationship

Exposure–response analysis was performed with all available efficacy and safety data from completed Phase II studies. The relationship analysis between T-DM1 exposure and response (partial response, stable disease, and progressive disease) was limited to a narrow range of T-DM1 exposure as most available data were limited to 3.6 mg/kg q3w dose regimen.

Tumor growth inhibition (TGI) and semi-mechanistic population PK/PD models were developed to characterize the effect of T-DM1 on longitudinal changes in tumor size assessed by sum of longest diameters (SLD) and platelet counts in clinical studies. In addition, exploratory correlation between T-DM1 exposure and efficacy/safety variables were performed.

A semi-mechanistic population PK/PD model was developed to characterize the effect of T-DM1 on platelet counts in clinical studies as thrombocytopenia (TCP) was identified as the dose-limiting toxicity in Phase I study [14]. In this approach, a sequential exposure–response modeling approach was adopted to fit the PK (i.e., serum T-DM1 concentration–time) and PD (i.e., platelet–time) data to help identify PK parameters that may be responsible for TCP. The model consisted of a proliferative platelet pool compartment, three transit compartments, and a circulating platelet compartment, mimicking platelet development and circulation. The PK/PD model developed accurately reflected and quantified clinical observations of platelet counts during T-DM1 treatment. The model also supported the hypothesis of a partial depletion of the proliferating platelet pool as a mechanism for the downward drift in some platelet–time profiles. This was further supported by data from in vitro mechanistic studies with hematopoietic stem cells, megakaryocytes, and platelets. T-DM1 did not have a direct effect on platelet function but did impair megakaryocyte and platelet production [21]. Further, the model

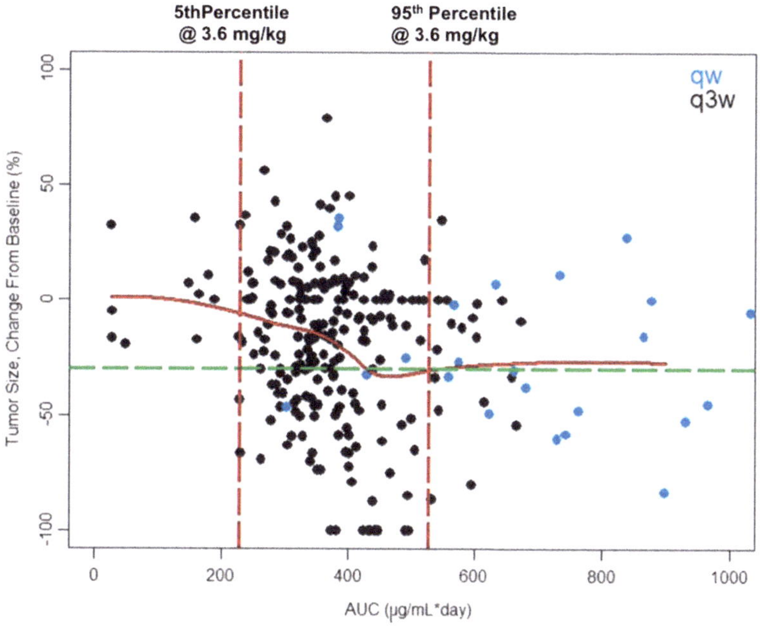

Fig. 4.6 Exposure–response relationship

also suggested the presence of a nondepletable platelet pool that appears to maintain safe platelet levels in most patients. The results of the modeling analyses supported single-agent T-DM1 dosing at 3.6 mg/kg q3w in patients with HER2-positive breast cancer; this dose of T-DM1 is well tolerated, requiring minimal dose delays and reductions for TCP.

Additionally, a tumor growth inhibition (TGI) model was developed, which describes the sum of longest diameters (SLD) of target lesions, as a function of time and area under the concentration–time curve using all the data with different doses tested in Phase I/II studies thus far [20]. The model accounts for natural (first-order) tumor growth rate, antitumor drug effect (i.e., cell-kill rate driven by drug exposure), and drug resistance. The model predicted that median ORR was in alignment with observed ORR from Phase II studies. Also, in an exploratory analysis, measured efficacy and safety endpoints were plotted against exposure measures for any correlative trends. Correlation between steady state T-DM1 exposure (AUC) at all doses tested (1.2–2.7 mg/kg qw and 0.3–4.8 mg/kg q3w) and TGI at Week 12 is shown in Fig. 4.6. Higher exposure, as achieved with weekly regimen, did not translate to greater decrease in tumor size from baseline at week 12. Further, low exposures (at doses less than 2.4 mg/kg) did not meaningfully decrease the tumor size. In the 5th and 95th percentile range for 3.6 mg/kg q3w schedule, a trend in exposure and tumor shrinkage was observed. However this relationship in T-DM1 exposure did not translate to ORR as the endpoint following 3.6 mg/kg q3w T-DM1 dosing across Phase II studies. Further assessments will be done to identify tentative relationships between T-DM1 exposure and time to tumor progression, progression free survival, and overall survival as data become available for larger pivotal trials.

No obvious relationships were observed between T-DM1 exposure (by AUC quartiles) and platelet, AST, or ALT levels during the course of T-DM1 treatment across the Phase II studies [17].

Impact of ATA response to T-DM1 on PK/PD

Overall, ATA formation was observed in 4.5% (13 of 286) of patients after repeated dosing of T-DM1 across four Phase I/II clinical studies but no obvious changes were observed in the PK, safety profiles, or efficacy outcomes of patients who developed antibodies to T-DM1 compared with patients who tested negative for antibodies to T-DM1. The clinical significance of antibody development against T-DM1 is therefore not perceptive.

Metabolic Fate of T-DM1

To gain a better understanding of the disposition of T-DM1 and its catabolites, preclinical radiolabeled studies of absorption, distribution, metabolism, and excretion (ADME) were conducted in rats [8, 22]. In addition, the T-DM1 catabolites, MCC–DM1 and Lysine–MCC–DM1, were analyzed in the plasma of patients with MBC receiving treatment with single-agent T-DM1 in a phase II clinical study (TDM4688g) [12, 17]. The integrated results from radiolabeled studies, together with additional data from the clinical study, helped to characterize the catabolism of T-DM1. As supported by radiolabeled studies in rats, the majority of T-DM1 remains conjugated with one or more DM1 molecules in systemic circulation. As with trastuzumab, T-DM1 undergoes receptor-mediated and nonspecific endocytosis, followed by trafficking to the lysosomal compartment where proteolytic degradation/catabolism to amino acids occurs [12, 17, 18]. Very low levels of catabolites/metabolites, including lysine–MCC–DM1, MCC–DM1, and DM1, were observed in vivo in rat and human plasma following T-DM1 administration [12, 17, 22].

In rats, catabolites, including DM1 adducts, lysine–MCC–DM1, and MCC–DM1, have been predominantly observed in bile with minimal elimination in urine [17, 22]. In both preclinical and clinical pharmacology studies T-DM1 catabolites MCC–DM1 levels were found to peak immediately after dosing, and a lag time was associated with the formation of Lysine–MCC–DM1, as higher levels of this catabolite were observed at later time points [17].

Additionally, in vitro metabolism and radiolabeled studies were conducted with DM1, a component of T-DM1 [22]. DM1 undergoes metabolism by CYP450 enzymes, specifically by CYP3A4 and to a lesser extent by CYP3A5. Further, at clinically relevant concentrations DM1 is not a CYP450 inhibitor.

The fecal/biliary route appears to be the major pathway of elimination of DM1-containing catabolites in rats. Up to 80% of radioactivity was recovered in bile and less than 5% was recovered in urine primarily as DM1 and DM1-containing catabolites (MCC–DM1, Lysine–MCC–DM1) in both bile and urine samples. MCC–DM1 and Lys–MCC–DM1 were higher than DM1 levels in both matrices. Given the current understanding of the ADME profile of T-DM1 in rats, hepatic function, but not renal function, may have an impact on T-DM1 disposition.

Organ Dysfunction Studies

Renal Impairment

No formal study was conducted in patients with renal impairment. Though limited, this assessment is based on available data from a POP PK model that has been developed using clinical PK data across three clinical studies (TDM3569g, TDM4258g, and TDM4374g) [12]. The effect that renal impairment has on the PK of T-DM1 was evaluated on the basis of calculated creatinine clearance as a surrogate of renal function. Creatinine clearance was included as a potential continuous covariate in the POP PK model with pooled data from Phase I and two Phase II studies. The results showed that creatinine clearance had no impact on T-DM1 PK (Fig. 4.7). The impact of renal function on T-DM1 PK was also assessed by categorizing patients on the basis of their calculated creatinine clearance (normal: creatinine clearance > 80 mL/min; mild: creatinine clearance = 50–80 mL/min; moderate: creatinine clearance = 30–50 mL/min; severe: creatinine clearance < 30 mL/min). Renal function was found to have no influence on T-DM1 clearance. Only a limited assessment was possible in patients with moderate and severe renal impairment: nine and three patients were studied with moderate and severe renal impairment, respectively. In spite of the small numbers, given this analysis and the fact that renal route is a minor elimination route in preclinical radiolabeled studies with T-DM1 and DM1, renal function is unlikely to affect the systemic exposure of T-DM1 [12, 17, 22].

Hepatic Impairment

Collectively there appears to be no clinically significant relationship between ALT/AST, total bilirubin, and albumin levels (indicators of hepatic function) and T-DM1 exposure [17, 20]. Furthermore, receptor-mediated endocytosis and nonspecific endocytosis and catabolism to amino acid products are expected, and clearance mechanisms similar to other mAbs are expected to be the major route. Therefore, hepatic impairment as such is not expected to impact T-DM1 exposure. However, the impact on DM1 and DM1 containing metabolites remains unclear. Also based on the May 2003 FDA guidance document (PK in Patients with Impaired Hepatic Function), a study is recommended even if a drug and/or active metabolite

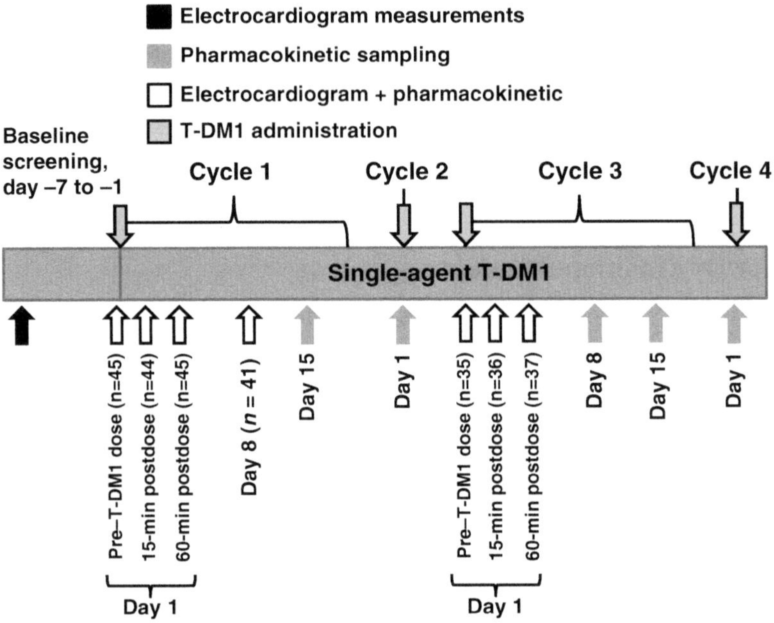

Fig. 4.7 QTc study design. *n* in parenthesis refers to pharmacokinetic- and electrocardiogram-evaluable patients

(i.e., DM1) is eliminated to a lesser extent (<20%) when there is evidence to suggest a narrow therapeutic drug range [23]. A study is therefore under way to fully understand the relationship of varying degrees of liver impairment on PK, safety, and appropriate dosing, as the DM-1 component of T-DM1 is primarily metabolized and eliminated as DM1-containing catabolites through the biliary route.

QTc Strategy

Current regulatory guidelines [24] for QT studies were developed to assess small molecules and as such do not provide specific guidance for evaluating large molecules or an ADC for oncology indications. It has been shown that mAbs have very low potential to interact with the extracellular or intracellular (pore) domains on hERG channel based on their targeted, specific binding properties and large molecular weight [25, 26]. Therefore mAbs are highly unlikely to inhibit hERG channel activity and it is not appropriate to conduct an in vitro hERG assay for assessing the heart rate corrected QT interval (QTc) prolongation risk of mAbs [25].

Erdman et al. performed a systemic review of all 21 approved mAbs, and no QTc prolongation or Torsades de Pointes risk was identified in any label for approved mAbs [27]. A recent white paper published on the QTc for biologics [28] recommends that no thorough QT study is required for mAbs, although it might be required for some proteins of smaller size (e.g., non-mAb biologics).

Therefore for ADCs, a hybrid approach for QT assessment can be used. Sufficient, good quality ECG data should be collected in early development to assess any potential clinically important QT effect. In the absence of direct hERG inhibition, triplicate 12-lead ECG monitoring is generally recommended at the maximal peak concentrations, delayed time points, and after successive doses at steady state. Typically, it is only possible to analyze baseline-matched ECGs, as the use of long placebo periods is logistically difficult, and positive controls are difficult to use in oncology indications.

A dedicated QT study was conducted for T-DM1 in clinical development to rule out any clinically meaningful QT prolongation in 51 patients. A strategy was developed (Fig. 4.7) to assess the effects of the HER2-directed ADC, T-DM1, on QTc in a multicenter phase II study [17, 20]. The effect of T-DM1 (3.6 mg/kg q3w) on corrected QT interval (QTc) was assessed and exposure–response relationships between the primary endpoint and each T-DM1 analyte [T-DM1 conjugate, TT (conjugated and unconjugated), and DM1] concentrations were evaluated using linear mixed-effects modeling [20].

In this study, serum and plasma samples were analyzed for T-DM1 conjugate, TT, and DM1 in cycles 1 and 3 (steady state). Triplicate 12-lead electrocardiograms were time matched with pharmacokinetic sampling. The primary endpoint was the change in the QTc interval from baseline to each post-baseline time point, adjusted for heart rate using Fridericia's correction (ΔQTcF).

The upper limit of the 95% one-sided confidence interval of the estimated average prolongation in QTcF at the T-DM1 maximum plasma concentration (C_{max}) of 75.6 μg/mL was 2.3 ms in cycle 1 and 6.8 ms in cycle 3. Similar results were observed at the median DM1 and TT C_{max} concentrations in cycles 1 and 3. Therefore, in the proposed therapeutic regimen T-DM1 had no clinically relevant effect on QTc interval. The observed upper limit of the 95% one-sided confidence interval was below the 10 ms threshold of regulatory concern.

Potential for Therapeutic Protein–Drug Interactions (TP-DI)

In oncology, TP-DI evaluation is usually not a stand-alone study due to logistical constraints. It is critical to have a question-based risk assessment of the PK-based TP-DI and build a clinical pharmacology strategy during development of combination treatment to ensure safe and effective use of therapeutics [29]. A systematic approach to answering the question of "Can a therapeutic protein (TP) be either a

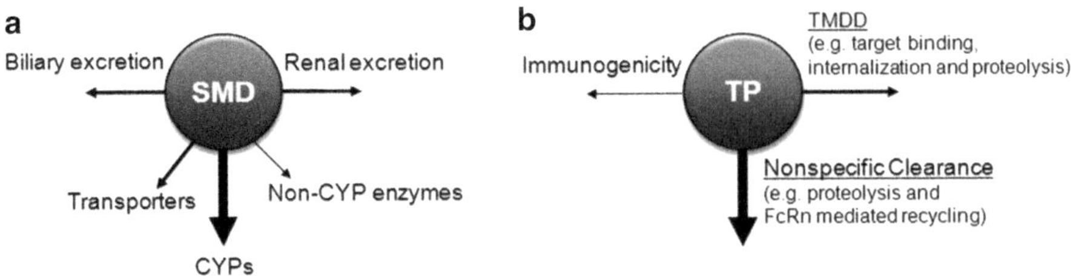

Fig. 4.8 Factors affecting small molecule drug (*SMD*) and protein therapeutic (*TP*)

victim or a perpetrator of a TP-DI?" assesses the clearance mechanisms of a particular TP and evaluates whether coadministered drugs can affect these clearance processes (Figs. 4.8 and 4.9).

A similar risk assessment approach was adopted for T-DM1 in combination with taxanes and pertuzumab [13, 18, 29]. Collective in vitro metabolism and preclinical data suggest that T-DM1 is unlikely to be a perpetrator of a DI. Although the risk for a PK-based DI was considered low based on the predominantly nonoverlapping clearance mechanisms, low systemic DM1 levels, it was not possible to rule out whether T-DM1 could be a victim of TP-DI in combination with other drugs. Therefore, in Phase Ib/II combination studies a drug interaction strategy was included. For T-DM1 in combination with taxanes (Taxol® and Taxotere®) a staggered dosing design was adopted and for T-DM1 in combination with antibody like pertuzumab a sequential dosing was adopted [13, 18]. A PK sampling schedule to quantify the levels of T-DM1, TT and DM1, pertuzumab, paclitaxel, and docetaxel were included in protocols. PK parameters from combination treatment were either compared to historical single-agent data or within study (Cycle 1; Taxane PK in absence of T-DM1 vs. Cycle 2; Taxane PK in presence of T-DM1). These results confirm the low potential for PK-based drug interactions. The PK of these agents (taxane, pertuzumab) was not altered in the presence of T-DM1 or vice versa.

Summary and Conclusions

A unique and customized clinical pharmacology strategy was applied towards clinical development of T-DM1, Genentech's first ADC molecule in late stage clinical development. Clinical pharmacology strategies, including bioanalytical, M&S, PK characterization, metabolic fate, organ dysfunction studies, exposure–response analysis, QTc, and TP-DI, were conceived and implemented early in clinical development. This case study can likely serve as a foundation for future ADC clinical development. Furthermore, clinical pharmacology data from all these studies are likely to be an integral part of the package insert and can provide useful information to oncologists and patients. Additional data in ongoing late stage studies will guide further development of T-DM1.

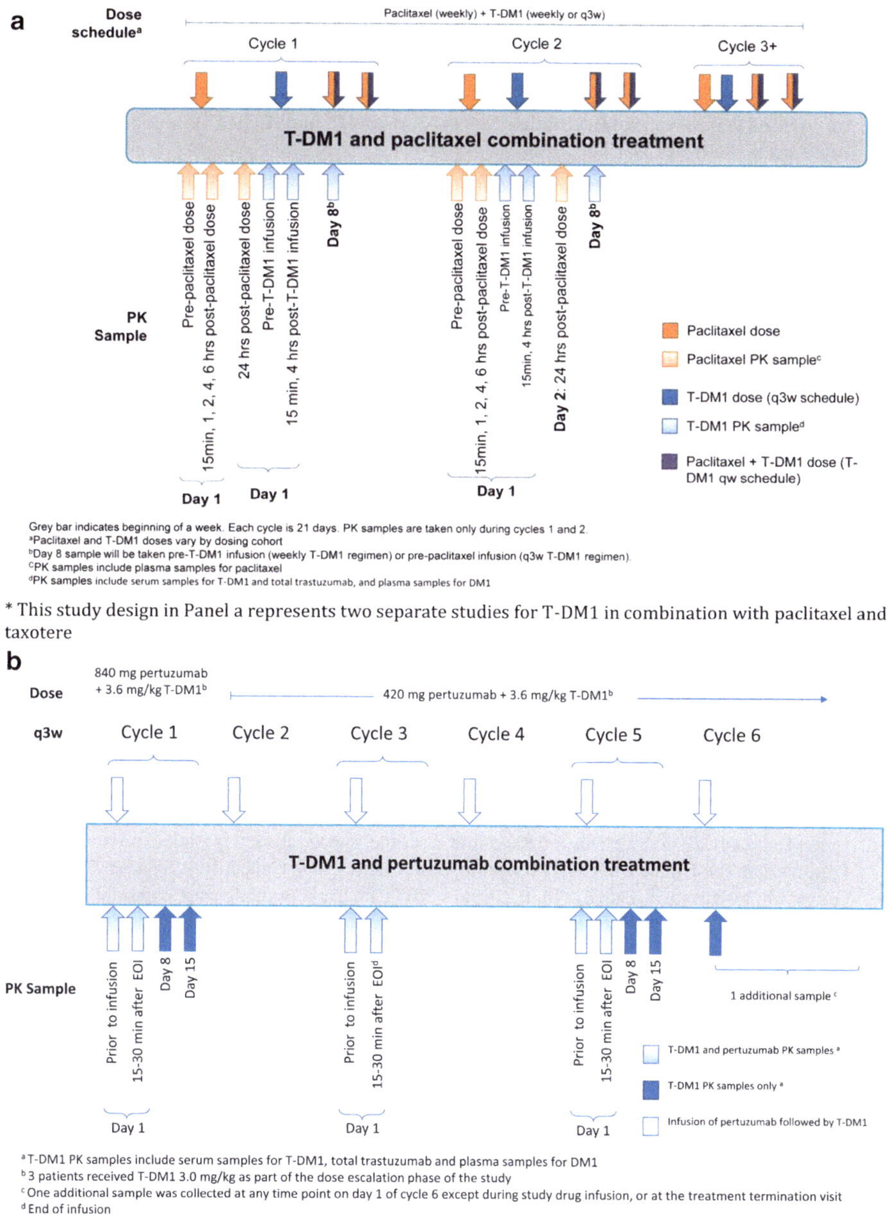

Fig. 4.9 Drug–drug interaction studies design. This study design in panel (**a**) represents two separate studies for T-DM1 in combination with paclitaxel and taxotere

References

1. FDA (2010) Mylotarg® (Gemtuzumab Ozogamicin): market withdrawal. http://www.fda.gov/Safety/MedWatch/SafetyInformation/SafetyAlertsforHumanMedicalProducts/ucm216458.htm. Accessed 10 Feb 2012
2. BEXXAR® (tositumomab and iodine I 131 tositumomab) Prescribing Information - GlaxoSmithKline
3. ZEVALIN® (ibritumomab tiuxetan) Prescribing Information
4. Adcetris® (2011) (Brentuximab Vedotin, SGN-35) [Package Insert]. Seattle Genetics Inc., Bothell, WA
5. LoRusso PM, Weiss D, Guardino E et al (2011) Trastuzumab emtansine: a unique antibody-drug conjugate in development for human epidermal growth factor receptor 2-positive cancer. Clin Cancer Res 17(20):6437–6447
6. Younes A, Bartlett NL, Leonard JP et al (2010) Brentuximab Vedotin (SGN-35) for relapsed CD30-positive lymphomas. N Engl J Med 363(19):1812–1821
7. Krop IE, Beeram M, Modi S et al (2010) Phase I study of trastuzumab-DM1, an HER2 antibody-drug conjugate, given every 3 weeks to patients with HER2-positive metastatic breast cancer. J Clin Oncol 28(16):2698–704
8. Girish S, Gupta M, Wang B et al (2011) Clinical pharmacology of T-DM1: a novel antibody-drug conjugate (ADC) in development for the treatment of HER2-positive (HER2+) cancer. Clin Pharmacol Ther 89(1):PI–11, S12
9. Burris HA III, Lu D, Dees EC et al (2010) Pharmacokinetic (PK) interaction potential of trastuzumab-DM1 (T-DM1) and pertuzumab in patients with HER2-positive, locally advanced or metastatic breast cancer (MBC): results from a phase 1b/2 study. Cancer Res 70(Suppl 24):Abstr P3-14-06
10. Burris HA III, Rugo HS, Vukelka SJ et al (2011) Phase II study of the antibody drug conjugate trastuzumab-DM1 (T-DM1) for the treatment of HER2-positive breast cancer following prior HER2-directed therapy. J Clin Oncol 29(4):398–405. doi:10.1200/JCO.2010.29.5865
11. Krop IE, LoRusso PM, Miller KD (2010) A Phase II Study of trastuzumab-DM1 (T-DM1), a novel HER2 antibody–drug conjugate, in patients with HER2+ metastatic breast cancer who were previously treated with an anthracycline, a taxane, capecitabine, lapatinib, and trastuzumab. Presented at The Breast Cancer Symposium, San Antonio, TX. Cancer Res 70:Abstr 710
12. Gupta M, LoRusso P, Burris HA III, et al (2011) Pharmacokinetic and pathophysiological covariates influencing treatment outcomes with T-DM1 in patients with HER2-positive metastatic breast cancer (MBC). J Clin Oncol 29(Suppl):Abstract 633
13. Lu D, Gupta M, Wang B et al (2011) An integrated population pharmacokinetic model for a first-in-class HER2-targeted antibody–drug conjugate trastuzumab-DM1 (T-DM1): simultaneous modeling of T-DM1 and total trastuzumab pharmacokinetics in heavily pretreated HER2+ metastatic breast cancer patients. Clin Pharmacol Ther (89):PII–51
14. Bender B, Schaedeli-Stark F, Joshi A et al (2011) A semi-physiologic population pharmacokinetic/pharmacodynamic (PK/PD) model of thrombocytopenia (TCP) characterizing the effect of trastuzumab-DM1 (T-DM1) on platelet counts in patients with HER2-positive MBC. J Clin Oncol 29(Suppl):Abstr 605
15. Chudasama VL, Harrold JM, Stark FS et al (2011) Semi-mechanistic population pharmacokinetic model of multivalent trastuzumab-DM1 (T-DM1) in patients with metastatic breast cancer. Clin Pharmacol Ther 89(1):PIII–67, S89
16. Gupta M, Lorusso PM, Wang B et al (2011) Clinical implications of pathophysiological and demographic covariates on the population pharmacokinetics of trastuzumab emtansine, a HER2-targeted antibody-drug conjugate, in patients with HER2-positive metastatic breast cancer. J Clin Pharmacol. doi:10.1177/0091270011403742
17. Girish S, Gupta M, Wang B et al (2012) Clinical pharmacology of trastuzumab emtansine (T-DM1): an antibody-drug conjugate in development for the treatment of HER2-positive cancer. Cancer Chemother Pharmacol. doi:10.1007/s00280-011-1817-3

18. Lu D, Krop I, Modi S et al (2010) Pharmacokinetics (PK) of trastuzumab-DM1 (T-DM1) and paclitaxel (T) in patients with HER2-positive locally advanced or metastatic breast cancer (MBC) previously treated with a trastuzumab-containing regimen. Presented at the Breast Cancer Symposium, San Antonio, TX. Cancer Res 70:Abstr P3-14-22
19. Lu D, Joshi A, Agarwal P et al (2012) Assessment of drug interaction potential of an antibody drug conjugate with other therapeutic agents: case studies of trastuzumab emtansine (T-DM1) in combination with pertuzumab or taxane. Presented at 113th Annual Meeting of the American Society for Clinical Pharmacology and Therapeutics (ASCPT), National Harbor, MD, PIII-44
20. Gupta M, Wang B, Carrothers TJ, et al (2011) Exposure-response analysis in patients with HER2-positive (HER2+) metastatic breast cancer (MBC) to assess the effect of T-DM1 on Qtc prolongation. Clin Pharmacol Ther 89:PII–64, S58
21. Mahapatra K, Darbonne W, Bumbaca D et al (2011) T-DM1-induced thrombocytopenia results from impaired platelet production in a HER2-independent manner. Presented at Molecular Targets and Cancer Therapeutics, San Francisco, CA. Molecular Cancer Therapeutics 10(11):Suppl 1
22. Shen B, Bumbaca D, Saad O et al (2011) Metabolic fate and pharmacokinetic characterization of T-DM1: an emphasis on preclinical and clinical catabolism. Clin Pharmacol Ther 89(S1):Abstr S90 (Poster PIII-72)
23. FDA (2003) Guidance for industry: pharmacokinetics in patients with impaired hepatic function: study design, data analysis, and impact on dosing and labeling. http://www.fda.gov/downloads/Drugs/GuidanceComplianceRegulatoryInformation/Guidances/ucm072123.pdf. Accessed 18 Mar 2012
24. FDA (2005) International conference on harmonisation guidance for Industry: E14 clinical evaluation of QT/QTc interval prolongation and proarrhythmic potential for non-antiarrhythmic drugs. http://www.fda.gov/cder/guidance/index.htm. Accessed 10 Feb 2012
25. Vargas HM, Bass AS, Breidenbach A et al (2008) Scientific review and recommendations on preclinical cardiovascular safety evaluation of biologics. J Pharmacol Toxicol Methods 58(2):72–76
26. Gibbs M (2009) Clinical pharmacology of biotherapeutic proteins. QT analysis for biotherapeutic proteins. Presented at AAPS in Seatle, WA
27. Erdman A (2009) Monoclonal antibodies and QT prolongation—what is the risk? Presented at AAPS in Seatle, WA
28. Rodriguez I, Erdman A, Padhi D et al (2010) Electrocardiographic assessment for therapeutic proteins–scientific discussion. Am Heart J 160(4):627–634
29. Girish S, Martin SW, Peterson MC et al (2011) AAPS workshop report: strategies to address therapeutic protein-drug interactions during clinical development. AAPS J 13(3):405–416

Chapter 5
Predictive Biomarkers for Antibody–Drug Conjugates

David Dornan and Jeff Settleman

Introduction

For more than a decade, there has been growing interest in the possibility of directing chemotherapy drugs specifically to tumor cells, with the goal of sparing normal tissues from these generally toxic agents [1]. Although the road has been long and challenges have been plentiful, clear examples of successes have begun to emerge, and future efforts are likely to yield an abundance of potential new therapeutic options. Among the current successes exemplified by striking clinical activity are trastuzumab-emtansine (T-DM1; a Herceptin-cytotoxic drug conjugate) for the treatment of HER2-positive breast cancer [2, 3] and brentuximab vedotin (SGN-35; an anti-CD30-cytotoxic drug conjugate) administered to patients with CD30-positive lymphomas [4–6]. These agents have produced remarkable response rates in heavily pretreated patient populations, and many other ADCs are now being tested in earlier stage clinical trials, highlighting the excitement and promise for this therapeutic approach [7].

The rapidly emerging personalized medicine paradigm, that is, matching the right drug to the right patient, is critical to the success of most current and future targeted therapies in oncology given the plethora of genetic lesions and disease heterogeneity that contribute to the wide range in treatment response across the cancer patient population. In this chapter, we will discuss the potential role for predictive biomarkers in the context of ADCs to enable their successful clinical development, as well as the potential challenges associated with their implementation.

D. Dornan (✉)
Molecular Diagnostics and Cancer Cell Biology, Gilead Sciences, Inc., 333 Lakeside Dr, Foster City, CA 94404, USA
e-mail: david.dornan@gilead.com

J. Settleman (✉)
Molecular Diagnostics and Cancer Cell Biology, Genentech, Inc., 1 DNA Way, South San Francisco, CA 94080, USA
e-mail: settleman.jeffrey@gene.com

G.L. Phillips (ed.), *Antibody-Drug Conjugates and Immunotoxins: From Pre-Clinical Development to Therapeutic Applications*, Cancer Drug Discovery and Development, DOI 10.1007/978-1-4614-5456-4_5,

Predictive Biomarkers

Considering the substantial variation in clinical response and benefit that has been observed for virtually all of the current cancer treatments, the ability to identify the appropriate patient population for a novel therapeutic *a priori* is arguably one of the most important challenges in modern oncology practice. The plethora of genetic lesions in cancers that have been identified by approaches, such as targeted Sanger sequencing, next-generation whole-genome sequencing, transcriptome profiling, and comparative genomic hybridization array, highlights the complex nature of the genomic landscape in tumors [8–10]. Needless to say, in order to navigate such complexity with the goal of personalized cancer therapy, it is imperative to develop a deep understanding of a candidate drug's mechanism of action.

ADCs rely on five key factors to elicit an effect on the intended tumor cell: [1] generation of a selective high-affinity antibody that recognizes the intended cell surface target antigen, [2] a drug linker, [3] a potent cytotoxic drug, [4] internalization of the ADC by receptor-mediated endocytosis, and [5] release of the cytotoxic drug by a lysosomal-dependent process. Subsequently, the inherent properties of the tumor and molecular characteristics that determine the response to the delivered toxin are critical to its efficacy. The following are parameters that are likely to influence the response to an ADC.

Target Expression and Internalization Kinetics

For the majority of ADCs, the expression level of the intended target is likely to play a key role in defining the appropriate patient population for treatment. This is exemplified by the selection strategy for novel ADC targets, as most have been chosen based on their specific and relatively elevated expression in a specific cancer type or within a subpopulation of patients with a specific cancer type. T-DM1 is perhaps one of the best examples in that only HER2+ patients are selected for treatment since the target is not expressed in the majority of breast cancers. In contrast, other ADC targets have been selected because of their relatively high and broad expression across a particular tumor type. Inotuzumab ozogamicin is an ADC that targets CD22, an antigen that is specifically expressed across all cases of Hodgkin's lymphoma [4, 5]. In these examples, the very presence of the target appears to be sufficient to enrich for likely responders, as evidenced by the impressive response rates observed in recent trials where inotuzumab ozogamicin had an objective response rate of 50% (6 out of 12) in a phase I trial of heavily pretreated patients with Hodgkin's lymphoma in the maximum tolerated dose cohort. Furthermore, tumor regression was observed in 86% (36 out of 42) of all patients treated on this trial; however, these striking responses are unlikely to be the case for every ADC, and as clinical data accumulates, it may become clear that there are subpopulations of patients within these "high expressers" that do not demonstrate substantial benefit. At this current time, the clinical trial results from T-DM1, and inotuzumab ozogamicin studies suggest that patients indeed experience a wide range of clinical benefit, indicating that additional factors are likely to determine the efficacy of an ADC.

One of these factors is likely to be the extent to which the ADC is internalized by receptor-mediated endocytosis. Thus, an increased rate of internalization could potentially result in increased intracellular delivery of the cytotoxic agent. In this context, the selection of the ADC target with respect to its turnover on the cell surface may be important in order to maximize ADC efficacy. However, it is worth noting that some ADCs target poorly internalized antigens and elicit their effect by taking advantage of the tumor microenvironment rather than the intracellular machinery for release of the cytotoxic drug [11, 12]. In these examples, the use of a cleavable drug linker permits the release of a toxin under acidic conditions commonly found in the tumor microenvironment. This concept coupled with a membrane-permeable toxin results in the intended effect on surrounding tumor cells and mitigates the strict requirement for antibody internalization and lysosomal degradation for drug release. Therefore, there will be less dependence on target expression and internalization.

In-Cell Parameters of Sensitivity

Once an ADC is internalized, the next potential limitation to efficacy could be the rate and efficiency of lysosomal degradation of the antibody–drug linker to release the cytotoxic agent, which determines the concentration of free intracellular drug available to exert its biological effect. The lysosome contains a repertoire of enzymes and functions primarily as an "environmentally friendly" recycling machine by degrading macromolecules and organelles [13]. In addition, lysosomes have been implicated in programmed cell death processes including apoptosis and autophagy. Lysosomal activity and the expression of lysosomal-associated enzymes can vary across tumors [14] and can be an indicator of poor prognosis in certain cancers [15]. Intriguingly, key lysosomal enzymatic activities such as acid phosphatase and hexosaminidase have been found to be specifically altered in response to TNFα treatment, highlighting their potential to be modulated in the context of tumorigenesis and therapy [16]. In fact, lysosomal activity and lysosomal components are modulated by various classical tumor suppressor-inactivating and oncogenic-activating mutations such as those involving TP53 and RAS [17, 18], suggesting a potential role for tumor genetics in the response to ADCs. However, it is worth noting that reported preclinical studies have examined free drug release from CD22 and CD19 ADCs and found a poor correlation between the ability of the drug to be released and the observed in vitro efficacy [19, 20], suggesting that the inherent properties of the tumor cell that might constitute the critical determinants of efficacy.

One of the attractive features of the ADC strategy is that it provides the opportunity to conjugate the antibody with a wide array of toxins with various mechanisms of action and chemical properties. Thus far, most of ADCs that have been evaluated in clinical trials, or are about to enter clinical development, include the maytansines and auristatins as cytotoxic agents. These molecules exert their potent biological effect by interfering with microtubule dynamics by binding to the tubulin subunits. Mechanistically, microtubule-targeted agents either stabilize or destabilize microtubule polymerization, with auristatins and maytansines falling into the latter class. Regardless of the stabilization or destabilization mechanism of action, these agents ultimately promote G2/M arrest followed by programmed cell death [21].

Given the highly regulated nature of mitosis and the number of signaling pathways that converge on the key regulators, there are many potential modulators that could play a role in the response to such drugs and, therefore, to ADCs. With respect to in vitro sensitivity and resistance to microtubule-targeted agents, reports have suggested that mutations in TP53 confer sensitivity by virtue of increasing a G2/M arrest phenotype due to a defective G1 arrest that is normally regulated by p53-dependent induction of p21 [22]. Indeed, activity of the ADC CD79-vcMMAE was observed in TP53 mutant NHL cell lines [23], although activity was also present in some wild-type TP53 cases. Since TP53 mutations are common in multiple tumor types, this could provide an advantage for ADCs conjugated with microtubule-targeted agents, and it would be intriguing to test such a hypothesis in the clinic.

Aurora-A kinase overexpression has been associated with taxane resistance [24]. It is believed that Aurora-A overexpression drives cells to inappropriately enter anaphase, bypassing the spindle checkpoint. In addition, amplification of Aurora-A is prevalent in epithelial tumors—ranging from 12% to 50%—and can promote tumorigenesis in preclinical models [24]. Similarly, mutations in beta1-tubulin (TUBB) have also been reported to promote resistance to antimitotics in cell line models of acquired resistance [25]; however, the clinical relevance of these findings remains to be determined [26]. Single nucleotide polymorphisms (SNPs) in TUBB have also been identified that modulate the response to microtubule-targeted agents in cell line models [27]. Although the clinical significance of these findings has yet to be reported, the findings suggest that certain patients may inherently be less responsive to this class of anticancer agents.

Perhaps the most compelling evidence for resistance to microtubule-targeted agents comes from studies that describe overexpression of the beta3-tubulin (TUBB3) isoform. TUBB3 is normally expressed in the neurons and Sertoli cells and is associated with poor prognosis and resistance to taxanes as well as microtubule-destabilizing agents across multiple indications (reviewed in [28]). Importantly, depletion of TUBB3 by siRNA can revert cells demonstrating resistance to microtubule-targeted agents to a sensitive state, suggesting a direct link to the phenotype association observed [29]. In addition, microtubule-associated proteins (MAPs) such as MAP2, MAP4, and Tau, which function to stabilize microtubules and protect them from destabilization, have also been proposed to play a role in modulating sensitivity to antimitotics. Consistent with these observations, elevated Tau expression is associated with reduced response to paclitaxel in breast cancers due to its ability to block binding of taxanes to microtubules [30].

Intriguingly, microRNAs such as miR-200c have been shown to directly target the 3'UTR of TUBB3, and expression of this miRNA can restore sensitivity to paclitaxel in an inherently resistant cell line model [30]. Since miR-200c is a negative regulator of the epithelial to mesenchymal transition [32], which appears to yield a more chemoresistant stem cell-like phenotype, it is conceivable that repression of miR-200c expression would promote a resistant phenotype. In this instance, however, there is a direct connection to the mechanism of action elicited by microtubule-targeted agents, as opposed to a broader chemoresistance. It is worth noting though that overexpression of TUBB3 has been proposed to regulate resistance to other chemotherapies in addition to tubulin-binding agents [28].

Overall, it is clear that modulators of microtubule dynamics may play an important role in determining the response to ADCs that include a microtubule-targeted agent, and it is likely that biomarkers that define the status of several of these regulators will ultimately be required to predict response to these agents across the cancer population. In addition, the growth kinetics of tumors should be considered, and perhaps focusing on tumors with higher expression of proliferative markers, such as Ki-67, may be a consideration to further enrich for likely responders given the nature of microtubule-targeted drugs. Nonetheless, all of these potential markers certainly warrant further exploration in preclinical models and in the clinic, particularly in light of the many "flavors" of ADCs that are now entering clinical trials.

Regardless of the nature of the drug component of an ADC, it would be prudent to consider modulators of the apoptosis pathway in the response to treatment with these agents. For example, the anti-apoptotic proteins BCL-2, BCL-XL, MCL1, cIAP1/2, and XIAP have all been associated with resistance to various chemotherapies with distinct mechanisms of action in preclinical models [33–36]. These anti-apoptotic proteins function to either block caspase activation directly or protect the mitochondria from changes in mitochondrial outer membrane potential elicited by intrinsic or extrinsic apoptosis signals such as DNA damage and death receptor ligands, respectively. Multiple pro-survival signals, such as NFkB, and oncogenic lesions, such as PIK3CA mutations, promote the expression of multiple anti-apoptotic factors to tip the balance in favor of tumor cell survival. Considering that ADCs will most likely be administered to subsets of patients demonstrating activation of these signaling pathways, their potential role in predicting sensitivity to ADCs should certainly be considered. Consistent with a role for anti-apoptotic proteins in resistance to ADCs, it was reported that BCL-XL may constitute an important determinant of response to CD79b-vcMMAE [23]. Thus, increased levels of BCL-XL were correlated with reduced potency of this ADC above a specific threshold of CD79b on the cell surface. In addition, treatment with the BCL-2 family inhibitor, ABT-263, which targets BCL-XL, BCL-2, and BCL-W, was able to synergize with CD79b-vcMMAE to promote tumor regressions in a xenograft model. The potential role of anti-apoptotic proteins in the response to other ADCs remains to be determined and is likely to be assessed during the clinical testing of these agents.

As described above, there are multiple potential determinants of ADC efficacy, prompting the need to consider a variety of approaches to evaluate candidate predictive biomarkers. This could potentially demand a cadre of assays to evaluate clinical specimens, as will be further elucidated below. An alternative potential strategy would be to employ whole-genome expression signatures to identify likely responders to ADCs. A straightforward approach would be to determine expression profiles in preclinical efficacy models that display a dynamic range in sensitivity with the goal of defining a set of genes and classifiers in this "training set," followed by subsequent evaluation in a "test set" of additional preclinical models. Ideally, this signature would include genes that are biologically relevant to the drug response or at least encode components of cellular networks that could impact ADC efficacy to provide a foundation for further functional validation. Although this approach has yet to be clinically validated and therefore remains controversial, there have been some recent findings that support the potential utility of this strategy [37, 38]. Furthermore, mRNAs as well as miRNAs or other noncoding RNAs, which also are known to modulate pathways that may be important for ADC response, could be integrated into this methodology [31, 39, 40].

Acquired Resistance to ADC Therapy

Although ADC studies are already yielding proof-of-concept evidence in the clinic and are likely to define a paradigm shift in the treatment of a variety of cancers, it is perhaps inevitable that tumors that initially respond to ADCs will eventually become treatment-refractory and will continue to grow in the presence of ADC therapy. This acquired resistance phenomenon is widely observed in the context of other molecularly targeted therapies in the clinic and can often be modeled preclinically. Examples include the T790M mutation of EGFR in the context of erlotinib therapy [41], downregulation of CD20 in the setting of rituximab treatment [42, 43], overexpression of BCL-XL and BCL-A1 following ABT-263 therapy [44], and deletion of PTEN in the context of trastuzumab treatment [45]. Moreover, it is possible that intrinsic resistance and acquired resistance may involve similar mechanisms.

For any antibody therapeutic that targets a cell surface protein, one of the most likely mechanisms of resistance is downregulation of the antigen target. Preclinical models of acquired resistance to rituximab exemplify this. Thus, CD20 downregulation is a commonly observed mechanism of resistance [42, 43]. Furthermore, this has been observed in cases of rituximab-responsive patients who subsequently relapse [46]. The exact mechanism of CD20 receptor downregulation is unclear, but it may involve epigenetic suppression of the promoter region [43]. Since many of the ADCs are directed to surface targets that are not necessarily the oncogenic drivers of the disease, with the exception of trastuzumab-DM1 conjugate, it would not be surprising to find that tumor cells downregulate the ADC target without consequence for maintaining tumor cell growth and survival. Another potential mechanism of resistance is the increased expression of drug efflux pumps such as multidrug-resistant 1 (MDR1). Thus, cell lines conditioned to be resistant to chemotherapies such as colchicine, vinblastine, and adriamycin specifically demonstrate upregulation of MDR1 [47]. Clearly, measuring the expression of the surface target as well as candidate drug resistance genes could point to a clinically testable hypothesis regarding acquired resistance mechanisms, potentially leading to improved treatment strategies with these agents.

Thus far, there have been no published reports describing efforts to model acquired resistance to ADCs preclinically, and in light of the success of such efforts for other classes of antitumor drugs, this is likely to be pursued in the near future for ADCs. Conceptually, acquired resistance to ADCs could involve any of several components and processes—from receptor levels, internalization, drug release, and response to the associated chemotherapy drug. Given the plethora of potential mechanisms for acquired resistance, it would be important to implement broad discovery genomic efforts such as RNA-Seq and whole-genome analysis to reveal the specific molecular mechanisms underlying acquired resistance. This should also be explored as a "clinical experiment," and trials involving ADCs should probably be designed to ensure access to tumor specimens from patients who demonstrate disease progression following a clinical response. Ultimately, this approach would be expected to aid the development of therapeutic strategies to circumvent resistance associated with ADC treatment.

Predictive Diagnostic Implementation and Challenges

Key considerations in assessing the likelihood that a biomarker can be clinically implemented include, but are not limited to, [1] biomarker prevalence, [2] heterogeneity of target expression within a tumor, and [3] the feasibility of assays required to measure the biomarker endpoint from clinical tissue. Therefore, we shall consider each of these as it pertains to ADCs.

The prevalence of a predictive biomarker is a crucial first step in assessing the likelihood that a preclinically defined hypothesis can be clinically translated. In its simplest form, investigation of parameters of sensitivity and resistance might have revealed that the expression of MDR1, for example, was prevalent in about 40% of cell lines and accounted largely for the resistance phenotype to an ADC. However, if we were to assess such a biomarker in cancer patient samples and it revealed that the prevalence was <5%, then it would certainly reduce the likelihood of the biomarker having clinical utility, since there would be too few biomarker-positive cases represented in a standard clinical trial to reach statistical significance to test the hypothesis. Consequently, it becomes important to consider the caveats of preclinical models and to ensure that a broad spectrum of major cancer subtypes and mutations are represented in any experimental testing of ADCs. Furthermore, in the clinical setting, it also becomes important to consider the effect of prior treatments on the expression and prevalence of a candidate predictive biomarker. Prevalence studies conducted prior to assessment in the clinic are commonly carried out on clinical samples with poorly annotated clinical data, and it is becoming more common to report the prevalence of biomarkers in the context of clinical trials, as well as to analyze the presence of a biomarker in primary versus metastatic disease, with the latter more likely to be observed in phase I trials. As mentioned above, understanding the effect of biomarker expression and prevalence in response to standard of care therapies is a critical step in generating a robust clinical development plan.

It is often the case that new molecular entities (NMEs) enter clinical development in patients that have relapsed and/or are refractory to multiple prior therapies. By convention, archival fixed tissue is the most common form of tumor material available to assess the prevalence of a biomarker of interest and is usually obtained at the initial stages of disease presentation. However, we can speculate that the tumor biology is likely to have been significantly impacted by exposure to multiple treatment regimens, emphasizing the potential importance of establishing whether treatments have an effect on the prevalence of a biomarker. Once a patient progresses on therapy, it is not standard practice, regardless of cancer type, to re-biopsy tumors. One of the most challenging aspects of re-biopsying patients is tissue accessibility. For example, patients that have primary lesions in the breast or skin generally have more surgically accessible tumors than that those of non-small cell lung cancer or prostate cancer. However, this does not necessarily mean that it will not be possible to re-biopsy these less accessible tumors, and there is growing interest in implementing clinical protocols that include more invasive re-biopsy procedures.

A potential alternative to surgical re-biopsy to assess biomarker status is the isolation of circulating tumor cells (CTCs). CTCs are found in the bloodstream at very low frequency (~one tumor cell per one billion blood cells) and are believed to be derived from the primary tumor and to display similar genetic features (reviewed in [48]). This has been demonstrated, for example, in a study that examined CTCs in the context of EGFR mutation and gefitinib treatment, where 92% of patients demonstrated concordance of mutations when comparing the primary tumor and CTCs [49]. It is not yet clear whether more broad-based gene expression profiling of CTCs will reflect features corresponding to those seen in the primary lesion or that expression of various cell surface proteins would be similar; however, CTCs do provide a promising potential avenue to assess and characterize a patient's tumor through noninvasive means. CTC enrichment techniques generally rely upon antibodies to EpCam, which is specifically expressed on epithelial cells, and are amenable to downstream molecular assays such as qRT-PCR, mutation detection, and IHC [50]. In the context of ADCs, it would be important to determine if the expression of the ADC target is present on CTCs and if this is reflective of the primary tumor before relying solely on CTCs as an end point for patient selection or enrichment. Nonetheless, CTCs have enormous potential for the predictive biomarker field and clinical development, and future early stage clinical trials are soon expected to incorporate CTCs as exploratory end points.

Predictive Biomarker Assay Platforms

The most common assays performed on clinical samples are IHC, for the detection of protein expression, FISH for detecting DNA amplification, qPCR for mutation detection, qRT-PCR for measuring RNA expression, flow cytometry for assessing protein cell surface expression, and whole-genome expression profiling for evaluating the transcriptome. Collectively, these methodologies can capture the majority of biomarkers of interest; however, current clinical practice calls for tumor tissue to be fixed in formalin followed by embedding in paraffin, and this limits the sensitivity and robustness of many of these genomic assays.

For many years, genome-wide expression profiling of tumor material has been hampered by the fact that RNA derived from such samples tends to be highly degraded. Fortunately, in the past few years, there have been improvements in such analysis, made possible by the application of microarrays [51], DASL [52], and deep sequencing [53]. Ultimately, this affords the opportunity to assess the transcriptome of tumor samples and to interrogate a variety of biomarkers. A more focused approach using qRT-PCR has improved the yield of high-quality expression data from fixed tissue, not only in the research environment, but also as a diagnostic test for making treatment decisions in the setting of breast cancer [54]. The success of qRT-PCR for the analysis of RNA derived from fixed tissue is largely due to the predesigned small size of the amplicon for each transcript, thereby permitting efficient amplification of the mRNA of interest from highly degraded RNA. This makes this assay an attractive option for RNA expression, coupled with a well-defined regulatory approval route for this platform. Similarly, somatic mutations from tumor-derived DNA can be readily detected from fixed tissues using real-time PCR, pyrosequencing, and COLD-PCR approaches [55].

To assay protein expression, IHC is a well-established technique that can be applied to fixed tissue and has been used successfully for decades. It is commonly used to diagnose cancer subtypes and to select patients for targeted therapies [56, 57]. Moreover, from a regulatory standpoint, IHC is attractive in the context of regulatory approval in light of its track record. Although IHC is associated with a limited dynamic range in terms of signal to noise, it provides the advantage that it can be used to assess the heterogeneity within individual tumors, and this might be critical for decision making around specific assay cutoffs, as is exemplified by IHC criteria for trastuzumab use in the context of HER2+ breast cancer [58]. One of the main considerations regarding IHC assay development is to ensure that a biomarker of interest is preserved during fixation and that the epitope has not been masked. The use of alternative antibodies that recognize distinct epitopes may mitigate this concern. Unfortunately, flow cytometry cannot be performed on fixed tissue, and this limits the ability to assess cell surface protein expression in fixed tumors through means other than IHC. Furthermore, a trained pathologist is needed to interpret IHC data. Since a minimal level of target antigen on the cell surface is potentially required for ADC efficacy, this would be an important consideration. However, leukemias, such as CLL or AML, provide an opportunity to assess cell surface expression in real time by flow cytometry from fresh samples, thereby providing an attractive strategy to test a predictive biomarker hypothesis and to achieve clinical proof-of-concept without the concerns or challenges associated with fixed clinical specimens.

Conclusions

The ability to match the right drug to the right patient is a fundamental emerging paradigm in modern oncology practice. There are clear examples of successes in this arena, such as trastuzumab and imatinib, that have become the prototypic examples of personalized healthcare in action, with more recent examples

Table 5.1 Summary of potential predictive biomarkers for ADCs and potential assay platforms

Biomarker	Relationship to ADC mechanism of action	Assay platform
ADC target	Required for ADC activity	IHC, flow cytometry, qRT-PCR
Ki-67	Proliferative index of tumor may determine sensitivity to ADC with microtubule-targeted agent	IHC and qRT-PCR
Tubulin isoforms	Modulation of sensitivity to acquired resistance at ADC with microtubule-targeted agents	IHC and qRT-PCR
Anti-apoptosis regulators	Modulation of sensitivity and resistance to ADCs with chemotherapeutic agent	IHC and qRT-PCR
Drug efflux pumps	Modulation of ADC linker drug sensitivity	IHC and qRT-PCR
Oncogene and tumor suppressor mutations	Modulation of sensitivity and resistance to ADCs with chemotherapeutic agent	Real-time PCR, RNA-Seq
Microtubule modifiers and cell cycle regulators	Modulation of sensitivity to acquired resistance at ADC with microtubule-targeted agents	Multiple (qRT-PCR, IHC, etc.)
ADC target pathway	Negative and positive regulators of antibody internalization may modulate sensitivity to ADC	Multiple (qRT-PCR, IHC, etc.)
Others	Unknown from preclinical models and may require bedside to bench research	Broad exploratory platforms (e.g., RNA-Seq and whole-genome sequencing)

demonstrating clinical promise, such as vemurafenib for in the treatment of BRAF mutant melanoma [59], the ALK kinase inhibitor crizotinib in ALK-translocated NSCLC [60], and the ADC T-DM1 in Herceptin-refractory breast cancer [3]. The onslaught of a large number of ADCs approaching clinical development will potentially deliver novel promising treatment options for cancer patients, and the selection of the right treatment for individual patients will certainly play a role in this process. In this context, it will be crucial to consider testing biomarkers that encompass the various determinants of ADC efficacy, extending beyond target expression. With the plethora of potentially regulated steps related to antibody internalization, drug release, and toxin response, it would be prudent to develop a suite of testable biomarkers, such as those listed in Table 5.1, that encompass these potential modulators of ADC response. Whether or not a companion diagnostic test will eventually be featured as a component of an ADC drug label remains to be determined and will undoubtedly be context-dependent, but regardless of these unknowns, a sound diagnostic hypothesis generation and testing strategy will certainly contribute to securing the future of ADCs as a potential paradigm-shifting treatment option for cancer patients.

References

1. Garnett MC (2001) Targeted drug conjugates: principles and progress. Adv Drug Deliv Rev 53(2):171–216
2. Lewis Phillips GD, Li G, Dugger DL, Crocker LM, Parsons KL, Mai E, Blattler WA, Lambert JM, Chari RV, Lutz RJ, Wong WL, Jacobson FS, Koeppen H, Schwall RH, Kenkare-Mitra SR, Spencer SD, Sliwkowski MX (2008) Targeting HER2-positive breast cancer with trastuzumab-DM1, an antibody-cytotoxic drug conjugate. Cancer Res 68(22):9280–9290
3. Krop IE, Beeram M, Modi S, Jones SF, Holden SN, Yu W, Girish S, Tibbitts J, Yi JH, Sliwkowski MX, Jacobson F, Lutzker SG, Burris HA (2010) Phase I study of trastuzumab-DM1, an HER2 antibody-drug conjugate, given every 3 weeks to patients with HER2-positive metastatic breast cancer. J Clin Oncol 28(16):2698–2704
4. Francisco JA, Cerveny CG, Meyer DL, Mixan BJ, Klussman K, Chace DF, Rejniak SX, Gordon KA, DeBlanc R, Toki BE, Law CL, Doronina SO, Siegall CB, Senter PD, Wahl AF (2003) cAC10-vcMMAE, an anti-CD30-monomethyl auristatin E conjugate with potent and selective antitumor activity. Blood 102(4):1458–1465
5. Younes A, Forero-Tores A, Bartlett N, Leonard J, Lynch C, Kennedy D, Sievers E (2008) Multiple complete responses in a Phase 1 dose-escalation study of the antibody-drug conjugate SGN-35 in patients with relapsed or refractory CD30-positive lymphomas. Blood 112.
6. Younes A, Bartlett NL, Leonard JP, Kennedy DA, Lynch CM, Sievers EL, Forero-Torres A (2010) Brentuximab Vedotin (SGN-35) for relapsed CD30-positive lymphomas. N Engl J Med 363(19):1812–1821
7. Alley SC, Okeley NM, Senter PD (2010) Antibody-drug conjugates: targeted drug delivery for cancer. Curr Opin Chem Biol 14(4):529–537
8. Lee W, Jiang Z, Liu J, Haverty PM, Guan Y, Stinson J, Yue P, Zhang Y, Pant KP, Bhatt D, Ha C, Johnson S, Kennemer MI, Mohan S, Nazarenko I, Watanabe C, Sparks AB, Shames DS, Gentleman R, de Sauvage FJ, Stern H, Pandita A, Ballinger DG, Drmanac R, Modrusan Z, Seshagiri S, Zhang Z (2010) The mutation spectrum revealed by paired genome sequences from a lung cancer patient. Nature 465(7297):473–477
9. Hawkins RD, Hon GC, Ren B (2010) Next-generation genomics: an integrative approach. Nat Rev Genet 11(7):476–486
10. Meyerson M, Gabriel S, Getz G (2010) Advances in understanding cancer genomes through second-generation sequencing. Nat Rev Genet 11(10):685–696
11. Dijoseph JF, Dougher MM, Armellino DC, Kalyandrug L, Kunz A, Boghaert ER, Hamann PR, Damle NK (2007) CD20-specific antibody-targeted chemotherapy of non-Hodgkin's B-cell lymphoma using calicheamicin-conjugated rituximab. Cancer Immunol Immunother 56(7):1107–1117
12. Polson AG, Calemine-Fenaux J, Chan P, Chang W, Christensen E, Clark S, de Sauvage FJ, Eaton D, Elkins K, Elliott JM, Frantz G, Fuji RN, Gray A, Harden K, Ingle GS, Kljavin NM, Koeppen H, Nelson C, Prabhu S, Raab H, Ross S, Slaga DS, Stephan JP, Scales SJ, Spencer SD, Vandlen R, Wranik B, Yu SF, Zheng B, Ebens A (2009) Antibody-drug conjugates for the treatment of non-Hodgkin's lymphoma: target and linker-drug selection. Cancer Res 69(6):2358–2364
13. Kroemer G, Jaattela M (2005) Lysosomes and autophagy in cell death control. Nat Rev Cancer 5(11):886–897
14. Joyce JA, Hanahan D (2004) Multiple roles for cysteine cathepsins in cancer. Cell Cycle 3(12):1516–1619
15. Tandon AK, Clark GM, Chamness GC, Chirgwin JM, McGuire WL (1990) Cathepsin D and prognosis in breast cancer. N Engl J Med 322(5):297–302
16. http://www.ncbi.nlm.nih.gov/pubmed/2713856
17. Wu GS, Saftig P, Peters C, El-Deiry WS (1998) Potential role for cathepsin D in p53-dependent tumor suppression and chemosensitivity. Oncogene 16(17):2177–2183

18. Roshy S, Sloane BF, Moin K (2003) Pericellular cathepsin B and malignant progression. Cancer Metastasis Rev 22(2–3):271–286
19. Polson AG, Williams M, Gray AM, Fuji RN, Poon KA, McBride J, Raab H, Januario T, Go M, Lau J, Yu SF, Du C, Fuh F, Tan C, Wu Y, Liang WC, Prabhu S, Stephan JP, Hongo JA, Dere RC, Deng R, Cullen M, de Tute R, Bennett F, Rawstron A, Jack A, Ebens A (2010) Anti-CD22-MCC-DM1: an antibody-drug conjugate with a stable linker for the treatment of non-Hodgkin's lymphoma. Leukemia 24(9):1566–1573
20. Gerber HP, Kung-Sutherland M, Stone I, Morris-Tilden C, Miyamoto J, McCormick R, Alley SC, Okeley N, Hayes B, Hernandez-Ilizaliturri FJ, McDonagh CF, Carter PJ, Benjamin D, Grewal IS (2009) Potent antitumor activity of the anti-CD19 auristatin antibody drug conjugate hBU12-vcMMAE against rituximab-sensitive and -resistant lymphomas. Blood 113(18):4352–4361
21. Jordan MA, Wilson L (2004) Microtubules as a target for anticancer drugs. Nat Rev Cancer 4(4):253–265
22. Wahl AF, Donaldson KL, Fairchild C, Lee FY, Foster SA, Demers GW, Galloway DA (1996) Loss of normal p53 function confers sensitization to Taxol by increasing G2/M arrest and apoptosis. Nat Med 2(1):72–79
23. Dornan D, Bennett F, Chen Y, Dennis M, Eaton D, Elkins K, French D, Go MA, Jack A, Junutula JR, Koeppen H, Lau J, McBride J, Rawstron A, Shi X, Yu N, Yu SF, Yue P, Zheng B, Ebens A, Polson AG (2009) Therapeutic potential of an anti-CD79b antibody-drug conjugate, anti-CD79b-vc-MMAE, for the treatment of non-Hodgkin lymphoma. Blood 114(13):2721–2729
24. Anand S, Penrhyn-Lowe S, Venkitaraman AR (2003) AURORA-A amplification overrides the mitotic spindle assembly checkpoint, inducing resistance to Taxol. Cancer Cell 3(1):51–62
25. Cabral F, Abraham I, Gottesman MM (1981) Isolation of a taxol-resistant Chinese hamster ovary cell mutant that has an alteration in alpha-tubulin. Proc Natl Acad Sci USA 78(7):4388–4391
26. Berrieman HK, Lind MJ, Cawkwell L (2004) Do beta-tubulin mutations have a role in resistance to chemotherapy? Lancet Oncol 5(3):158–164
27. Yin S, Bhattacharya R, Cabral F (2010) Human mutations that confer paclitaxel resistance. Mol Cancer Ther 9(2):327–335
28. Kavallaris M (2010) Microtubules and resistance to tubulin-binding agents. Nat Rev Cancer 10(3):194–204
29. Gan PP, Pasquier E, Kavallaris M (2007) Class III beta-tubulin mediates sensitivity to chemotherapeutic drugs in non small cell lung cancer. Cancer Res 67(19):9356–9363
30. Tanaka S, Nohara T, Iwamoto M, Sumiyoshi K, Kimura K, Takahashi Y, Tanigawa N (2009) Tau expression and efficacy of paclitaxel treatment in metastatic breast cancer. Cancer Chemother Pharmacol 64(2):341–346
31. Cochrane DR, Howe EN, Spoelstra NS, Richer JK (2010) Loss of miR-200c: a marker of aggressiveness and chemoresistance in female reproductive cancers. J Oncol 2010:821717
32. Gregory PA, Bert AG, Paterson EL, Barry SC, Tsykin A, Farshid G, Vadas MA, Khew-Goodall Y, Goodall GJ (2008) The miR-200 family and miR-205 regulate epithelial to mesenchymal transition by targeting ZEB1 and SIP1. Nat Cell Biol 10(5):593–601
33. Lestini BJ, Goldsmith KC, Fluchel MN, Liu X, Chen NL, Goyal B, Pawel BR, Hogarty MD (2009) Mcl1 downregulation sensitizes neuroblastoma to cytotoxic chemotherapy and small molecule Bcl2-family antagonists. Cancer Biol Ther 8(16):1587–1595
34. Petersen SL, Peyton M, Minna JD, Wang X (2010) Overcoming cancer cell resistance to Smac mimetic induced apoptosis by modulating cIAP-2 expression. Proc Natl Acad Sci USA 107(26):11936–11941
35. Reed JC (1995) Regulation of apoptosis by bcl-2 family proteins and its role in cancer and chemoresistance. Curr Opin Oncol 7(6):541–546
36. Sasaki H, Sheng Y, Kotsuji F, Tsang BK (2000) Down-regulation of X-linked inhibitor of apoptosis protein induces apoptosis in chemoresistant human ovarian cancer cells. Cancer Res 60(20):5659–5666
37. Huang EP, Fridlyand J, Lewin-Koh N, Yue P, Shi X, Dornan D, Burington B (2010) Statistical techniques to construct assays for identifying likely responders to a treatment under evaluation from cell line genomic data. BMC Cancer 10:586

38. O'Brien C, Wallin JJ, Sampath D, GuhaThakurta D, Savage H, Punnoose EA, Guan J, Berry L, Prior WW, Amler LC, Belvin M, Friedman LS, Lackner MR (2010) Predictive biomarkers of sensitivity to the phosphatidylinositol 3′ kinase inhibitor GDC-0941 in breast cancer preclinical models. Clin Cancer Res 16(14):3670–3683
39. Cimmino A, Calin GA, Fabbri M, Iorio MV, Ferracin M, Shimizu M, Wojcik SE, Aqeilan RI, Zupo S, Dono M, Rassenti L, Alder H, Volinia S, Liu CG, Kipps TJ, Negrini M, Croce CM (2005) miR-15 and miR-16 induce apoptosis by targeting BCL2. Proc Natl Acad Sci USA 102(39):13944–13949
40. Huarte M, Guttman M, Feldser D, Garber M, Koziol MJ, Kenzelmann-Broz D, Khalil AM, Zuk O, Amit I, Rabani M, Attardi LD, Regev A, Lander ES, Jacks T, Rinn JL (2010) A large intergenic noncoding RNA induced by p53 mediates global gene repression in the p53 response. Cell 142(3):409–419
41. Kobayashi S, Boggon TJ, Dayaram T, Janne PA, Kocher O, Meyerson M, Johnson BE, Eck MJ, Tenen DG, Halmos B (2005) EGFR mutation and resistance of non-small-cell lung cancer to gefitinib. N Engl J Med 352(8):786–792
42. Olejniczak SH, Hernandez-Ilizaliturri FJ, Clements JL, Czuczman MS (2008) Acquired resistance to rituximab is associated with chemotherapy resistance resulting from decreased Bax and Bak expression. Clin Cancer Res 14(5):1550–1560
43. Hiraga J, Tomita A, Sugimoto T, Shimada K, Ito M, Nakamura S, Kiyoi H, Kinoshita T, Naoe T (2009) Down-regulation of CD20 expression in B-cell lymphoma cells after treatment with rituximab-containing combination chemotherapies: its prevalence and clinical significance. Blood 113(20):4885–4893
44. Vogler M, Butterworth M, Majid A, Walewska RJ, Sun XM, Dyer MJ, Cohen GM (2009) Concurrent up-regulation of BCL-XL and BCL2A1 induces approximately 1000-fold resistance to ABT-737 in chronic lymphocytic leukemia. Blood 113(18):4403–4413
45. Nagata Y, Lan KH, Zhou X, Tan M, Esteva FJ, Sahin AA, Klos KS, Li P, Monia BP, Nguyen NT, Hortobagyi GN, Hung MC, Yu D (2004) PTEN activation contributes to tumor inhibition by trastuzumab, and loss of PTEN predicts trastuzumab resistance in patients. Cancer Cell 6(2):117–127
46. Davis TA, Czerwinski DK, Levy R (1999) Therapy of B-cell lymphoma with anti-CD20 antibodies can result in the loss of CD20 antigen expression. Clin Cancer Res 5(3):611–615
47. Shen DW, Fojo A, Chin JE, Roninson IB, Richert N, Pastan I, Gottesman MM (1986) Human multidrug-resistant cell lines: increased mdr1 expression can precede gene amplification. Science 232(4750):643–645
48. Maheswaran S, Haber DA (2010) Circulating tumor cells: a window into cancer biology and metastasis. Curr Opin Genet Dev 20(1):96–99
49. Maheswaran S, Sequist LV, Nagrath S, Ulkus L, Brannigan B, Collura CV, Inserra E, Diederichs S, Iafrate AJ, Bell DW, Digumarthy S, Muzikansky A, Irimia D, Settleman J, Tompkins RG, Lynch TJ, Toner M, Haber DA (2008) Detection of mutations in EGFR in circulating lung-cancer cells. N Engl J Med 359(4):366–377
50. Punnoose EA, Atwal SK, Spoerke JM, Savage H, Pandita A, Yeh RF, Pirzkall A, Fine BM, Amler LC, Chen DS, Lackner MR (2010) Molecular biomarker analyses using circulating tumor cells. PLoS One 5(9):e12517
51. Williams PM, Li R, Johnson NA, Wright G, Heath JD, Gascoyne RD (2010) A novel method of amplification of FFPET-derived RNA enables accurate disease classification with microarrays. J Mol Diagn 12(5):680–686
52. Hoshida Y, Villanueva A, Kobayashi M, Peix J, Chiang DY, Camargo A, Gupta S, Moore J, Wrobel MJ, Lerner J, Reich M, Chan JA, Glickman JN, Ikeda K, Hashimoto M, Watanabe G, Daidone MG, Roayaie S, Schwartz M, Thung S, Salvesen HB, Gabriel S, Mazzaferro V, Bruix J, Friedman SL, Kumada H, Llovet JM, Golub TR (2008) Gene expression in fixed tissues and outcome in hepatocellular carcinoma. N Engl J Med 359(19):1995–2004
53. Weng L, Wu X, Gao H, Mu B, Li X, Wang JH, Guo C, Jin JM, Chen Z, Covarrubias M, Yuan YC, Weiss LM, Wu H (2010) MicroRNA profiling of clear cell renal cell carcinoma by whole-genome small RNA deep sequencing of paired frozen and formalin-fixed, paraffin-embedded tissue specimens. J Pathol 222(1):41–51

54. Gianni L, Zambetti M, Clark K, Baker J, Cronin M, Wu J, Mariani G, Rodriguez J, Carcangiu M, Watson D, Valagussa P, Rouzier R, Symmans WF, Ross JS, Hortobagyi GN, Pusztai L, Shak S (2005) Gene expression profiles in paraffin-embedded core biopsy tissue predict response to chemotherapy in women with locally advanced breast cancer. J Clin Oncol 23(29):7265–7277
55. Zuo Z, Chen SS, Chandra PK, Galbincea JM, Soape M, Doan S, Barkoh BA, Koeppen H, Medeiros LJ, Luthra R (2009) Application of COLD-PCR for improved detection of KRAS mutations in clinical samples. Mod Pathol 22(8):1023–1031
56. Choi WW, Weisenburger DD, Greiner TC, Piris MA, Banham AH, Delabie J, Braziel RM, Geng H, Iqbal J, Lenz G, Vose JM, Hans CP, Fu K, Smith LM, Li M, Liu Z, Gascoyne RD, Rosenwald A, Ott G, Rimsza LM, Campo E, Jaffe ES, Jaye DL, Staudt LM, Chan WC (2009) A new immunostain algorithm classifies diffuse large B-cell lymphoma into molecular subtypes with high accuracy. Clin Cancer Res 15(17):5494–5502
57. Hammond ME, Hayes DF, Dowsett M, Allred DC, Hagerty KL, Badve S, Fitzgibbons PL, Francis G, Goldstein NS, Hayes M, Hicks DG, Lester S, Love R, Mangu PB, McShane L, Miller K, Osborne CK, Paik S, Perlmutter J, Rhodes A, Sasano H, Schwartz JN, Sweep FC, Taube S, Torlakovic EE, Valenstein P, Viale G, Visscher D, Wheeler T, Williams RB, Wittliff JL, Wolff AC (2010) American Society of Clinical Oncology/College of American Pathologists guideline recommendations for immunohistochemical testing of estrogen and progesterone receptors in breast cancer. J Clin Oncol 28(16):2784–2795
58. Sauter G, Lee J, Bartlett JM, Slamon DJ, Press MF (2009) Guidelines for human epidermal growth factor receptor 2 testing: biologic and methodologic considerations. J Clin Oncol 27(8):1323–1333
59. Flaherty KT, Puzanov I, Kim KB, Ribas A, McArthur GA, Sosman JA, O'Dwyer PJ, Lee RJ, Grippo JF, Nolop K, Chapman PB (2010) Inhibition of mutated, activated BRAF in metastatic melanoma. N Engl J Med 363(9):809–819
60. http://www.ncbi.nlm.nih.gov/pubmed/20979469

Part III
Selection of Cytotoxic Agents

Chapter 6
Factors Involved in the Design of Cytotoxic Payloads for Antibody–Drug Conjugates

Wayne C. Widdison and Ravi V.J. Chari

Introduction

Selective targeting of cancer can be accomplished by the use of monoclonal antibodies (mAbs) that bind to tumor-associated antigens expressed preferentially on the surface of cancer cells. Several of these non-derivatized antibodies, or naked antibodies, have been approved for the treatment of various cancer types. However, compelling single agent activity has only been demonstrated in the treatment of hematological malignancies. For example, the anti-CD20 mAb rituximab (Rituxan) is widely used in the treatment of B-cell lymphomas. Also, the anti-CD52 antibody alemtuzumab (Campath) is used in the treatment of some leukemias. However, antibodies targeting solid tumors, such as trastuzumab (Herceptin) for breast cancer, anti-EGF receptor antibodies cetuximab (Erbitux) and panitumumab (Vectibix) for head and neck and colon cancers, and the anti-angiogenic agent bevacizumab (Avastin), display only modest antitumor activity as single agents. Thus, these antibodies are most often used in combination with conventional anticancer drugs, thus retaining the high systemic toxicity of standard chemotherapy. In an alternative approach, the efficacy of a naked antibody can be greatly enhanced by attachment of a cytotoxic molecule to give an antibody–drug conjugate (ADC).[1] The selection of the optimal cytotoxic effector, linker, and antibody component of the ADC can be facilitated by an understanding of the environments to which the ADC will be exposed to once it is administered to a patient and also through the knowledge gained from the development of previous ADCs. Most of the current ADCs under development are for the

[1] Because each ADC is itself a drug or drug candidate, the attached cytotoxic effector will not be referred to as a "drug" in this chapter unless it is, on its own, an FDA-approved therapeutic agent (e.g., doxorubicin).

W.C. Widdison (✉) • R.V.J. Chari
ImmunoGen, Inc., 830 Winter St., Waltham, MA 02451, USA
e-mail: wayne.widdison@immunogen.com

G.L. Phillips (ed.), *Antibody-Drug Conjugates and Immunotoxins: From Pre-Clinical Development to Therapeutic Applications*, Cancer Drug Discovery and Development, DOI 10.1007/978-1-4614-5456-4_6,

treatment of cancer; however, ADCs are also being investigated for the treatment of autoimmune diseases [1]. This chapter will deal with the selection of an appropriate cytotoxic effector for the preparation of anticancer ADCs, but much of the discussion is relevant to ADCs for the treatment of autoimmune diseases as well.

Overview of ADC Delivery to Target Cells

Ideally, an ADC should be designed so that it is non-immunogenic and remains nontoxic in circulation in vivo until it reaches its target site. After binding to the target cell, the conjugate is internalized by a mechanism called receptor-mediated endocytosis. The extent of internalization, or endocytosis of an antibody, depends on the nature of the cell surface antigens to which the antibody binds and on the abundance of these antigens. After internalization one or more active forms of the cytotoxic effector are released from the ADC in endosomes or lysosomes, these metabolites can then diffuse into the cytoplasm of the cell. Once in the cytoplasm, the metabolites can bind to an intracellular target such as microtubules or DNA and induce cell death. An ADC must deliver a given threshold concentration of cytotoxic metabolite to the cytoplasm of a cell in order to kill it. This threshold level can be reduced if higher potency metabolites are released.

In principle, a cytotoxic metabolite can be cleaved from an ADC, while the ADC is bound to the surface of a targeted cell. This would require the ADC linkage to be labile, at least to the conditions on the surface of the targeted cell. The extracellular environment of tumors has been reported to be slightly acidic (pH~6) in which case an ADC employing an acid-labile linkage could release active metabolite on the tumor cell surface [2,3]. Some tumor cell lines are also known to express various proteases on their surface such as cathepsins and metalloproteases, which could potentially cleave the effector molecule from ADCs that utilize peptide linkers [4]. Protein disulfide isomerases [5], which cause disulfide cleavage/interchange, are present on the surface of some tumor cells and have the potential to release active metabolite from ADCs possessing disulfide-bearing linkers. Once an active form of the effector is released at the surface of the targeted cell, the effector could diffuse into the targeted cell or into a nearby cell in order to cause cell death. The effectiveness of such cell surface release for the various linkage systems however is unclear.

Structure of ADCs

A structural representation of an ADC is shown in Fig. 6.1. Typically, an average of 2–5 molecules of the effector (depicted as orange spheres) is linked per molecule of antibody. Ideally, the effectors are linked at the Fc or constant region of the antibody which does not participate in binding to the antigen. The antigen-binding complementarity-determining region loops are shown in yellow and green.

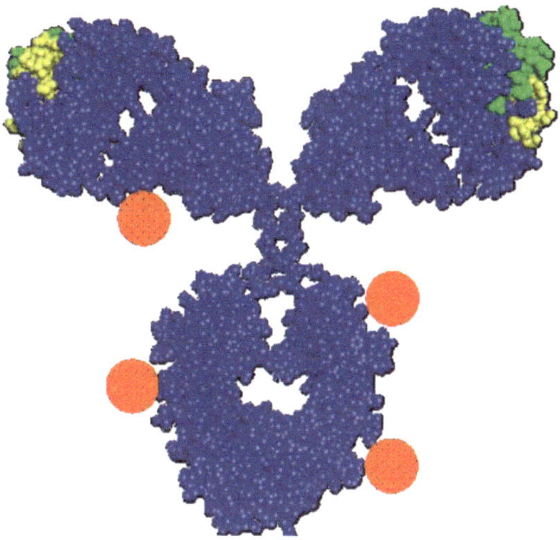

Fig. 6.1 Antibody bearing cytotoxic effectors randomly linked on lysine residues

The effector is most often linked to the antibody via lysine or cysteine residues on the antibody. In the case of lysine attachment, linkage of effector molecules to the antibody could theoretically occur through the ε-amino group of any one of the ~80 lysine residues present on an antibody, but typically a much fewer number of lysines (~10) are preferentially accessible for chemical modification. In the case of cysteine attachment, the effector can be linked to reactive cysteine residues, generated by reduction of internal hinge region cystine disulfide bonds of the antibody or cystine disulfides linking the heavy chains to the light chains of the antibody. Complete reduction of all four cystines enables the linkage of 8 effector molecules per antibody in defined locations. Carefully controlled reaction conditions are required to reduce just two cystines to enable linkage of 4 effector molecules, and often variable amounts of higher and lower effector incorporation may be obtained [6]. Thus, both conjugation methods described above give a heterogeneous distribution of effector molecules linked to the antibody molecule. The reported number of effectors per antibody for these ADCs is therefore usually given as an average derived from all of the formed species.

Genetically engineered antibodies can also be produced in which two or more reactive cysteine residues are incorporated into the antibody at known locations, typically in the Fc region [7]. Such antibodies have been used to prepare ADCs for preclinical testing, but it is not yet clear if this engineered linkage method will improve the therapeutic window of ADCs.

Linkage of more than five molecules of the effector by any of these methods is often not achievable, since the cytotoxic effectors are usually hydrophobic, which can impair the aqueous solubility of the ADC. In addition, linkage of a large number of effectors may not be desirable since it could adversely alter the pharmacokinetics of the antibody component *in vivo* or diminish the binding affinity of the antibody to the antigen on the target cell [8].

Knowledge Gained from First-Generation ADCs

The concept of ADCs evolved from the hope that targeted delivery of approved anticancer drugs by using mAbs would confer some degree of tumor selectivity and thus improve their therapeutic index. Early ADCs were comprised of a tumor-specific mAb covalently linked to several molecules of a clinically used anticancer drug such as doxorubicin, vinblastine, or methotrexate. In the targeting of solid tumors, it was believed that the conjugate could deliver a clinically relevant dose of the effector to the tumor while sparing cells of noncancerous tissue. These early conjugates were evaluated in human clinical trials but were found to have little or no activity. Several shortcomings of these early ADCs have since been identified.

Immune Response

mAbs used in the early conjugates were either of murine origin or partly murine and partly human (chimeric), resulting in an immune response and the generation of human anti-murine antibodies that prevented repeat cycles of therapy.

Insufficient Potency of the Effector

Linkage of the cytotoxic effector to an antibody often resulted in poorer *in vitro* potency for the ADC than the parent compound. Since the effectors used in early ADCs were only modestly potent (IC_{50} values ~10^{-8} M), a large number of molecules had to be internalized to achieve a lethal effect. While cytotoxic compounds are usually hydrophobic and can freely diffuse into the cell, the extent of ADC delivery into cells is limited by antigen expression resulting in diminished potency. Thus, the circulating serum concentration of ADCs in patients was not in the therapeutic range.

Limited Expression of the Antigen

Tumor cells typically express only a limited number of antigen molecules on the cell surface (typically $<1 \times 10^5$ receptors/cell); the number of effector molecules that can be delivered by an antibody may not achieve the intracellular threshold concentration required to cause cell death in the case of the early modestly potent effectors that were used [9].

Internalization

Internalization mechanisms of antibodies can be inefficient; the actual number of conjugate molecules that are delivered into endocytic vesicles of a cell is often lower than the number of molecules that were bound to the cell surface. The route by which ADC is internalized can potentially impact ADC processing. For instance, caveolae vesicle-mediated internalization, at least in some cases, has been reported to traffic material to the Golgi or endoplasmic reticulum instead of endosomes or lysosomes [10]. Other modes of internalization appear to traffic vesicles to proteolytic compartments. Caveolae-mediated trafficking therefore may not efficiently generate cytotoxic metabolites from internalized ADCs when proteolysis is required [11].

Processing

Once internalized into endocytic vesicles of a cell, the ADC must release a metabolite that is capable of diffusing or being transported into the cytoplasm. At this point, the metabolite must either be active or undergo further processing to give an active metabolite that can kill the cell. As previously mentioned, internalization of an ADC to non-proteolytic compartments may impede proteolytic metabolite release.

Tumor Localization (Tumor Penetration)

The localization rate of mAbs at the tumor in patients has been measured for a number of different tumor types using radiolabeled antibodies and found to be low (0.003–0.08% of the injected dose/g tumor) [12]. In contrast, much higher accumulation rates (~15–20% injected dose/g tumor) were measured in tumor xenografts in mice [13].

Linker Stability

The antibody component of an ADC is typically of an IgG type that can be bound by the neonatal Fc receptor (FcRn) at low pH. During circulation, naked antibodies and ADCs are taken up by cells of the reticuloendothelial system (RES) [14]. FcRn in the low-pH (pH ~6) RES endosomes then binds to most of the antibody, including ADCs, and recycles them back into the blood. Any ADC that did not bind to FcRn would be degraded in lysosomes of the RES cells to release one or more cytotoxic metabolites. Blood plasma also contains some hydrolytic enzymes which can potentially cleave an effector from an ADC during circulation. Thus, circulating ADC is exposed to various hydrolytic plasma enzymes as well as to the acidic environment in the endosomes of RES cells which can cleave the payload from the ADC depending on the chemistry of the utilized linker (see Chap. 7). This nontargeted release of effector may contribute to systemic toxicity and also, over time, diminish the load of effector on the ADC resulting in poorer potency to the targeted cancer cells.

Payload Requirements for an ADC

Potency

Some of the problems facing the first generation of ADCs can be addressed by employing ADCs bearing more highly potent effectors. The problems of limited antigen expression and poor antigen internalization ideally would be addressed by targeting surface antigens that are highly expressed on cancer cells and to which the bound ADC is efficiently internalized. This however may not be possible for a given cancer indication, but the use of ADCs bearing more highly potent effectors will increase the probability of delivering a therapeutic dose to tumor cells that have low antigen expression or have poor processing. Also because ADCs are likely to have limited tumor penetration, they require a highly potent effector component to achieve sufficient killing of tumor cells. The problem of poor tumor penetration is less of an obstacle for the treatment of predominantly liquid tumors, such as acute myeloid leukemia. Thus, liquid tumors are generally considered to be more accessible to ADCs than solid tumors.

Since only a fraction of an administered ADC is actually taken up by targeted cancer cells, the ADC ideally should be equipped with an effector, or an effector-linker combination, that induces higher potency against cancerous cells than noncancerous cells. Cancer cells often divide more rapidly than noncancerous cells; thus, an agent which preferentially kills rapidly dividing cells could have higher potency against targeted cancer cells than many noncancerous cells. Some cancer cells are reported to have elevated levels of reduced glutathione (GSH) or enzymes that reduce disulfide adducts of GSH [15]. GSH can react with DNA-alkylating agents to lower their potency against these cancer cells. GSH can also attack and cleave disulfide bonds. It has been suggested that disulfide-linked ADCs may have higher potency against GSH-rich cancer cells due to enhanced reductive cleavage [5]. Some cancer cells are also multidrug resistant (MDR) because they possess proteins, referred to as MDR pumps, which can efflux hydrophobic molecules from the cell [16, 17]. Cancer cells possessing MDR pumps are often more resistant to ADCs than other cells. ADCs that release hydrophilic metabolites that are poor substrates for the MDR1 pump have recently been developed and shown to have improved efficacy against such MDR cancers in preclinical evaluation [18]. Solid tumor cells are reported to have low oxygen levels; the cells are hypoxic [19]. Some anticancer drugs, such as doxorubicin, mitoxantrone, and etoposide, are known to have lower activity under hypoxic conditions which may impair the efficacy of such compounds when they are utilized in ADCs targeting solid tumors [20, 21].

Stability

Besides the requirement for high potency, the effector component of an ADC should also be stable during preparation or storage and during circulation in a patient. Effector components that are not fully stable during the preparation or storage of the ADC can potentially be converted to more stable prodrug forms prior to antibody conjugation. The antibody-linked prodrug can then be converted to its active form in circulation or during cellular internalization. However, the use of a prodrug in ADCs adds a level of complexity since the ADC itself could be viewed as a targeted prodrug of the effector. In addition, the activation of a prodrug may be different across species, and what is observed in preclinical models (e.g., mice or rats) may not translate to the human situation. For example, mouse and human cathepsin B proteases were found to be very similar, while differences were found in the catalytic regions of human and mouse cathepsin K proteases [22]. A review comparing mouse and human degradative enzymes, some of which could potentially be used to release effectors from ADCs, has been published [23].

If the effector component of an ADC is not stable in lysosomes, then the effector would need to be cleaved on the cell surface or during cellular internalization but before the ADC is subjected to prolonged exposure to lysosomal enzymes. Cytotoxic effectors which for instance bear esters, two or more directly attached alpha-amino acids, or glycosidic bonds are potentially labile to lysosomal enzymes. For example, the highly potent antimitotic agents, dolastatin 15 and cemadotin, can be cleaved by intracellular proteases to first give the potent metabolite P5, which is further cleaved to give the much less potent metabolite P4 (Fig. 6.2 [24]). A non-cleavable linkage would not be appropriate for ADCs that utilize protease-labile effector components. The stability of an effector or linkage system to lysosomal enzymes can be determined by HPLC analyses derived from (a) incubation of ADCs bearing radiolabeled effector with cells [25, 26] or (b) incubation of free unconjugated effector with isolated lysosomes [27].

Solubility and Membrane Permeability

Because an antibody is a protein, the conjugation reactions used to covalently attach an effector to an antibody are done in aqueous solutions. Water-miscible organic cosolvents can be used in these reactions; however, excessive amounts of organic solvent may be required to conjugate a very hydrophobic molecule, which can damage the antibody. Extremely hydrophobic effectors also have the potential to change the pharmacokinetic properties of a conjugate or to cause hydrophobic aggregation of conjugate. Thus, the effector and linkage system used to prepare an ADC should be reasonably soluble in aqueous solutions with minimal organic cosolvents. If an effector has poor aqueous solubility, then a more soluble prodrug form can be employed. Also if the ADC utilizes a cleavable linker, then it may be preferable for

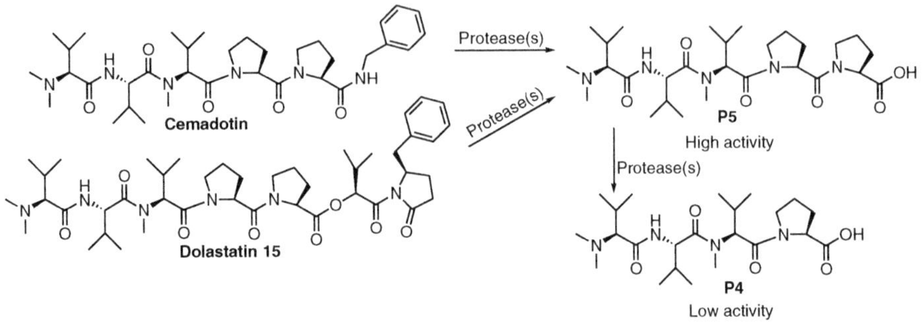

Fig. 6.2 Protease cleavage of cemadotin and dolastatin 15

the linker to be hydrophilic to aid in ADC aqueous solubility [28]. Again if a prodrug form of an effector is chosen, it should be efficiently activated in circulation or during cellular internalization.

The membrane permeability of the cytotoxic metabolites released from an ADC is an important factor to consider. When a non-charged relatively hydrophobic metabolite is released from an ADC in a cell, the metabolite will not only be able to kill the target cell, but it may also diffuse into and kill a neighboring cell, a process known as bystander killing. This may be beneficial if the metabolite is released in an intentionally targeted tumor cell because bystander killing may also kill a neighboring tumor cell that is less accessible to the ADC. Bystander killing however also has the potential to affect noncancerous cells, possibly contributing to systemic toxicity. For a given indication, the decision on whether an ADC should employ bystander killing may rely on several factors including (a) homogeneity of antigen expression on the tumor; (b) tumor type, liquid tumors may gain little or no benefit from bystander killing; (c) efficacy in animal studies and therapeutic index; and (d) known target antigen expression in noncancerous human tissue.

Attributes of ADCs in Clinical Trials

There are many ADCs currently in clinical trials, each utilizing one of the following linker types: non-cleavable, peptide cleavable, disulfide cleavable, or acid cleavable. The lysosomes of cells are rich in proteolytic enzymes which can degrade the antibody portion of an ADC or cleave the peptide moiety of peptide-linked ADCs to release one or more cytotoxic metabolites. The concentrations of proteases in blood however are much lower than in lysosomes, which often allows these conjugates to be stable in circulation. Thiols can reductively cleave disulfide bonds. Concentrations of glutathione, the predominant thiol compound in cells, have been found to be in

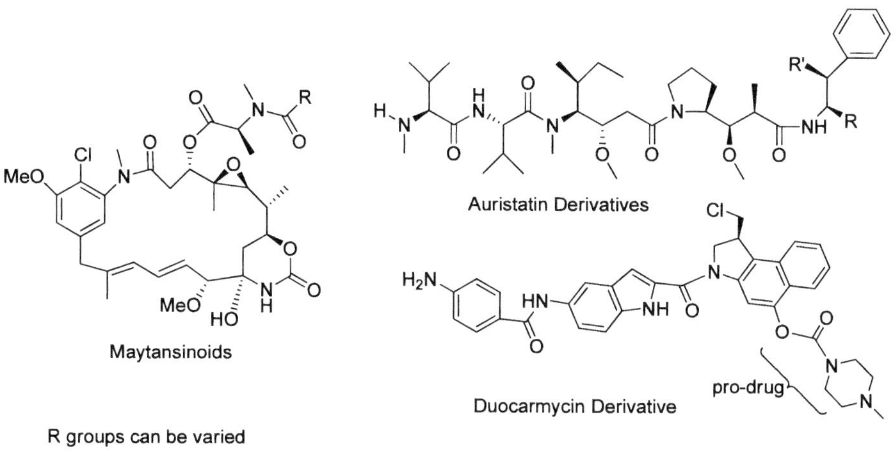

Fig. 6.3 Structures of effectors utilized by ADCs currently in clinical trials

the millimolar range in the cytoplasm, while the concentration of reductive thiols in blood is approximately 1,000-fold lower [29, 30]. This difference in reductive potential allows disulfide-linked ADCs to be stable in circulation, while efficiently releasing cytotoxic metabolites once the conjugate is internalized by cells.

Each of the ADCs currently in clinical trials also utilizes one of five distinct classes of effectors: the tubulin-interacting agents comprised of maytansinoids or auristatins or the DNA-damaging agents calicheamicin, duocarmycin, or doxorubicin derivatives (Fig. 6.3). The first four effectors are highly potent against cells in vitro, with IC_{50} values in the sub-nanomolar range: maytansinoids (10–100 pM) [31, 32], auristatins (10–500 pM) [33], *N*-acetyl γ calicheamicin (~1 nM) [34], and duocarmycin (40–100 pM) [35], while doxorubicin is 100–1,000 times less potent.

Microtubule-Binding Agents

Microtubules are tube-shaped polymers of alpha and beta tubulin dimers that are important components of the cytoskeleton, which gives the cell its defined shape and also acts as a scaffold to which organelles are attached and transported within a cell. Microtubules are the main component of mitotic spindles which precisely segregate chromosomes during cell division. To function properly, microtubules must be able to readily grow and contract at their ends, a process referred to as microtubule dynamics. Cytotoxic compounds such as the taxanes bind to tubulin to cause the formation of an altered form of microtubules which are stabilized and cannot contract properly [36]. Other compounds such as vincristine and vinblastine

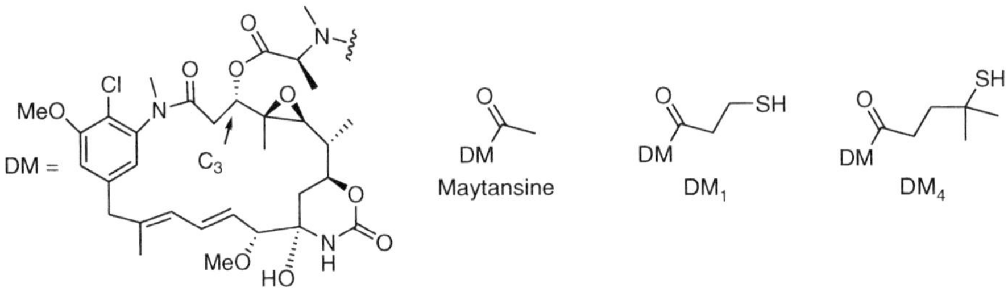

Fig. 6.4 Structures of maytansine, DM1 and DM4 maytansinoids

inhibit the formation of microtubules [37]. These effects of microtubule stabilization or the suppression of microtubule assembly generally have a greater impact on dividing cells than nondividing cells presumably because mitotic spindle function is impaired causing cells to arrest in the G2/M phase and subsequently die. Thus, microtubule-binding agents may be an ideal choice for use in ADCs because their mechanism of action provides an inherent selectivity for killing dividing cells, such as cancer cells. Microtubule-binding agents however have been found to impair the function of peripheral neurons resulting in neuropathy [36, 38].

Maytansinoids

Maytansine is a benzoansamacrolide that was first isolated from the bark of the African shrub *Maytenus ovatus* (Fig. 6.4). Maytansine binds with high affinity to tubulin near the vinca alkaloid binding site. Maytansinoids were found to bind with high affinity to the ends of microtubules and also to bind with lower affinity to sites distributed throughout the microtubules resulting in the suppression of microtubule dynamics [39]. Maytansine was extensively tested in preclinical and clinical settings but failed to demonstrate a therapeutic benefit at tolerable doses. The unusually high cytotoxic activity of the maytansinoids however makes them attractive candidates for antibody-targeted delivery. In addition, maytansine met other key criteria, such as good aqueous stability and reasonable aqueous solubility, for use as a payload for ADCs.

Several maytansinoid ADCs have been developed to utilize a disulfide linkage between the maytansinoid and the antibody in order to exploit the higher glutathione levels in cells vs. blood and the even higher levels of glutathione in many drug-resistant cancer cells. Conjugates having different disulfide bond strengths were desired in order to optimize the activity of the ADC for a given indication. It is known that the strength of a disulfide bond can be increased by incorporating methyl groups on the carbon bearing the sulfur atoms in order to sterically hinder nucleophilic attack (Fig. 6.5). Structure–activity relationship (SAR) studies on

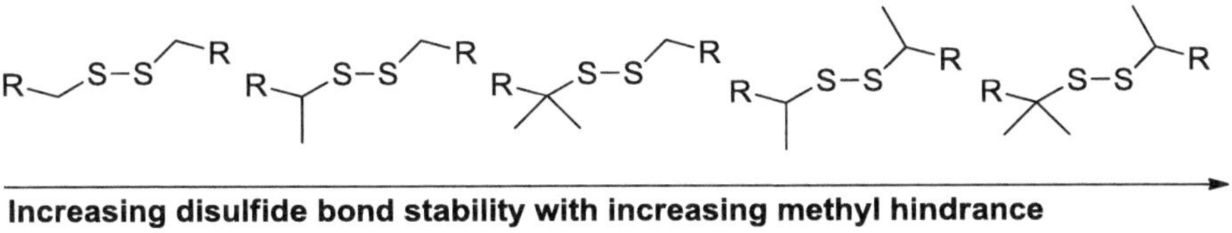

Fig. 6.5 Effect of hindrance on disulfide bond stability

maytansinoids showed that the C3 side chain is required for biological activity but that the structure of this side chain can be varied without a significant loss of activity (Fig. 6.4 [40]).

Incorporation of methyldisulfide substituents into the C3 ester side chain resulted in maytansinoids that retained or exceeded the in vitro potency of the parent compound maytansine. Reduction of the methyldisulfides then provided thiol-containing maytansinoids. Two of these maytansinoid compounds, DM1, bearing a thiol on a primary carbon, and DM4, which has two methyl groups on the carbon atom bearing the thiol, were selected for evaluation in ADCs. These maytansinoids were linked to antibodies via cleavable disulfide bonds or non-cleavable thioether links [41]. ADCs bearing an average of 3–4 maytansinoids linked per antibody are presently in clinical trials.

Linkage of DM1 to the lysine residues of a mAb via a non-cleavable linker such as SMCC gives a non-cleavably linked maytansinoid ADC (mAb–SMCC–DM1) (Fig. 6.6). When such a mAb–SMCC–DM1 conjugate is internalized by a cell, the antibody portion is degraded in a lysosome to release a sole metabolite consisting of DM1 attached via the linker to a lysine residue (Fig. 6.7 [25]). This metabolite then diffuses into the cytoplasm of the cell to induce cell death.

DM1 has also been linked to a mAb via the SPP linker to give an ADC with a cleavable disulfide bond, mAb–SPP–DM1 (Fig. 6.8). Similarly, DM4 has been linked to a mAb via the SPDB linker to give mAb–SPDB–DM4; the disulfide bond of which is approximately seven times more stable to thiol attack in vitro than that of mAb–SPP–DM1 conjugates [42]. The antibody component of disulfide cleavable maytansinoid conjugates is generally cleaved in lysosomes to give a lysine-bearing metabolite with the linker and maytansinoid still attached. This metabolite diffuses into the cytoplasm where the disulfide bond is cleaved, presumably by GSH, to release non-charged, membrane-permeable DM1 or DM4 (Fig. 6.9). The DM4 metabolite can also be *S*-methylated, presumably by enzymes in the cytoplasm of cells, to give the corresponding sulfide *S*-methyl-DM4. DM1 can also be *S*-methylated by cells but to a lower extent. Thus, both mAb–SPP–DM1 and mAb–SPDB–DM4 conjugates produce membrane-permeable metabolites that can diffuse into, and kill, neighboring cells. This bystander killing enhances the potency of these conjugates against solid tumors in vivo [43]. Studies employing ADCs with non-cleavable linkers bearing isotopically labeled maytansinoids have confirmed that the

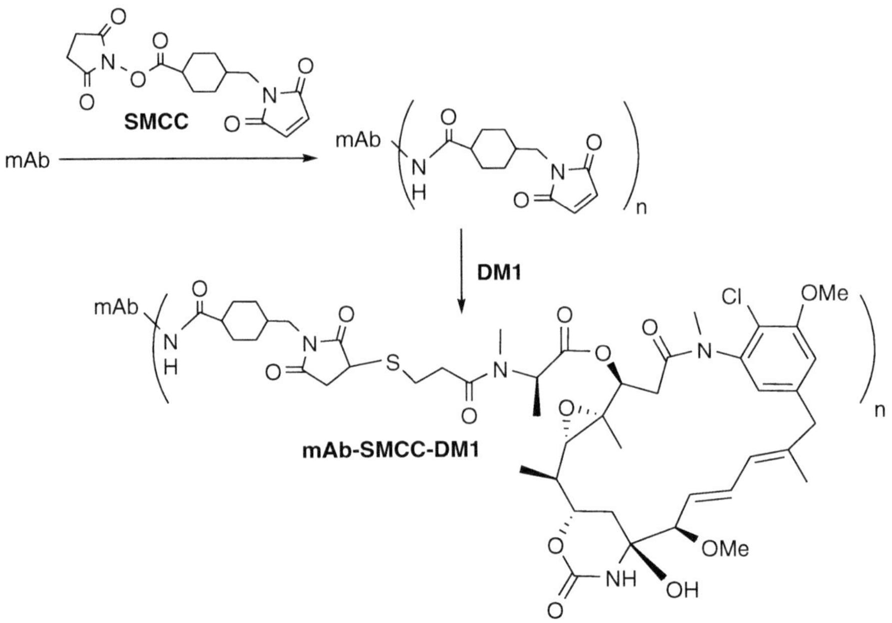

n indicates the average number of effectors linked per antibody (usually 3-5)

Fig. 6.6 Preparation of non-cleavable SMCC-based maytansinoid ADCs. *n* indicates the average number of effectors linked per antibody (usually 3–5)

maytansinoid component is fully stable to endosomal and lysosomal conditions during internalization into targeted cells [25]. Also, as expected, maytansinoid ADCs suppress microtubule dynamics in a similar manner to unconjugated maytansinoids [44]. Clinical results of selected maytansinoid ADCs are described in separate chapters of this book.

Auristatins

Dolastatin 10 is a highly potent antimitotic agent which was isolated from the sea hare *Dolabella auricularia* found in the Indian Ocean and the coastal waters of Japan (Fig. 6.10 [45]). Dolastatin 10 and its derivatives were found to have the following properties: inhibition of tubulin-dependent GTP binding, noncompetitive inhibition of vincristine binding to tubulin, and inhibition of microtubule dynamics. The synthetic auristatin series of antimitotic agents were identified by SAR studies based on dolastatin 10 [46]. The dolaphenine residue of dolastatin 10 could be replaced with phenethylamine or substituted phenethylamine moieties without loss

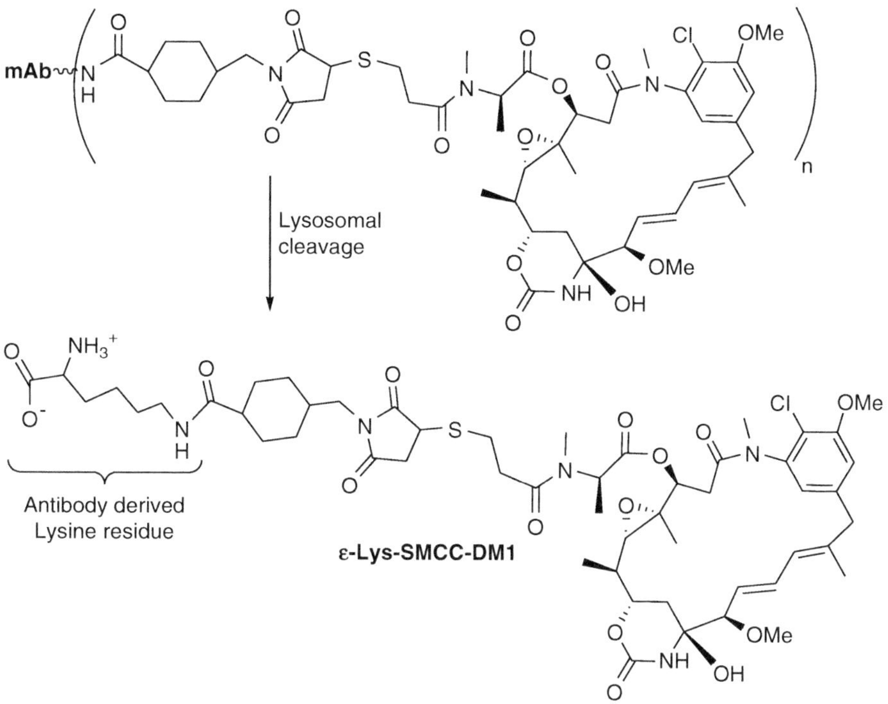

Fig. 6.7 Cellular processing of non-cleavable SMCC-linked maytansinoid ADCs

of potency. It was also found that potency was retained when the terminal tertiary amine moiety of dolastatin was replaced with a primary or secondary amine.

There are two forms of auristatin presently employed in ADCs under clinical evaluation, auristatin E (MMAE) which can diffuse through cell membranes to kill cells and auristatin F (MMAF) which bears a carboxylic acid that impedes diffusion into cells. MMAE is conjugated to antibodies through a peptide-cleavable self-immolating linkage system. The resulting ADCs release MMAE in cells by first cleaving the amide bond between the peptide and the aromatic amine, followed by self-immolation of the para-aminobenzyl moiety and loss of carbon dioxide (Fig. 6.11). MMAF is conjugated to the antibody through a non-cleavable linker. The antibody portion of the resulting ADC is degraded once internalized by cells to release a metabolite containing MMAF linked to a cysteine residue (Fig. 6.12). MMAE conjugates have been shown to induce bystander killing, while MMAF conjugates do not [47]. Studies employing non-cleavable ADCs bearing isotopically labeled auristatin F have shown that the released metabolite is stable in vitro during cellular internalization and exposure to lysosomes [26]. Clinical results of selected ADCs containing auristatins are described in separate chapters of this book.

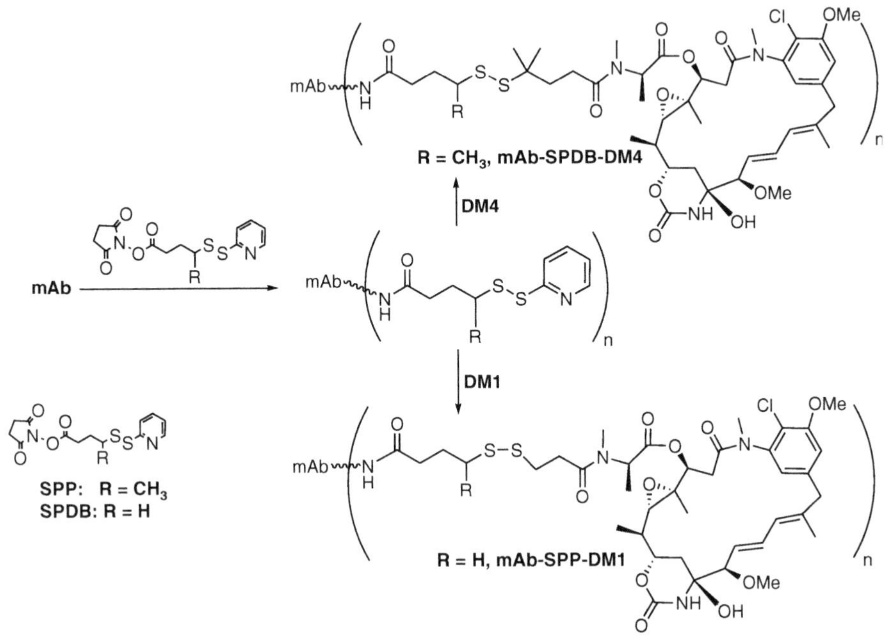

n indicates the average number of effectors linked per antibody (usually 3-5)

Fig. 6.8 Preparation of disulfide cleavable maytansinoid ADCs. *n* indicates the average number of effectors linked per antibody (usually 3–5)

DNA-Targeting Agents

There are cancer indications where low-molecular-weight antimitotic drugs, including tubulin binding agents, are not effective, and in such cases, it is not yet clear if antimitotic agents will be the best choice of effector component for an ADC. Chemotherapeutic agents targeting DNA can cause damage by several mechanisms: base alkylation, induction of single or double-strand cleavage, or the agent can intercalate into the DNA minor grove to alter the DNA's three dimensional structure [48]. In many cases, DNA repair enzymes can fix the damage as long as it is not too extensive. DNA agents are also toxic to noncancerous cells but in many cases have been reported to show a greater selectivity toward killing rapidly dividing cells than slowly dividing cells. Two possible rationales for this selectivity have been proposed: (i) during replication, regions of chromatin decondense to become more accessible to DNA agents [49], and (ii) rapidly dividing cells have little time to repair DNA damage before encountering G2 phase checkpoints that can trigger cell death [50]. Antimitotic agents however appear to be more selectively potent against rapidly dividing cells compared to slowly or nondividing cells than DNA-damaging agents [48].

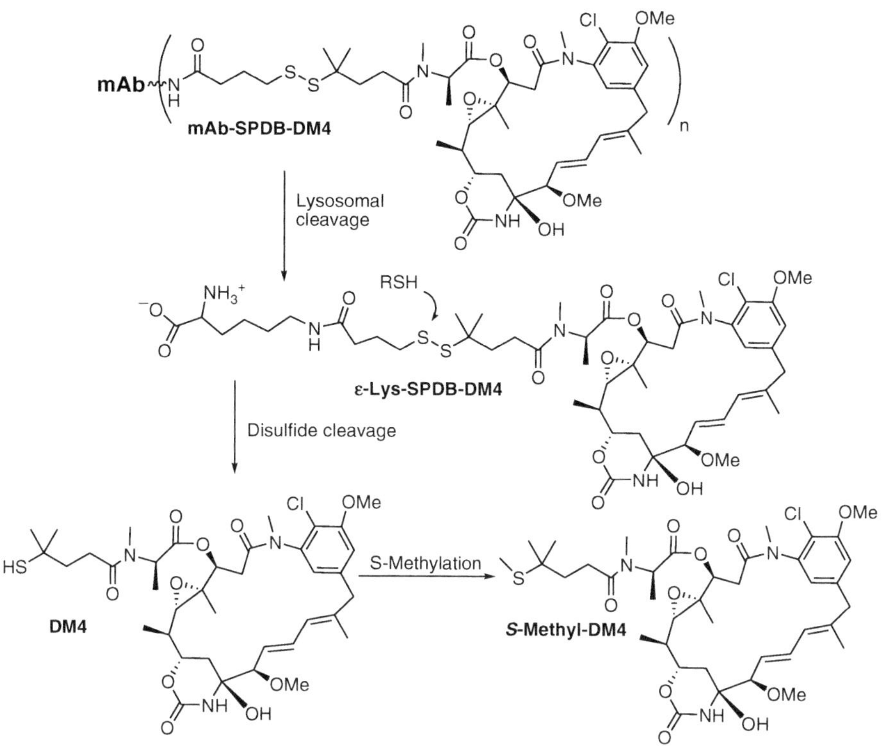

n indicates the average number of effectors linked per antibody (usually 3-5)

Fig. 6.9 Cellular processing of DM4 disulfide cleavable ADCs. *n* indicates the average number of effectors linked per antibody (usually 3–5)

Doxorubicin

Doxorubicin, also known as Adriamycin, is a DNA-intercalating anthracycline antibiotic. It can kill cells in the manner described for DNA-damaging agents, but it also appears to induce toxicity due to binding and interference with the enzyme topoisomerase, which is required for DNA replication [51]. Milatuzumab–doxorubicin is an ADC which targets CD74 antigens for the treatment of multiple myeloma and is currently in phase I clinical trials. In spite of its relatively modest potency, milatuzumab–doxorubicin is being investigated because the targeted cells are reported to have a very high uptake and catabolic processing of bound anti-CD74, up to 8×10^6 anti-CD74 per day; thus, cells treated with this ADC could be exposed to high levels of cytotoxic metabolite [52]. However it may be difficult for milatuzumab–doxorubicin to penetrate into tumor cells which are located in the bone marrow [53].

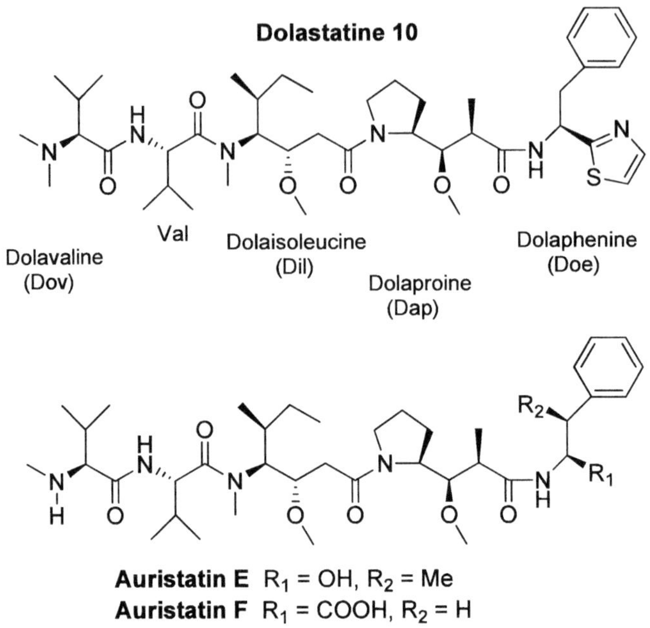

Fig. 6.10 Structures of dolastatin 10, auristatin E, and auristatin F

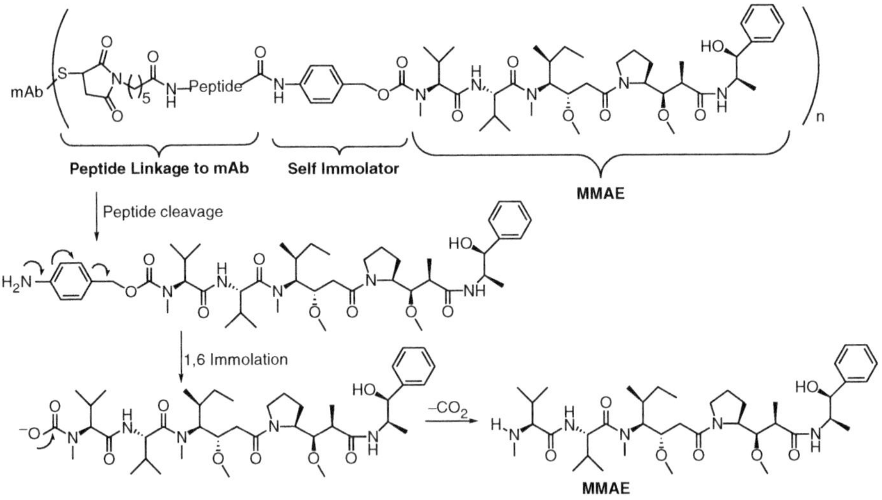

n indicates the average number of effectors linked per antibody (usually 3-5)

Fig. 6.11 Cellular processing of peptide-cleavable auristatin E ADCs. *n* indicates the average number of effectors linked per antibody (usually 3–5)

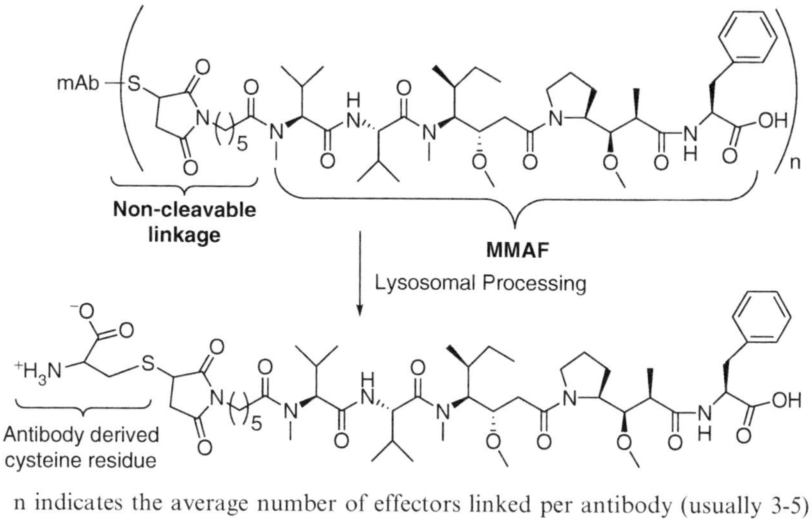

Fig. 6.12 Cellular processing of non-cleavably linked auristatin F ADCs. *n* indicates the average number of effectors linked per antibody (usually 3–5)

Calicheamicin

Calicheamicin γ1 is an enediyne-containing molecule produced by the bacterium *Micromonospora echinospora* and is approximately 4,000-fold more potent than doxorubicin (Fig. 6.3 [54]). Calicheamicin γ1 was likely thought to be too toxic for use in ADCs, and hence, *N*-acetyl-γ-calicheamicin, which is 20-fold less potent, was utilized instead. The natural trisulfide moiety was also replaced with a disulfide to simplify the synthesis of the effector. Once internalized by a target cell, *N*-acetyl-γ-calicheamicin induces DNA damage via a diradical mechanism (Fig. 6.13). First, *N*-acetyl-γ-calicheamicin binds, via its oligosaccharide moiety, to the minor groove of DNA, followed by cleavage of the disulfide moiety, presumably by intracellular glutathione in the cytoplasm, to release a thiol which intramolecularly attacks the bridgehead double bond of the enediyne causing diradical formation. In the presence of oxygen, this diradical can then abstract two hydrogen atoms from the same or separate strands of DNA ultimately resulting in single- or double-strand cleavage.

N-acetyl-γ-calicheamicin is typically linked to antibodies through an acid-labile hydrazone bond, and the resulting ADCs are highly potent. ADCs of *N*-acetyl-γ-calicheamicin that contain a non-cleavable linker instead of the hydrazone linkage have also been shown to be active in vitro on some cell lines [55].

Mylotarg, an acid-labile hydrazone-linked ADC utilizing an anti-CD33 antibody and *N*-acetyl-γ-calicheamicin, was developed by Wyeth but was recently withdrawn from the market because of its poor therapeutic index. The dose-limiting toxicity (DLT) was cited as hepatic sinusoidal obstruction. It has been speculated that the

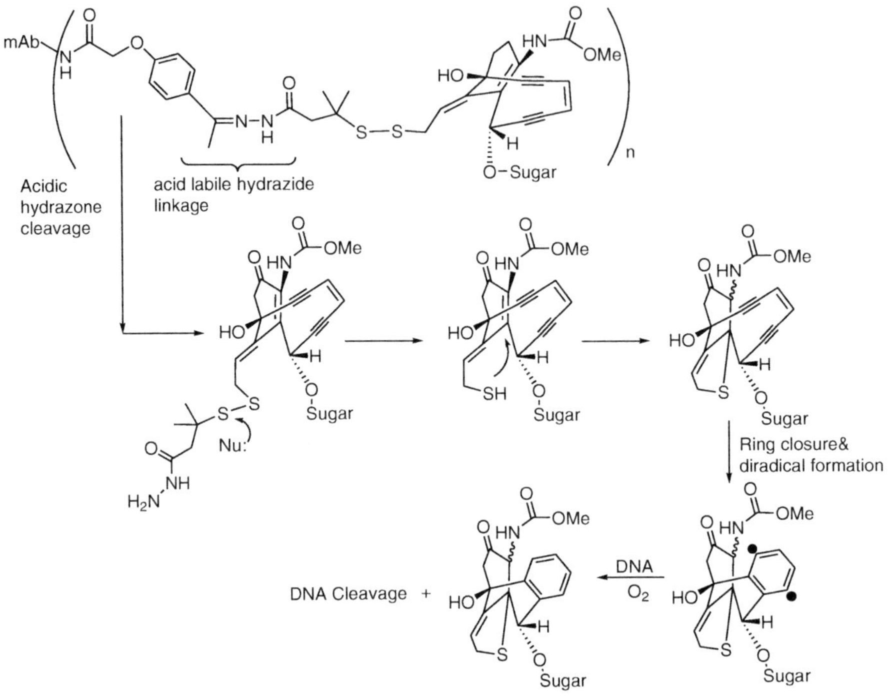

n indicates the average number of effectors linked per antibody (usually 3-5)

Fig. 6.13 Cellular processing of ADCs that utilize *N*-acetyl-γ-calicheamicin. *n* indicates an average number of effectors linked per antibody (usually 3–5)

conjugate undesirably targeted CD33+ cells in the hepatic sinusoids of human liver to induce the dose-limiting toxicity and that ADCs utilizing *N*-acetyl-γ-calicheamicin with other antibodies would not necessarily have this problem [56]. The more recent *N*-acetyl-γ-calicheamicin ADC inotuzumab ozogamicin, which targets CD22+ cells, is presently in phase III and phase II clinical trials for aggressive non-Hodgkin's lymphoma (A-NHL) and indolent non-Hodgkin's lymphoma, respectively (I-NHL). Reversible thrombocytopenia was identified as the main DLT, with few occurrences of liver DLTs [57], although the maximum tolerated dose was quite low (1.8 mg/m^2). An I-NHL study has recently shown a 50% overall response rate with 19% complete responses [58].

Duocarmycin

Duocarmycins are naturally occurring antibacterial agents isolated from *Streptomyces* [59]. They are DNA minor groove alkylators, and synthetic analogs have been prepared in both the "active" cyclopropyl ring-closed form and in the

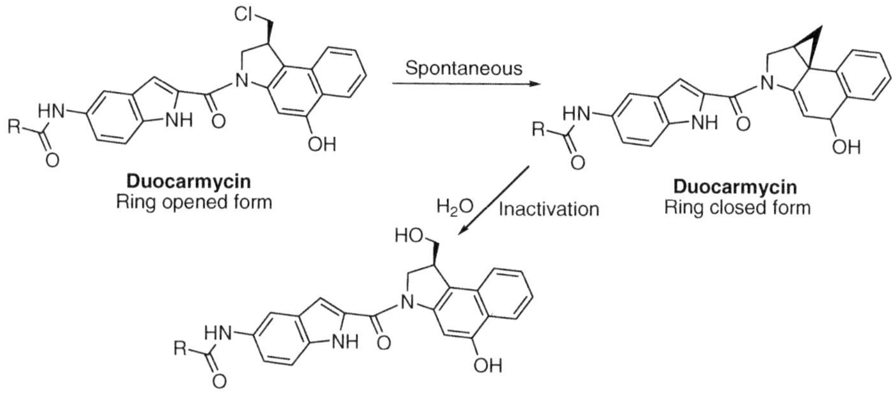

Fig. 6.14 Open and closed structures of duocarmycin and inactivation

ring-opened form (Fig. 6.14 [35]). The ring-opened form can be converted to the ring-closed cyclopropyl form in the presence of mild base, and this ring-closed form reacts with adenine residues on DNA causing alkylation. However, the ring-closed form is prone to inactivation by water or other nucleophiles. For the purpose of preparing an ADC, it was desirable to prevent inactivation of the effector. This was achieved by converting the hydroxyl group of the phenolic moiety in the ring-opened form to a methyl piperazinyl carbamate prodrug prior to conjugation with an antibody. The amine moiety of the carbamate, which is charged in aqueous solution, may also improve the effector's aqueous solubility. The ADC MDX-1203 which utilizes a human anti-CD70 antibody linked to a synthetic duocarmycin derivative is currently undergoing phase I clinical evaluation in patients with clear cell renal cell carcinoma (ccRCC) or B-cell non-Hodgkin's lymphoma (B-NHL). Once internalized by antigen-positive CD-70 cells, the valine–citrulline linkage of MDX-1203 is cleaved in an endosome or lysosome to release the aniline-bearing duocarmycin, followed by cleavage of the phenolic carbamate by carboxyl esterase (Fig. 6.15). Once the phenolic hydroxyl is freed, cyclopropane ring closure occurs to give the active cytotoxic metabolite. The metabolite can then diffuse into the minor groove of DNA where it alkylates preferentially on the N3 adenine of AT-rich regions. Data on the stability of duocarmycin derivatives to lysosomal enzymes has not been reported.

Conclusion

The lessons learned from the failure of the first-generation ADCs have led to improvements in almost every aspect of ADC design. Most of the new-generation ADCs employ humanized antibodies that are not immunogenic and cytotoxic effectors that are highly potent such that the low amount of ADC typically delivered to tumor cells in vivo can induce cell death. Both antimitotic and

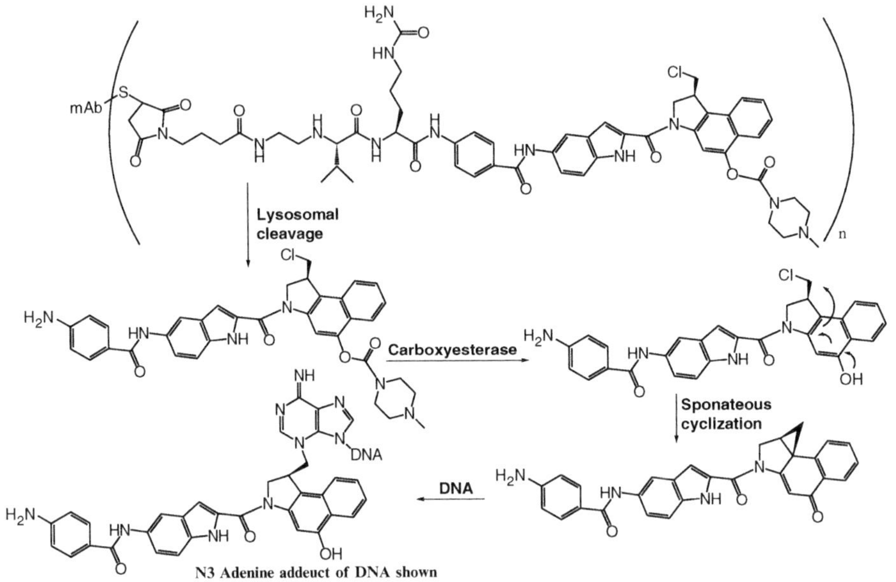

n indicates an average number of effectors linked per antibody (usually 3-5)

Fig. 6.15 Cellular processing of ADCs bearing a duocarmycin prodrug. *n* indicates an average number of effectors linked per antibody (usually 3–5)

DNA-damaging agents have been used as effectors in the preparation of clinically effective ADCs. However, in some cases, attributes of the effector, such as poor aqueous solubility or low stability in circulation, have been problematic. Conversion of the cytotoxic agent into a prodrug form has been shown to solve many of these problems, although such derivatizations can increase complexity. An understanding of the mechanism of cellular activation of ADCs had led to the design of linkers that are stable in circulation, yet release active metabolite inside the cell.

The current generation of ADCs represents a new paradigm in cancer therapy, and the recent clinical successes have rejuvenated interest in this field. New cytotoxic effectors or effector/linker combinations are actively being evaluated, some of which may invoke novel mechanisms of action. However, the properties of high potency, stability in circulation, reasonable aqueous solubility, and efficient metabolite release in targeted cells will likely continue to be highly important in designing effectors for ADCs. There will also be a continued emphasis on widening the therapeutic index, while also addressing other needs, such as ways to treat tumors with low antigen expression and those that are multidrug resistant.

References

1. Zheng B, Fuji RN, Elkins K, Yu SF, Fuh FK, Chuh J et al (2009) In vivo effects of targeting CD79b with antibodies and antibody-drug conjugates. Mol Cancer Ther 8:2937–2946
2. Kraus M, Severin T, Wolf B (1994) Relevance of microenvironmental pH for self-organized tumor growth and invasion. Anticancer Res 14:1573–1583
3. Kraus M, Wolf B (1996) Implications of acidic tumor microenvironment for neoplastic growth and cancer treatment: a computer analysis. Tumour Biol 17:133–154
4. Madri JA (2003) The evolving roles of cell surface proteases in health and disease: implications for developmental, adaptive, inflammatory, and neoplastic processes. Curr Top Dev Biol 54:391–410
5. Saito G, Swanson JA, Lee KD (2003) Drug delivery strategy utilizing conjugation via reversible disulfide linkages: role and site of cellular reducing activities. Adv Drug Deliv Rev 55:199–215
6. Stephan JP, Chan P, Lee C, Nelson C, Elliott JM, Bechtel C et al (2008) Anti-CD22-MCC-DM1 and MC-MMAF conjugates: impact of assay format on pharmacokinetic parameters determination. Bioconjug Chem 19:1673–1683
7. Junutula JR, Flagella KM, Graham RA, Parsons KL, Ha E, Raab H et al (2010) Engineered thio-trastuzumab-DM1 conjugate with an improved therapeutic index to target human epidermal growth factor receptor 2-positive breast cancer. Clin Cancer Res 16:4769–4778
8. Hamblett KJ, Senter PD, Chace DF, Sun MM, Lenox J, Cerveny CG et al (2004) Effects of drug loading on the antitumor activity of a monoclonal antibody drug conjugate. Clin Cancer Res 10:7063–7070
9. Chari Ravi VJ (2008) Targeted cancer therapy: conferring specificity to cytotoxic drugs. Acc Chem Res 41:98–107
10. Le PU, Nabi IR (2003) Distinct caveolae-mediated endocytic pathways target the Golgi apparatus and the endoplasmic reticulum. J Cell Sci 116:1059–1071
11. Katz J, Janik JE, Younes A (2011) Brentuximab Vedotin (SGN-35). Clin Cancer Res 17:6428–6436
12. Sedlacek HH et al (1992) Antibodies as carriers of cytotoxicity in contributions to oncology 43, 1–145, H. Huber, W. Queisser eds, Karger, Basel
13. Uadia P, Blair AH, Ghose T (1984) Tumor and tissue distribution of a methotrexate-anti-EL4 immunoglobulin conjugate in EL4 lymphoma-bearing mice. Cancer Res 44:4263–4266
14. Tabrizi MA, Tseng CM, Roskos LK (2006) Elimination mechanisms of therapeutic monoclonal antibodies. Drug Discov Today 11:81–88
15. Shen H, Kauvar L, Tew KD (1997) Importance of glutathione and associated enzymes in drug response. Oncol Res 9:295–302
16. Ishikawa T, Kuo MT, Furuta K, Suzuki M (2000) The human multidrug resistance-associated protein (MRP) gene family: from biological function to drug molecular design. Clin Chem Lab Med 38:893–897
17. Nooter K, Stoter G (1996) Molecular mechanisms of multidrug resistance in cancer chemotherapy. Pathol Res Pract 192:768–780
18. Kovtun YV, Audette CA, Mayo MF, Jones GE, Doherty H, Maloney EK et al (2010) Antibody-maytansinoid conjugates designed to bypass multidrug resistance. Cancer Res 70:2528–2537
19. Vaupel P, Mayer A (2007) Hypoxia in cancer: significance and impact on clinical outcome. Cancer Metastasis Rev 26:225–239
20. Sullivan R, Paré GC, Frederiksen LJ, Semenza GL, Graham CH (2008) Hypoxia-induced resistance to anticancer drugs is associated with decreased senescence and requires hypoxia-inducible factor-1 activity. Mol Cancer Ther 7:1961–1973
21. Teicher BA (1994) Hypoxia and drug resistance. Cancer Metastasis Rev 13:139–168
22. Caglic D, Kosec G, Bojic L, Reinheckel T, Turk V, Turk B (2009) Murine and human cathepsin B exhibit similar properties: possible implications for drug discovery. Biol Chem 390:175–179

23. Puente XS, Sanchez LM, Overall CM, Lopez-Otin C (2003) Human and mouse proteases: a comparative genomic approach. Nat Rev Genet 4:544–558
24. Bai R, Edler MC, Bonate PL, Copeland TD, Pettit GR, Luduena RF et al (2009) Intracellular activation and deactivation of tasidotin, an analog of dolastatin 15: correlation with cytotoxicity. Mol Pharmacol 75:218–226
25. Erickson HK, Park PU, Widdison WC, Kovtun YV, Garrett LM, Hoffman K et al (2006) Antibody-maytansinoid conjugates are activated in targeted cancer cells by lysosomal degradation and linker-dependent intracellular processing. Cancer Res 66:4426–4433
26. Doronina SO, Mendelsohn BA, Bovee TD, Cerveny CG, Alley SC, Meyer DL et al (2006) Enhanced activity of monomethylauristatin F through monoclonal antibody delivery: effects of linker technology on efficacy and toxicity. Bioconjug Chem 17:114–124
27. Dubowchik GM, Firestone RA, Padilla L, Willner D, Hofstead SJ, Mosure K et al (2002) Cathepsin B-labile dipeptide linkers for lysosomal release of doxorubicin from internalizing immunoconjugates: model studies of enzymatic drug release and antigen-specific in vitro anticancer activity. Bioconjug Chem 13:855–869
28. Zhao RY, Wilhelm SD, Audette C, Jones G, Leece BA, Lazar AC et al (2011) Synthesis and evaluation of hydrophilic linkers for antibody-maytansinoid conjugates. J Med Chem 54:3606–3623
29. Wu G, Fang YZ, Yang S, Lupton JR, Turner ND (2004) Glutathione metabolism and its implications for health. J Nutr 134:489–492
30. Mills BJ, Lang CA (1996) Differential distribution of free and bound glutathione and cyst(e)ine in human blood. Biochem Pharmacol 52:401–406
31. Kupchan SM, Komoda Y, Court WA, Thomas GJ, Smith RM, Karim A et al (1972) Maytansine, a novel antileukemic ansa macrolide from Maytenus ovatus. J Am Chem Soc 94:1354–1356
32. Remillard S, Rebhun LI, Howie GA, Kupchan SM (1975) Antimitotic activity of the potent tumor inhibitor maytansine. Science 189:1002–1005
33. Gerber HP, Kung-Sutherland M, Stone I, Morris-Tilden C, Miyamoto J, McCormick R et al (2009) Potent antitumor activity of the anti-CD19 auristatin antibody drug conjugate hBU12-vcMMAE against rituximab-sensitive and -resistant lymphomas. Blood 113:4352–4361
34. Thorson JS, Sievers EL, Ahlert J, Shepard E, Whitwam RE, Onwueme KC et al (2000) Understanding and exploiting nature's chemical arsenal: the past, present and future of calicheamicin research. Curr Pharm Des 6:1841–1879
35. Boger D (1994) Design, synthesis, and evaluation of DNA minor groove binding agents: the duocarmycins. Pure Appl Chem 66:837–844
36. Gascoigne KE, Taylor SS (2009) How do anti-mitotic drugs kill cancer cells? J Cell Sci 122:2579–2585
37. Jordan MA, Himes RH, Wilson L (1985) Comparison of the effects of vinblastine, vincristine, vindesine, and vinepidine on microtubule dynamics and cell proliferation in vitro. Cancer Res 45:2741–2747
38. Hadfield JA, Ducki S, Hirst N, McGown AT (2003) Tubulin and microtubules as targets for anticancer drugs. Prog Cell Cycle Res 5:309–325
39. Lopus M, Oroudjev E, Wilson L, Wilhelm S, Widdison W, Chari R et al (2010) Maytansine and cellular metabolites of antibody-maytansinoid conjugates strongly suppress microtubule dynamics by binding to microtubules. Mol Cancer Ther 9:2689–2699
40. Cassady JM, Chan KK, Floss HG, Leistner E (2004) Recent developments in the maytansinoid antitumor agents. Chem Pharm Bull (Tokyo) 52:1–26
41. Widdison WC, Wilhelm SD, Cavanagh EE, Whiteman KR, Leece BA, Kovtun Y et al (2006) Semisynthetic maytansine analogues for the targeted treatment of cancer. J Med Chem 49:4392–4408
42. Kellogg BA, Garrett L, Kovtun Y, Lai KC, Leece B, Miller M et al (2011) Disulfide-linked antibody-maytansinoid conjugates: optimization of in vivo activity by varying the steric hindrance at carbon atoms adjacent to the disulfide linkage. Bioconjug Chem 22:717–727
43. Kovtun YV, Audette CA, Ye Y, Xie H, Ruberti MF, Phinney SJ et al (2006) Antibody-drug conjugates designed to eradicate tumors with homogeneous and heterogeneous expression of the target antigen. Cancer Res 66:3214–3221

44. Oroudjev E, Lopus M, Wilson L, Audette C, Provenzano C, Erickson H et al (2010) Maytansinoid-antibody conjugates induce mitotic arrest by suppressing microtubule dynamic instability. Mol Cancer Ther 9:2700–2713
45. Pettit RK, Pettit GR, Hazen KC (1998) Specific activities of dolastatin 10 and peptide derivatives against Cryptococcus neoformans. Antimicrob Agents Chemother 42:2961–2965
46. Pettit GR, Srirangam JK, Barkoczy J, Williams MD, Boyd MR, Hamel E et al (1998) Antineoplastic agents 365. Dolastatin 10 SAR probes. Anticancer Drug Des 13:243–277
47. Okeley NM, Miyamoto JB, Zhang X, Sanderson RJ, Benjamin DR, Sievers EL et al (2010) Intracellular activation of SGN-35, a potent anti-CD30 antibody-drug conjugate. Clin Cancer Res 16:888–897
48. Silverman RB (2004) The organic chemistry of drug design and drug action, 2nd edn. Elsevier Academic Press, Amsterdam/Boston
49. Reich Z, Ghirlando R, Arad T, Weinberger S, Minsky A (1990) Extensive interference of DNA packaging processes affected by chemotherapeutic drugs. J Biol Chem 265:16004–16006
50. Leijen S, Beijnen JH, Schellens JH (2010) Abrogation of the G2 checkpoint by inhibition of Wee-1 kinase results in sensitization of p53-deficient tumor cells to DNA-damaging agents. Curr Clin Pharmacol 5:186–191
51. Burden DA, Osheroff N (1998) Mechanism of action of eukaryotic topoisomerase II and drugs targeted to the enzyme. Biochim Biophys Acta 1400:139–154
52. Sapra P, Stein R, Pickett J, Qu Z, Govindan SV, Cardillo TM et al (2005) Anti-CD74 antibody-doxorubicin conjugate, IMMU-110, in a human multiple myeloma xenograft and in monkeys. Clin Cancer Res 11:5257–5264
53. Mitsiades CS, Mitsiades NS, Munshi NC, Richardson PG, Anderson KC (2006) The role of the bone microenvironment in the pathophysiology and therapeutic management of multiple myeloma: interplay of growth factors, their receptors and stromal interactions. Eur J Cancer 42:1564–1573
54. Lee MD, Dunne TS, Chang CC, Ellestad GA, Siegel MM, Morton GO, McGahren WJ, Borders DB (1987) Calichemicins, a novel family of antitumor antibiotics. 2. Chemistry and structure of calichemicin gamma 1. J Am Chem Soc 109:3466–3468
55. Hamann PR, Hinman LM, Beyer CF, Greenberger LM, Lin C, Lindh D et al (2005) An anti-MUC1 antibody-calicheamicin conjugate for treatment of solid tumors. Choice of linker and overcoming drug resistance. Bioconjug Chem 16:346–353
56. Rajvanshi P, Shulman HM, Sievers EL, McDonald GB (2002) Hepatic sinusoidal obstruction after gemtuzumab ozogamicin (Mylotarg) therapy. Blood 99:2310–2314
57. Advani A, Coiffier B, Czuczman MS, Dreyling M, Foran J, Gine E et al (2010) Safety, pharmacokinetics, and preliminary clinical activity of inotuzumab ozogamicin, a novel immunoconjugate for the treatment of B-cell non-Hodgkin's lymphoma: results of a phase I study. J Clin Oncol 28:2085–2093
58. Fuerst M (2011) NHL: Inotuzumab ozogamicin shows activity both alone & combined with rituximab. Oncol Times 33:52–53
59. Ichimura M, Ogawa T, Katsumata S, Takahashi K, Takahashi I, Nakano H (1991) Duocarmycins, new antitumor antibiotics produced by Streptomyces; producing organisms and improved production. J Antibiot (Tokyo) 44:1045–1053

Chapter 7
Linker Technology and Impact of Linker Design on ADC Properties

Victor S. Goldmacher, Rajeeva Singh, Thomas Chittenden, and Yelena Kovtun

Introduction

The function of a linker in an ADC is to covalently connect its effector moiety, the cytotoxic drug, with its targeting moiety, the antibody. A conjugate, following its binding to the target cell surface antigen and uptake, degrades in the tumor cell with the release of an active cytotoxic moiety, often called a metabolite. Depending on the design of the linker, this metabolite may consist of either the cytotoxic drug in its original form or that agent with some or all of the linker attached. Linkers are intended to provide sufficient stability to keep the ADC intact during formulation, storage, and in circulation following administration to the patient and yet allow for efficient (i.e., with a high enough yield and fast enough) release of an active, cytotoxic moiety in the tumor. In addition, recently some linkers have been designed to overcome multidrug resistance.

Several types of linkers have been developed that take advantage of differences between the extracellular and intracellular environments, so that the release of the active cytotoxic moiety would happen only following the antigen-mediated internalization of the ADC into a tumor cell. (1) Disulfide-containing linkers are used in ADCs to exploit the abundance of intracellular thiols, which can facilitate the cleavage of their disulfide bonds. The intracellular concentrations of the most plentiful intracellular thiol, reduced glutathione, are typically in the range of 1–10 mM [1], which is about 1,000-fold higher than that of the most abundant low-molecular thiol in the blood, cysteine, at about 5 μM [2]. The thiol group in serum albumin, which has a relatively high concentration in the blood of ~0.6 mM [3], is buried and relatively inaccessible to thiol–disulfide interchange [4]. The intracellular enzymes of the protein disulfide isomerase family [5] may also contribute to the intracellular cleavage

V.S. Goldmacher (✉) • R. Singh • T. Chittenden • Y. Kovtun
ImmunoGen, Inc., 830 Winter Street, Waltham, MA 02451, USA
e-mail: victor.goldmacher@immunogen.com

G.L. Phillips (ed.), *Antibody-Drug Conjugates and Immunotoxins: From Pre-Clinical Development to Therapeutic Applications*, Cancer Drug Discovery and Development,
DOI 10.1007/978-1-4614-5456-4_7,

of the disulfide linkers. (2) Hydrazone linkers, which undergo acid-catalyzed hydrolysis, are used with a goal of remaining intact in the near-neutral pH environments in circulation and other extracellular compartments and be cleaved in the acidic environments of the late endosomes and lysosomes [6]. (3) Peptide-based linkers are designed to be cleaved via peptide bond hydrolysis catalyzed by lysosomal and, possibly, by endosomal or cytoplasmic proteases [7]. Conjugates with non-cleavable linkers may also be considered belonging to this category, since the antibody moiety of the ADC undergoes proteolysis inside the cell, presumably in lysosomes, releasing the cytotoxic moiety attached to the linker and the single remaining amino acid derived from the antibody [8].

In the conjugates now in clinical development, two main approaches have been used to attach the linkers to the antibody: (1) conjugation with thiol groups of cysteine residues in the antibody that are generated by reduction of interchain disulfide bonds and (2) conjugation with amino groups of surface lysine residues. These approaches will be covered below. In addition, new approaches to engineer-specific sites of modification, such as introduced cysteine residues, are also being evaluated [9].

In this chapter, we will review various ADC linkers that have been reported and the effects of these linkers on the properties of the resulting ADCs. A separate chapter in this volume discusses the intracellular metabolism of ADCs with alternative linkers.

Linker Structures and Preparations of Antibody–Drug Conjugates

This section describes the structures of linkers and conjugates that have been reported for the various ADCs in clinical and advanced preclinical programs. To prepare ADCs, reactive functional groups are incorporated in the cytotoxic moiety and the antibody molecule for facile conjugation with a linker in aqueous conditions compatible with antibody. Other design requirements for ADCs include a relatively water-soluble cytotoxic moiety and use of heterofunctional reactive groups in the cytotoxic moiety and the antibody to minimize the formation of cytotoxin–cytotoxin and antibody–antibody conjugates. Several types of linkers have been used to make ADCs, including non-cleavable linkers, and cleavable linkages, such as disulfide, cleavable peptide, and hydrazone.

Non-cleavable Linkers

Thioether is the linkage that is most commonly used in non-cleavable linkers. It is prepared by the conjugation of a thiol group on the cytotoxic compound or the antibody with the maleimide or haloacetamide group on antibody or cytotoxic moiety,

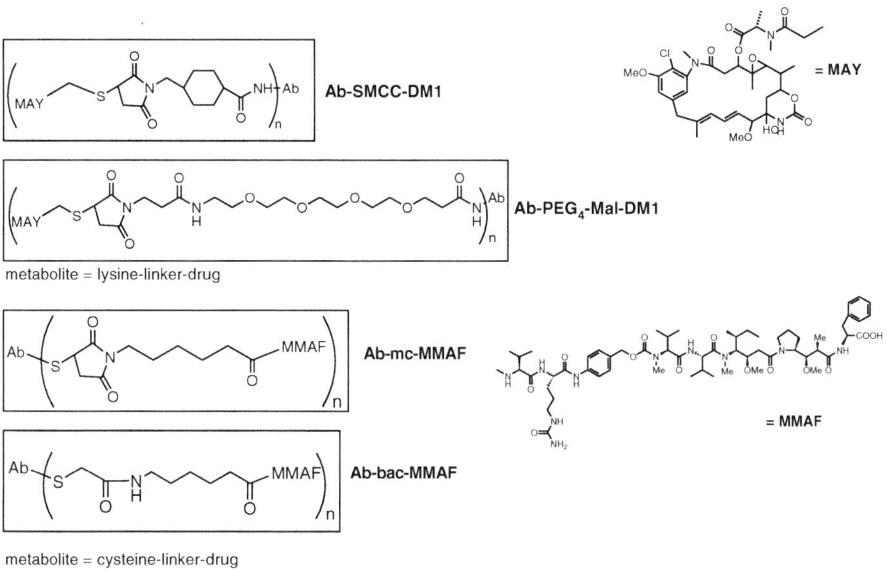

Fig. 7.1 Non-cleavable linkers

respectively. Figure 7.1 shows the structures of representative thioether non-cleavable linkers, which include the SMCC–DM1 linkage (also known as MCC–DM1) formed by reaction of *N*-succinimido 4-(*N*-maleimidomethyl)cyclohexane-1-carboxylate (SMCC) with DM1 employed in the trastuzumab emtansine (T-DM1) conjugate [10] and the mc–MMAF linkage, maleimidocaproyl–monomethyl auristatin F, employed in the anti-CD70–mc–MMAF conjugate [11]. Both types of ADCs are currently in clinical trials.

The trastuzumab–SMCC–DM1 conjugate is prepared by the modification of lysine amino groups on the antibody with the *N*-hydroxysuccinimide ester reactive moiety on the heterobifunctional linker SMCC. This linker also bears a maleimide reactive group, which is conjugated with the thiol-containing maytansinoid, DM1. The trastuzumab–SMCC–DM1 conjugate bears approximately 3.5 maytansinoid molecules per antibody molecule. In target cells, the intracellular cytotoxic metabolite of antibody–SMCC–DM1 is lysine–SMCC–DM1 [12]. An analogous linker where the hydrophobic cyclohexane moiety of SMCC was replaced by a hydrophilic tetraethylene glycol (PEG_4) group which results in a hydrophilic link between the antibody and the payload (Fig. 7.1) enhances the potency of the conjugate against pgp-expressing multidrug-resistant cancer cells [13]. The intracellular metabolite derived from the PEG_4 thioether-linked conjugate is lysine–PEG_4–DM1, which is more hydrophilic than the lysine–SMCC–DM1 metabolite. Another conjugation format has been reported where a cysteine-engineered antibody (termed Thiomab) bearing two nonnative cysteine groups introduced into specific locations on the heavy chain is conjugated with the thiol of DM1 using a PEG_4-containing bis-maleimide (1,11-bis-maleimidotetraethyleneglycol) [9].

The maleimidocaproyl–monomethyl auristatin F (mc–MMAF) conjugate contains a thioether linkage derived from conjugation with cysteine residues generated by reduction of native, interchain disulfide bonds in the antibody [14]. Conjugates bearing an average of 4 and 8 MMAF molecules per antibody molecule have been prepared [14], and the anti-CD70–mc–MMAF conjugate in clinical development has an average of about four MMAF molecules per antibody molecule [11]. In lysosomes of target cells, the cysteine-linked mc–MMAF conjugate is processed to the cysteine-linker-MMAF metabolite [14].

Cleavable Disulfide Linkers

A number of antibody–maytansinoid conjugates with sterically hindered disulfide linkers are undergoing clinical evaluation for an array of cancers. The disulfide linker designs shown in Fig. 7.2 incorporate increasing steric hindrance of methyl groups on carbon atoms adjacent to either side of the disulfide linkage. For a simple abbreviation, the hindered disulfide conjugates are denoted by the number of methyl groups on the antibody side and the cytotoxic agent side, respectively, for example, the SPP–DM1 conjugate with monomethyl hindrance on the antibody side and no hindrance on the cytotoxic agent side is abbreviated as 1:0, and the SPDB–DM4 conjugate with no hindrance on antibody side and double methyl hindrance on cytotoxic agent side is abbreviated as 0:2. The rate of cleavage via thiol/disulfide exchange of the different hindered disulfide linkages was first analyzed in vitro using dithiothreitol. The results showed that the 2:2 hindered conjugate was reduced at a rate more than 22,000-fold slower than the unhindered 0:0 conjugate (Fig. 7.2b). The disulfide cleavage rate of the 0:2 hindered SPDB–DM4 conjugate (or the 2:0 hindered conjugate) was about 20-fold slower than that of the 0:0 conjugate, whereas the 1:2 hindered conjugate was reduced at a rate about 1,000-fold slower than that of the 0:0 conjugate. The relative rates of reduction of the hindered disulfide conjugates observed with dithiothreitol in vitro were similar to their relative plasma stabilities in mice [15].

The cytotoxicity in vitro of conjugates made with these diverse disulfide linkers was similar in antigen-expressing cells and comparable to the cytotoxicity of the non-cleavable SMCC–DM1 conjugate, presumably due to their efficient lysosomal processing. A large difference, however, was observed among the in vivo activities of the hindered disulfide-linked conjugates in tumor xenograft studies. In an in vivo study using anti-CanAg maytansinoid conjugates in COLO 205 xenografts (which express CanAg homogenously on all cells) and HT29 xenografts (which express CanAg heterogeneously, only on a fraction of cells), the 0:2 SPDB–DM4 conjugate was the most active. Its activity was greater than that of the 0:1 conjugate, which in turn was greater than that of the 1:0 or 2:0 conjugate. The even more hindered 1:1 and 1:2 conjugates were, however, less active than the 1:0 and 0:2 conjugates. The greater in vivo activities of the less hindered conjugates could be explained by their bystander cytotoxic activities [15, 16], stemming from the abilities of their metabolites

a

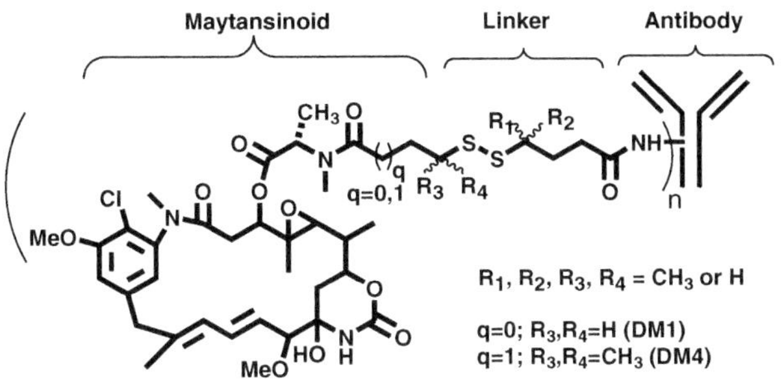

b

Sterichindrance in linker (Ab side; drug side)	Abbreviation of linker (number of CH_3 substituents)	Relative stability to disulfide bond cleavage[1]
R_1,R_2=H; R_3,R_4=H	0:0	1
R_1=CH_3, R_2=H; R_3,R_4=H	1:0 (SPP-DM1)	7
R_1,R_2=H; R_3=CH_3, R_4=H	0:2 (SPDB-DM4)	22
R_1=CH_3, R_2=H; R_3=CH_3, R_4=H	1:1	170
R_1=CH_3, R_2=H; R_3,R_4=CH_3	1:2	980
R_1,R_2=CH_3; R_3,R_4=CH_3	2:2	>22000

[1]Rates of reduction of disulfide-linked conjugates by dithiothreitol were measured at 37°C, pH 6.5. Relative disulfide stability normalized to the unhindered (0:0) conjugate.

Fig. 7.2 Cleavable disulfide linkers. (**a**) Hindered disulfide linkers, (**b**) rates of disulfide-bond cleavage in conjugates with sterically hindered disulfide linkers

DM4 and DM3 and their *S*-methylated forms to diffuse from target cancer cells in which the conjugates were processed into neighboring tumor cells, irrespective of whether the latter express the target antigen or not, thus enhancing the antitumor activity of the conjugate [16, 17]. In an in vivo study targeting anti-α_v integrin in HT29 and A549 xenograft models, the activity trend observed was 0:2 > 1:0 > 1:2 [18], similar to that observed in the anti-CanAg antibody/COLO 205 test system. Both the anti-CanAg conjugate made with the non-cleavable SMCC–DM1 linker and the anti-α_v integrin conjugate made with the highly hindered 1:2 disulfide linker were not active, consistent with the predicted lack of the bystander activities of conjugates made with slowly cleavable or uncleavable linkers [15].

Cleavable Peptide Linkers

Figure 7.3 shows the structures of valine–citrulline (often denoted as val–cit or vc) dipeptide-containing protease-cleavable linkers employed in clinical-stage ADCs with both microtubule-targeting (MMAE) and DNA-targeting (a duocarmycin analog)

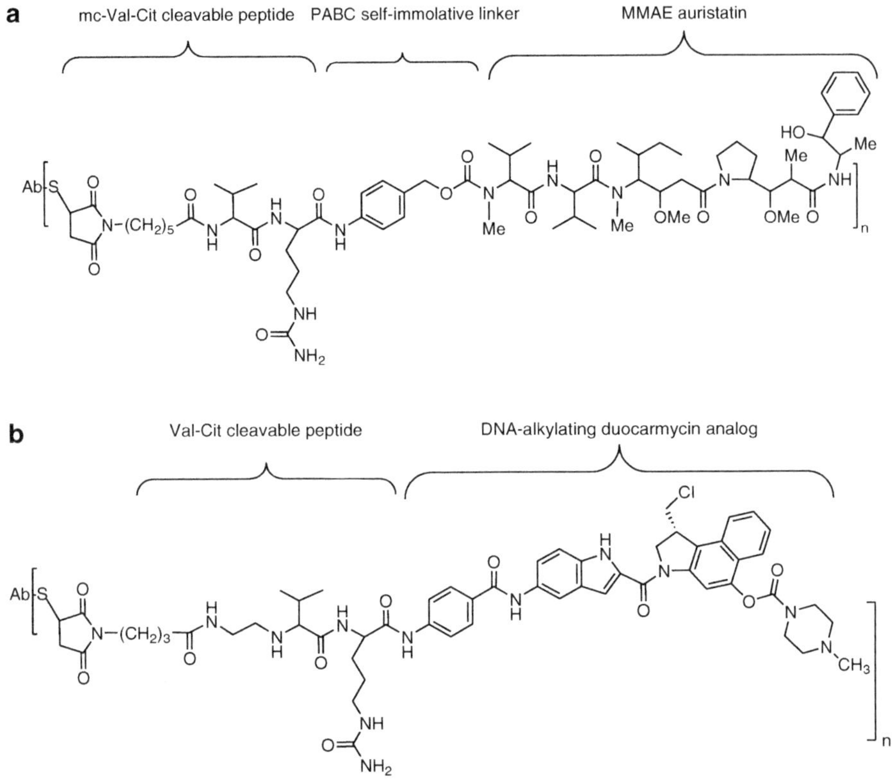

Fig. 7.3 Cleavable peptide linkers. (**a**) Val–Cit–PABC–MMAE, (**b**) Val–Cit–DNA–alkylating agent

effector molecules. The vc–MMAE linker contains a valine–citrulline dipeptide and a self-immolative *p*-aminobenzyloxycarbonyl linkage (PABC). Upon endosomal trafficking of the ADC via the lysosomal route, cleavage of the val–cit peptide by lysosomal proteases releases PABC–MMAE that undergoes self-immolation at the PABC site, further releasing the cytotoxic MMAE molecule that has potential bystander effect on neighboring tumor cells [19, 20]. The anti-CD30–vc–MMAE conjugate currently in clinical testing has an average of about 4 linked MMAE molecules per antibody molecule, derived from the reduction of native interchain disulfide bonds to cysteine and its conjugation with maleimide-containing mc–MMAE [20]. Cysteine-engineered antibodies (Thiomabs) have been conjugated with mc–MMAE to generate ADCs with two MMAE molecules per antibody molecule [21]. The duocarmycin analog is an esterase-cleavable prodrug that is attached via a val–cit linker to the antibody. Following esterase-catalyzed cleavage, the prodrug converts into a DNA alkylator (Fig. 7.3b).

Acid-Cleavable Hydrazone Linkers

The hydrazone linkage is designed to be hydrolyzed in the acidic environment of the endosomes. Two types of hydrazone-linked DNA-targeting cytotoxic effector conjugates currently (or formerly) in the clinic are shown in Fig. 7.4. The highly potent DNA-alkylating *N*-acetyl-γ_1^{I}-calicheamicin is linked via an acid-cleavable hydrazone linkage to antibodies targeting CD33, MUC1, and CD22, of which the CD22 conjugate is currently in clinical trials [22]. Antibody–calicheamicin conjugates were prepared using the *N*-hydroxysuccinimide ester of *N*-acetyl-γ-calicheamicin dimethyl hydrazide 4-(4′-acetylphenoxy)butanoic acid, which reacts with lysine residues on the antibody with an average incorporation of 5–7 calicheamicin molecules per antibody molecule. The acid-hydrolyzable 4-(4′-acetylphenoxy)butanoic acid hydrazone linker contains a disulfide linkage, which needs to be metabolically

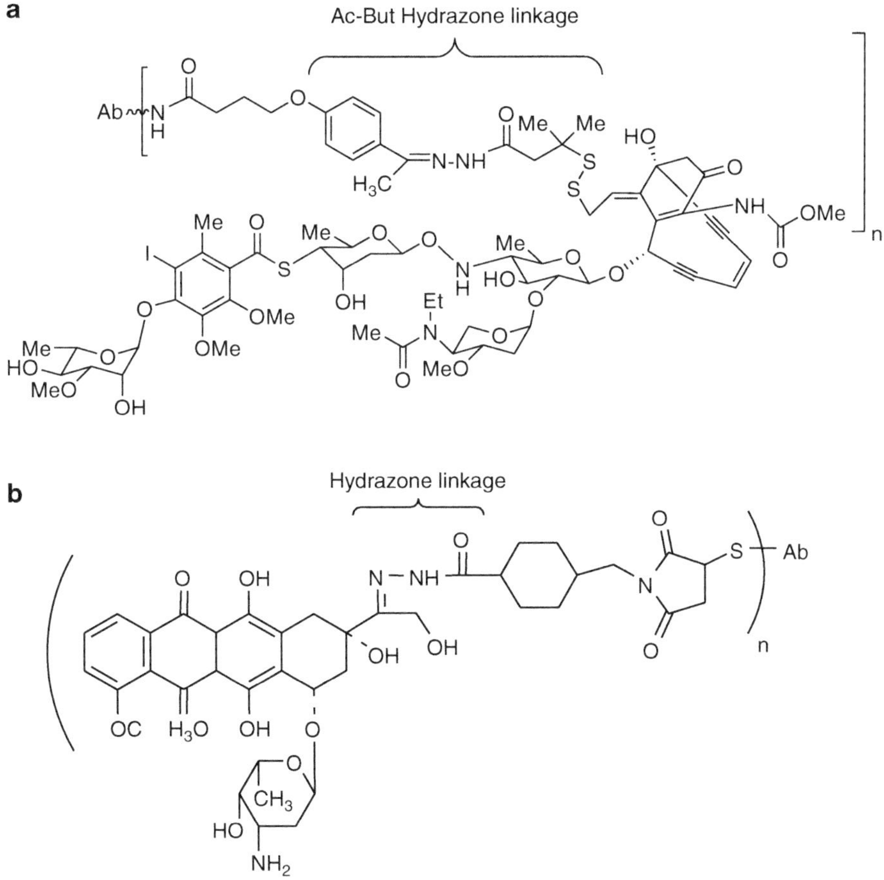

Fig. 7.4 Cleavable hydrazone linkers. (**a**) Calicheamicin conjugate with hydrazone linkage, (**b**) doxorubicin conjugate with hydrazone linkage

cleaved to release the thiol form of calicheamicin. The latter undergoes a Bergman cyclization reaction generating a *p*-benzyne biradical that causes sequence-specific double-stranded DNA cleavage in target cancer cells. Another hydrazone-linked ADC in clinical testing consists of the cytotoxic agent doxorubicin conjugated to an anti-CD74 antibody [23]. The doxorubicin containing 4-(*N*-maleimidomethyl) cyclohexane-1-carboxyhydrazide is conjugated to cysteine residues in the antibody generated by interchain disulfide reduction, with an average incorporation of 6–8 doxorubicin molecules per antibody molecule.

Stability of ADCs with Various Linkers in Circulation and Tissues

The pharmacokinetics of immunoconjugates from the bloodstream is controlled by two concurrent phenomena, clearance of the intact immunoconjugate from circulation and release (cleavage) of the cytotoxic effector moiety from the antibody in the circulation and during the diffusion of the conjugate through tissues from the bloodstream to the tumor cells. The former process has been reviewed previously [24] and is also covered in a separate chapter of this volume. Here, we will focus on the effects of the linker on the rate of decrease of the cytotoxic drug per antibody ratio (DAR) while the immunoconjugate is in circulation or on its way from circulation to the tumor site.

Linkers are designed to hold the conjugate together in circulation for a reasonably long period of time (days) and stable enough not to cleave upon conjugate exposure to tissues on its way from circulation to the tumor while allowing rapid release of the cytotoxic linker in its active form following uptake of the conjugate by the target cell. The accomplishment of these objectives is complicated by several factors: (1) a variety of proteases are present in extracellular matrix, interstitial fluids, on extracellular surface of plasma membranes, and in the blood (although the latter are mostly present as proenzymes) [13, 17, 25, 26]; some of these enzymes may, in principle, degrade the antibody moiety or cleave the linker if it contains a peptide bond; (2) the thiol groups of cysteine and serum albumin which are present in the bloodstream (see above), and of cell surface protein disulfide isomerase [5], may contribute to the cleavage of disulfide-containing linkers; (3) acid-sensitive linkers that cleave at a sufficient rate at pH 5–6 in endosomal or lysosomal compartments in cancer cells will also hydrolyze at neutral pH, for example, just tenfold slower at pH 7 than pH 6; and (4) while in the bloodstream, antibodies continuously recirculate in and out of endothelial cells [8], and as discussed above, while in the endosome, conjugates are exposed to low pH which may enhance hydrolysis of acid-labile linkers, glutathione which may cleave the disulfide bond of the linker, and, possibly, to proteases which may cleave peptide bonds of the linker or degrade the antibody. The relative importance of each of these mechanisms is at present unclear.

A variety of linkers have been designed to keep the conjugate intact in the circulation while affording the release of the cytotoxic effector moiety inside the target cell. These linkers have been described above in more detail: the acid-labile hydrazone functionality [2, 27, 28], lysosomal-protease-cleavable dipeptide-containing linkers [5, 29], thiol-labile hindered (to a varying degree) disulfide, and non-cleavable thioethers. Among antibody–maytansinoid conjugates connected by disulfide-containing linkers, a strong correlation was found between the degree of their steric hindrance, resistance to thiol-mediated cleavage in vitro, and the relative role of cleavage in circulation in mice [15]. The two disulfide linker-maytansinoid combinations used in conjugates in clinical development, SPP–DM1 and SPDB–DM4, were found to release maytansinoids from the ADC slowly in circulation in mice, with the half-degradation periods[1] of 2.4 and 6.9 days, respectively [15]. The trastuzumab–SMCC–DM1 conjugate linked via the non-cleavable thioether was found to be stable in circulation in preclinical studies in mice with the half-life being longer than 7 days [10] and similarly stable in patients [30]. The plasma stability of a thioether-linked MMAF conjugate, bromoacetamidocaproyl–MMAF (bc–MMAF), was found to be better than that of the maleimidocaproyl–MMAF (mc–MMAF) in circulation in mice [31, 32], despite the fact that both conjugates have nominally non-cleavable linkers (Fig. 7.1). It appears that the reaction between cysteine thiol of antibody and maleimido group of mc–MMAF can be slowly reversed in circulation [31]. An auristatin dipeptide-linked immunoconjugate (valine–citrulline–MMAE) was reported to be stable with a linker half-life of 6 days and 9.6 days in circulation of mice and cynomolgus monkeys, respectively [33].

There is another phenomenon, in addition to the linker cleavage, that may contribute to the apparent decrease in the DAR value of an ADC in circulation. ADCs typically consist of mixtures of species with different DAR values [34], and, in principle, conjugates with different DAR values may have different circulation lifetimes. Indeed, it was found that the clearance rate of an antibody–auristatin conjugate depended on its DAR. An anti-CD30–vc–MMAE conjugate preparation was separated using hydrophobic interaction chromatography into fractions containing conjugates with approximately two, four, and eight cytotoxic drugs per antibody (E2, E4, and E8, respectively), and the blood clearance rates of these conjugates and of the nonconjugated antibody were investigated in mice. E2 and E4 fractions cleared with rates only modestly faster than that of the nonconjugated antibody, but E8 cleared dramatically faster [35]. In contrast, anti-CD70–mc–MMAF conjugates bearing 4 and 8 MMAF molecules per antibody were reported to have similar clearance rates, with terminal half-lives of 12.8 and 14.1 days in mice, respectively [11]. One caveat here is that interpretation of the terminal half-life of an ADC may, sometimes, reflect the behavior of only a small fraction of initially injected material, not representative of the bulk conjugate. From an unusually low C_{max} reported in Table

[1] Half-degradation period is defined as the period of the twofold decrease of the average DAR value.

S1 [11] for the dose injected (in our experience with maytansinoid ADCs, approximately threefold lower than a typical C_{max}), this may well be the case. Then, since according to [35], the conjugate with high DAR would clear faster than that with low DAR, the remaining material might consist mostly of the latter, irrespective of what the initial DAR was.

Effect of Linker Design on the Extent of the Cytotoxicity of ADCs Toward Bystander Cells

In addition to killing antigen-positive cells, some ADCs also kill other cells in their vicinity, irrespective of whether these neighboring cells express the antigen or not, a phenomenon that was termed "bystander cytotoxicity" or "bystander effect" [16]. For example, antibody–maytansinoid conjugates linked via a reducible disulfide-bond-containing linker have the bystander effect, whereas similar conjugates linked via a non-reducible thioether link exhibited no bystander killing [15, 16, 36]. We found that the ability of a given conjugate to induce bystander killing depends on the nature of the maytansinoid derivative(s) into which it is converted inside the target cell. Lysosomal proteases proteolytically degrade the antibody and release maytansinoid attached to the linker which is attached to lysine [12]. The newly formed maytansinoid-linker-lysine derivatives diffuse into cytoplasm where they target microtubules, leading to mitotic arrest and cell death [37]. The maytansinoid-thioether linker-lysine is the terminal metabolite of thioether-linked conjugates, whereas maytansinoid-disulfide linker-lysine is further metabolized to the maytansinoid thiol, which either remains free or is *S*-methylated [12]. The cytotoxicity of these maytansinoid metabolites, prepared as synthetic compounds, was tested in vitro. The maytansinoid-linker-lysine derivatives were found to be only modestly cytotoxic, presumably due to their hydrophilicity, which likely inhibited their diffusion across the plasma membrane into the cell, while lipophilic maytansinoid thiols and *S*-methyl maytansinoid compounds were highly cytotoxic, implicating the latter in the bystander killing [12, 17].

We found that the degree of the bystander cytotoxicity of a given antibody–maytansinoid conjugate depended on the steric hindrance of maytansinoid thiol derivatives. The in vitro bystander activity of conjugates of the hindered maytansinoids DM3 or DM4 was found to be superior compared to those of the conjugates of unhindered DM1 [15]. This can be explained by the higher reactivity of the DM1 thiol compared to the DM3 thiol or the DM4 thiol in disulfide interchange with cystine, with the likely enhanced formation of a hydrophilic, poorly cytotoxic mixed disulfide (cysteine-DM1). In addition, the thiols of DM3 and DM4 are readily *S*-methylated inside the cell, forming stable, lipophilic, and highly cytotoxic

S-methyl maytansinoid compounds [17]. The thiol of DM1 appears to be a poor substrate for such *S*-methyl transferase activity in cancer cells [17].

There is some evidence that these phenomena are not limited to ADCs made with maytansinoids and that lipophilicity of metabolites of other cytotoxic agents released from their respective ADCs may also affect the degree of the bystander activity of these ADCs. A conjugate of an anti-CD30 antibody with auristatin MMAE linked via protease-cleavable linker containing valine–citrulline dipeptide is metabolized to a lipophilic auristatin derivative [19] and induces potent bystander killing [20]. A conjugate of the same antibody with auristatin MMAF linked via a non-cleavable linker is metabolized to a hydrophilic auristatin derivative, which has only modest cytotoxicity [14], and therefore is presumably incapable of the bystander killing. A disulfide-linked conjugate of the CC1065 analog DC1 induced a prominent bystander effect, while a similar "non-cleavable" conjugate of DC1 did not kill bystander cells [16], most likely because the former was metabolized to a lipophilic compound, while the latter to its hydrophilic lysine derivative.

The bystander cytotoxicity can enhance the potency of ADCs against solid tumors. Many tumors express the target cell surface antigen in a heterogeneous fashion and consist of a mixture of antigen-positive and antigen-negative cancer cells [38, 39]. Our experiments with heterogeneous xenograft tumors in mice suggest that ADCs that induce the bystander effect may be more effective in eradicating such tumors [16] than ADCs that lack this activity. ADCs that induce bystander effect may also be more potent in eradicating solid tumors that express the target antigen homogenously. Poor and nonuniform penetration of antibodies into tumors has been reported [40–42], and some cells within the tumor might be relatively inaccessible to ADCs due to the barriers to macromolecule delivery and their slow diffusion. The small cytotoxic molecules released from ADCs inside such tumors may be able to penetrate the solid tumors deeper than the antibodies, killing additional cells. In addition, the bystander activity may effect local damage to the tissues involved in supporting tumor growth, such as endothelial cells and pericytes of the tumor neovasculature, or tumor stromal cells.

The bystander effect may add a degree of nonselective killing activity to the target-cell-restricted cytotoxicity of ADCs. Potentially, this could be a drawback if normal cells in tissues surrounding the tumor are affected. This potential collateral toxicity might, however, be well tolerated if it is limited only to a small number of cells in the immediate proximity of the tumor tissues. Indeed, if active cytotoxic metabolites are released from an accessible cancer cell, the concentration of the released cytotoxin will decrease with distance from the cancer cell (assuming no barriers to free diffusion of the small molecule compounds), and because of this concentration gradient, only the proximal bystander cells are likely to be exposed to the concentration of the cytotoxic agent sufficient for cell killing. Also, the potential toxicities contributed by the bystander effect to normal tissues might be mitigated by the inherent insensitivity of nondividing cells to some cytotoxic compounds, including DNA- and microtubule-targeting agents, in particular, maytansine [43, 44].

Effect of Linker Design on Activity of ADCs Against Multidrug-Resistant Cells

Multidrug resistance (MDR) of cancers is one of the main reasons for clinical failures of chemotherapies. Overexpression of ATP-dependent drug transporters MDR1, MRP1, and BCRP is the best studied and the most commonly observed mechanisms of cancer-related MDR [45]. A majority, if not all cytotoxic drugs that are currently used in ADCs, are substrates of at least one of these three transporters. For example, all three transporters effectively mediate efflux of anthracyclines, such as doxorubicin [45], and accordingly, immunoconjugates of doxorubicin are ineffective in killing MDR cell lines [46]. MDR1 [47], and to a lesser degree MRP1 [48], mediates efflux of the enediyne antibiotic calicheamicin used in gemtuzumab ozogamicin. MDR1 mediates efflux of taxanes [45], dolastatin 10 [49], and CC-1065 [50, 51]. Recently, it was reported that MDR1 mediates resistance of cancer cells to maytansinoids and antibody–maytansinoid conjugates, while MRP1 and BCRP do not [13, 52].

Since MDR1 favors hydrophobic substrates [53], we developed linkers that contained either a polar or a negatively charged group and used these linkers in antibody–maytansinoid conjugates with the hope that the conjugates would escape MDR1-mediated efflux and would be able to kill MDR1-expressing cells. A polar ethylene glycol tetramer (PEG_4) was incorporated into a thioether-containing non-cleavable linker. The observed ADC metabolite, lysine-PEG_4Mal-DM1, was retained inside MDR1-expressing cells better than the lysine–SMCC–DM1 metabolite from an analogous SMCC-linked conjugate [13], and in accord, PEG_4Mal-linked conjugates had a greater antimitotic and cytotoxic potency in vitro against MDR-expressing cells and a greater antitumor activity against MDR1-expressing xenograft tumors in mice [13]. To enhance the potency of disulfide-linked conjugates against multidrug-resistant cells, a negatively charged sulfonate group was added to the SPDB linker (sulfo-SPDB linker). The sulfo-SPDB-linked conjugate was more potent than an analogous SPDB-linked conjugate against MDR1-expressing cells in cell culture and in a xenograft tumor model, while the two conjugates had similar activities in vitro and in vivo toward MDR1-negative cells [54].

The polar nature of the released metabolite possibly contributed to the enhanced cytotoxicity of two non-maytansinoid ADCs to MDR cells. Hamann et al. reported that substitution of a hydrazide group by an amide in the linker of an antibody–calicheamicin conjugate rendered this ADC more efficacious against MDR cells [46]. Although the authors did not explain the mechanism of this phenomenon, we speculate that the conjugate with the pH-sensitive hydrazide linker released a hydrophobic calicheamicin via hydrolysis, whereas the non-cleavable amide-linked conjugate was processed to a polar amino acid-containing derivative that might be a poor MDR1 substrate. In another study, an ADC of a polar version of the cytotoxic compound auristatin was able to kill MDR cells [14]. However, it is not clear if the potency of this conjugate could be attributed to the polarity of its cytotoxic moiety since the potency of ADC of the original, nonpolar auristatin was not reported.

Clinical Experience with ADCs Made with Different Linkers

There are presently over a dozen ADCs in clinical testing, employing a diverse set of linkers and cytotoxic agents. Compounds which have clinical data reported to date, along with their respective linker designs, are summarized in Table 7.1. Several different cleavable linkers, designed to allow release of the payload upon internalization into tumor cells through disulfide reduction, protease activity, or acid hydrolysis, have now been evaluated in cancer patients. Many of these compounds are still in early phases of clinical testing, and the diversity of different targets, antibodies, payloads, and disease indications makes it difficult to attribute particular clinical findings uniquely to the linker component of the ADCs. Nevertheless, the emerging data can provide useful information and important lessons on the clinical performance of these linker designs.

For disulfide-linked maytansinoid conjugates, the contribution of linker design to ADC pharmacokinetics in patients has proven to be predictable from preclinical studies (see above) and reflects the inherent chemical stability of the disulfide bond,

Table 7.1 ADC linker formats currently in clinical development

Linker class	Linker–effector design	Compound	Status
Non-cleavable	SMCC–DM1, thioether—maytansinoid	Trastuzumab–DM1	Phase 2, 3
	mc–MMAF, thioether—auristatin	AGS-16M8F	Phase 1
	mc–MMAF, thioether—auristatin	SGN75	Phase 1
Cleavable, disulfide reduction	SPP–DM1, hindered disulfide—maytansinoid	IMGN901	Phase 1
	SPDB–DM4, highly hindered disulfide—maytansinoid	IMGN388	Phase 1
	SPDB–DM4, highly hindered disulfide—maytansinoid	BT062	Phase 1
	SPDB–DM4, highly hindered disulfide—maytansinoid	BAY94-9343	Phase 1
	SPDB–DM4, highly hindered disulfide—maytansinoid	SAR566658	Phase 1
	SPDB–DM4, highly hindered disulfide—maytansinoid	SAR3419	Phase 2
Cleavable, protease	vc–MMAE, dipeptide—auristatin	SGN35	Phase 1, 2, 3
	vc–MMAE, dipeptide—auristatin	CDX-011	Phase 1/2, 2
	vc–MMAE, dipeptide—auristatin	ASG-5ME	Phase 1
	vc–MMAE, dipeptide—auristatin	ASG-22ME	Phase 1
	vc–MMAE, dipeptide—auristatin	antiCD22 ADC	Phase 1
	vc–MMAE, dipeptide—auristatin	BAY79-4620	Phase 1
	vc–MMAE, dipeptide—auristatin	PSMA ADC	Phase 1
	dipeptide—duocarmycin derivative	MDX-1203	Phase 1
Cleavable, acid labile	Hydrazone—calicheamicin	CMC-544	Phase 3
	Hydrazone—doxorubicin	Milatuzumab–doxorubicin	Phase 1

with increasing bond resistance to thiol–disulfide exchange reactions extending the half-life of conjugate in circulation. In clinical studies, maytansinoid conjugates incorporating a highly hindered disulfide linkage, SPDB–DM4, with an important exception (see below) have achieved predictably longer circulating half-lives than conjugates with a less hindered disulfide bond, SPP–DM1. In the most direct comparison, two maytansinoid ADCs incorporating the same CanAg-targeting antibody, huC242, conjugated to either SPP–DM1 (cantuzumab mertansine) or SPDB–DM4 (IMGN242; cantuzumab ravtansine) were both evaluated in phase I studies. IMGN242 exhibited a significantly longer terminal half-life of 4–5 days (for patients with low CanAg plasma levels) compared to about 2 days reported for cantuzumab mertansine [55, 56] which mirrors similar differences in the pharmacokinetics of ADCs employing these cleavable linker formats in preclinical studies [24, 57]. A major confounding factor when assessing linker design and its role in pharmacokinetics in patients is the impact of target-mediated clearance of the antibody/conjugate ("antigen sink"). In the case of IMGN242, the clearance of the conjugate (and its huC242 antibody component) was greatly accelerated in a subset of patients with very high levels of circulating shed CanAg antigen resulting in a $t_{½}$ of less than 2 days (in some patients down to 0.6 days), whereas in patients with low circulating CanAg antigen levels, the half-life was about 4.6 days [55]. Another maytansinoid conjugate incorporating the SPDB–DM4 design, SAR3419, has a reported half-life of about 7 days in lymphoma patients with minimal target-mediated clearance of the CD19-targeting antibody component [58]. By contrast, an SPDB–DM4 conjugate targeting CD33 (AVE9633) exhibited a shorter half-life, ranging from 1 to 4 days, reflecting the accelerated clearance of the anti-CD33 antibody component of the compound in AML patients with high leukemic cell burdens [59]. Similarly, IMGN901, an SPP–DM1 conjugate that targets CD56, has a half-life of about 1 day in patients, which principally reflects the clearance of the antibody component of the conjugate via antigen-mediated clearance of the entire ADC rather than cleavage of the SPP–DM1 linkage [60].

The design of the linker in an ADC can have important consequences for the tolerability and/or nature of the dose-limiting toxicities ultimately observed in patients. Linker designs with respect to mechanism and rate of release of active payload both within cells and in the extracellular compartment are key parameters that affect the distribution and the pharmacokinetics (exposure) of the conjugate, or potentially the released payload, in patients. As discussed above, the choice of linker can have significant impact on the nature of the active metabolite produced after the conjugate is processed in targeted cells or metabolized through normal clearance mechanisms. By altering linker chemistries, conjugates can be designed to have improved antitumor activity (e.g., better retention of metabolites in multidrug-resistant cells or improved bystander activity in tumors with heterogeneous antigen expression) and/or potentially improved tolerability (e.g., yielding metabolites with less systemic toxicity).

Distinct clinical findings were reported in phase I studies of two maytansinoid ADCs incorporating the same CanAg-targeting huC242 antibody but differing in their disulfide linker design. Cantuzumab mertansine (huC242-SPP-DM1), which incorporated a more labile disulfide linker (1:0 format), reached a maximum tolerated dose (MTD) of 235 mg/m^2 (dosed every 3 weeks), with dose-limiting toxicities at 295 mg/m^2, associated with reversible elevation of hepatic transaminases [56]. Cantuzumab ravtansine (huC242-SPDB-DM4), with a more hindered disulfide linker (0:2), achieved an MTD of 168 mg/m^2 (in patients with low circulating CanAG antigen) with dose-limiting toxicities at 208 mg/m^2 associated with reversible ocular toxicity [55]. The significantly longer half-life in circulation of cantuzumab ravtansine relative to cantuzumab mertansine resulted in a greater exposure to the intact ADC at the MTD in patients despite the somewhat lower dose. However, the altered distribution of the payload (ADC vs. small molecule metabolite) and the different nature of the metabolites produced by these two conjugates in targeted (and nontargeted) cells [17] can both have an impact on their toxicity profiles. In general, while different maytansinoid conjugates to different targets made with three different maytansinoid-linker formats exhibit different DLTs at intolerable doses to define their MTDs, nevertheless, the MTDs for the 12 antibody–maytansinoid conjugates evaluated to date are in a similar range, from about 3.6 to 6.4 mg/kg [61]. For example, the maximum tolerated doses of trastuzumab-DM1 (noncleavable SMCC–DM1) [30] and SAR3419 (hindered disulfide SPDB–DM4) [58] were defined as 3.6 mg/kg and 160 mg/m^2 (~4.3 mg/kg), respectively, in phase 1 studies (dosed every 3 weeks).

Conclusion

Several different linkers have now been validated in clinical testing with respect to their intended performance, yielding ADCs that are stable in circulation and activated upon internalization into tumor cells. Linker design is critical for the optimal performance of an ADC and can impact virtually all key attributes of an ADC, including antitumor efficacy, pharmacokinetics, and tolerability. Understanding the mechanisms of ADC activation and metabolism in cells has provided opportunities to rationally develop new linker chemistries that can significantly alter the properties of the active metabolite (payload) ultimately released in cells. Linker research thus represents an important area for innovation in developing ADCs with improved therapeutic window.

References

1. Wu G, Fang YZ, Yang S, Lupton JR, Turner ND (2004) Glutathione metabolism and its implications for health. J Nutr 134:489–492
2. Mills BJ, Lang CA (1996) Differential distribution of free and bound glutathione and cyst(e)ine in human blood. Biochem Pharmacol 52:401–406
3. Turell L, Carballal S, Botti H, Radi R, Alvarez B (2009) Oxidation of the albumin thiol to sulfenic acid and its implications in the intravascular compartment. Braz J Med Biol Res 42:305–311

4. Wilson JM, Wu D, Motiu-DeGrood R, Hupe DJ (1980) A spectrophotometric method for studying the rates of reaction of disulfides with protein thiol groups applied to bovine serum albumin. J Am Chem Soc 102:359–363
5. Appenzeller-Herzog C, Ellgaard L (2008) The human PDI family: versatility packed into a single fold. Biochim Biophys Acta 1783:535–548
6. Pillay CS, Elliott E, Dennison C (2002) Endolysosomal proteolysis and its regulation. Biochem J 363:417–429
7. Ciechanover A (2006) Intracellular protein degradation: from a vague idea through the lysosome and the ubiquitin-proteasome system and onto human diseases and drug targeting. Hematol Am Soc Hematol Educ Prog 1–12:505–506
8. Singh R, Erickson HK (2009) Antibody-cytotoxic agent conjugates: preparation and characterization. Methods Mol Biol 525:445–467, xiv
9. Junutula JR, Flagella KM, Graham RA, Parsons KL, Ha E, Raab H, Bhakta S, Nguyen T, Dugger DL, Li G, Mai E, Lewis Phillips GD, Hiraragi H, Fuji RN, Tibbitts J, Vandlen R, Spencer SD, Scheller RH, Polakis P, Sliwkowski MX (2010) Engineered thio-trastuzumab-DM1 conjugate with an improved therapeutic index to target human epidermal growth factor receptor 2-positive breast cancer. Clin Cancer Res 16:4769–4778
10. Lewis Phillips GD, Li G, Dugger DL, Crocker LM, Parsons KL, Mai E, Blattler WA, Lambert JM, Chari RV, Lutz RJ, Wong WL, Jacobson FS, Koeppen H, Schwall RH, Kenkare-Mitra SR, Spencer SD, Sliwkowski MX (2008) Targeting HER2-positive breast cancer with trastuzumab-DM1, an antibody-cytotoxic drug conjugate. Cancer Res 68:9280–9290
11. Oflazoglu E, Stone IJ, Gordon K, Wood CG, Repasky EA, Grewal IS, Law CL, Gerber HP (2008) Potent anticarcinoma activity of the humanized anti-CD70 antibody h1F6 conjugated to the tubulin inhibitor auristatin via an uncleavable linker. Clin Cancer Res 14:6171–6180
12. Erickson HK, Park PU, Widdison WC, Kovtun YV, Garrett LM, Hoffman K, Lutz RJ, Goldmacher VS, Blattler WA (2006) Antibody-maytansinoid conjugates are activated in targeted cancer cells by lysosomal degradation and linker-dependent intracellular processing. Cancer Res 66:4426–4433
13. Kovtun YV, Audette CA, Mayo MF, Jones GE, Doherty H, Maloney EK, Erickson HK, Sun X, Wilhelm S, Ab O, Lai KC, Widdison WC, Kellogg B, Johnson H, Pinkas J, Lutz RJ, Singh R, Goldmacher VS, Chari RV (2010) Antibody-maytansinoid conjugates designed to bypass multidrug resistance. Cancer Res 70:2528–2537
14. Doronina SO, Mendelsohn BA, Bovee TD, Cerveny CG, Alley SC, Meyer DL, Oflazoglu E, Toki BE, Sanderson RJ, Zabinski RF, Wahl AF, Senter PD (2006) Enhanced activity of monomethylauristatin F through monoclonal antibody delivery: effects of linker technology on efficacy and toxicity. Bioconjug Chem 17:114–124
15. Kellogg BA, Garrett L, Kovtun Y, Lai KC, Leece B, Miller M, Payne G, Steeves R, Whiteman KR, Widdison W, Xie H, Singh R, Chari RV, Lambert JM, Lutz RJ (2011) Disulfide-linked antibody-maytansinoid conjugates: optimization of in vivo activity by varying the steric hindrance at carbon atoms adjacent to the disulfide linkage. Bioconjug Chem 22:717–727
16. Kovtun YV, Audette CA, Ye Y, Xie H, Ruberti MF, Phinney SJ, Leece BA, Chittenden T, Blattler WA, Goldmacher VS (2006) Antibody-drug conjugates designed to eradicate tumors with homogeneous and heterogeneous expression of the target antigen. Cancer Res 66:3214–3221
17. Erickson HK, Widdison WC, Mayo MF, Whiteman K, Audette C, Wilhelm SD, Singh R (2010) Tumor delivery and in vivo processing of disulfide-linked and thioether-linked antibody-maytansinoid conjugates. Bioconjug Chem 21:84–92
18. Chen Q, Millar HJ, McCabe FL, Manning CD, Steeves R, Lai K, Kellogg B, Lutz RJ, Trikha M, Nakada MT, Anderson GM (2007) Alphav integrin-targeted immunoconjugates regress established human tumors in xenograft models. Clin Cancer Res 13:3689–3695
19. Doronina SO, Toki BE, Torgov MY, Mendelsohn BA, Cerveny CG, Chace DF, DeBlanc RL, Gearing RP, Bovee TD, Siegall CB, Francisco JA, Wahl AF, Meyer DL, Senter PD (2003) Development of potent monoclonal antibody auristatin conjugates for cancer therapy. Nat Biotechnol 21:778–784

20. Okeley NM, Miyamoto JB, Zhang X, Sanderson RJ, Benjamin DR, Sievers EL, Senter PD, Alley SC (2010) Intracellular activation of SGN-35, a potent anti-CD30 antibody-drug conjugate. Clin Cancer Res 16:888–897
21. Dornan D, Bennett F, Chen Y, Dennis M, Eaton D, Elkins K, French D, Go MA, Jack A, Junutula JR, Koeppen H, Lau J, McBride J, Rawstron A, Shi X, Yu N, Yu SF, Yue P, Zheng B, Ebens A, Polson AG (2009) Therapeutic potential of an anti-CD79b antibody-drug conjugate, anti-CD79b-vc-MMAE, for the treatment of non-Hodgkin lymphoma. Blood 114:2721–2729
22. DiJoseph JF, Armellino DC, Boghaert ER, Khandke K, Dougher MM, Sridharan L, Kunz A, Hamann PR, Gorovits B, Udata C, Moran JK, Popplewell AG, Stephens S, Frost P, Damle NK (2004) Antibody-targeted chemotherapy with CMC-544: a CD22-targeted immunoconjugate of calicheamicin for the treatment of B-lymphoid malignancies. Blood 103:1807–1814
23. Stein R, Mattes MJ, Cardillo TM, Hansen HJ, Chang CH, Burton J, Govindan S, Goldenberg DM (2007) CD74: a new candidate target for the immunotherapy of B-cell neoplasms. Clin Cancer Res 13:5556s–5563s
24. Xie H, Blattler WA (2006) In vivo behaviour of antibody-drug conjugates for the targeted treatment of cancer. Expert Opin Biol Ther 6:281–291
25. Foidart J-M, Muschel RJ (2002) Proteases and their inhibitors in cancer metastasis. Kluwer Academic Publishers, Dordrecht/Boston
26. Lavie G, Zucker-Franklin D, Franklin EC (1980) Elastase-type proteases on the surface of human blood monocytes: possible role in amyloid formation. J Immunol 125:175–180
27. Ciechanover A (2007) Intracellular protein degradation from a vague idea through the lysosome and the ubiquitin-proteasome system and on to human diseases and drug targeting: Nobel Lecture, December 8, 2004. Ann N Y Acad Sci 1116:1–28
28. Jain RK, Baxter LT (1988) Mechanisms of heterogeneous distribution of monoclonal antibodies and other macromolecules in tumors: significance of elevated interstitial pressure. Cancer Res 48:7022–7032
29. Ciechanover A (2010) Intracellular protein degradation: from a vague idea through the lysosome and the ubiquitin-proteasome system and onto human diseases and drug targeting. Medicina (Buenos Aires) 70:105–119
30. Krop IE, Beeram M, Modi S, Jones SF, Holden SN, Yu W, Girish S, Tibbitts J, Yi JH, Sliwkowski MX, Jacobson F, Lutzker SG, Burris HA (2010) Phase I study of trastuzumab-DM1, an HER2 antibody-drug conjugate, given every 3 weeks to patients with HER2-positive metastatic breast cancer. J Clin Oncol 28:2698–2704
31. Alley SC, Benjamin DR, Jeffrey SC, Okeley NM, Meyer DL, Sanderson RJ, Senter PD (2008) Contribution of linker stability to the activities of anticancer immunoconjugates. Bioconjug Chem 19:759–765
32. Fishkin N, Maloney EK, Chari RV, Singh R (2011) A novel pathway for maytansinoid release from thioether linked antibody-drug conjugates (ADCs) under oxidative conditions. Chem Commun (Camb) 47:10752–10754
33. Sanderson RJ, Hering MA, James SF, Sun MM, Doronina SO, Siadak AW, Senter PD, Wahl AF (2005) In vivo drug-linker stability of an anti-CD30 dipeptide-linked auristatin immunoconjugate. Clin Cancer Res 11:843–852
34. Lazar AC, Wang L, Blattler WA, Amphlett G, Lambert JM, Zhang W (2005) Analysis of the composition of immunoconjugates using size-exclusion chromatography coupled to mass spectrometry. Rapid Commun Mass Spectrom 19:1806–1814
35. Hamblett KJ, Senter PD, Chace DF, Sun MM, Lenox J, Cerveny CG, Kissler KM, Bernhardt SX, Kopcha AK, Zabinski RF, Meyer DL, Francisco JA (2004) Effects of drug loading on the antitumor activity of a monoclonal antibody drug conjugate. Clin Cancer Res 10:7063–7070
36. Ikeda H, Hideshima T, Fulciniti M, Lutz RJ, Yasui H, Okawa Y, Kiziltepe T, Vallet S, Pozzi S, Santo L, Perrone G, Tai YT, Cirstea D, Raje NS, Uherek C, Dalken B, Aigner S, Osterroth F, Munshi N, Richardson P, Anderson KC (2009) The monoclonal antibody nBT062 conjugated to cytotoxic Maytansinoids has selective cytotoxicity against CD138-positive multiple myeloma cells in vitro and in vivo. Clin Cancer Res 15:4028–4037

37. Oroudjev E, Lopus M, Wilson L, Audette C, Provenzano C, Erickson H, Kovtun Y, Chari R, Jordan MA (2010) Maytansinoid-antibody conjugates induce mitotic arrest by suppressing microtubule dynamic instability. Mol Cancer Ther 9:2700–2713
38. Christiansen J, Rajasekaran AK (2004) Biological impediments to monoclonal antibody-based cancer immunotherapy. Mol Cancer Ther 3:1493–1501
39. Greiner JW (1986) Modulation of antigen expression in human tumor cell populations. Cancer Invest 4:239–256
40. Adams GP, Schier R, McCall AM, Simmons HH, Horak EM, Alpaugh RK, Marks JD, Weiner LM (2001) High affinity restricts the localization and tumor penetration of single-chain fv antibody molecules. Cancer Res 61:4750–4755
41. Rudnick SI, Adams GP (2009) Affinity and avidity in antibody-based tumor targeting. Cancer Biother Radiopharm 24:155–161
42. Saga T, Neumann RD, Heya T, Sato J, Kinuya S, Le N, Paik CH, Weinstein JN (1995) Targeting cancer micrometastases with monoclonal antibodies: a binding-site barrier. Proc Natl Acad Sci USA 92:8999–9003
43. Drewinko B, Patchen M, Yang LY, Barlogie B (1981) Differential killing efficacy of twenty antitumor drugs on proliferating and nonproliferating human tumor cells. Cancer Res 41:2328–2333
44. Rao PN, Freireich EJ, Smith ML, Loo TL (1979) Cell cycle phase-specific cytotoxicity of the antitumor agent maytansine. Cancer Res 39:3152–3155
45. Szakacs G, Paterson JK, Ludwig JA, Booth-Genthe C, Gottesman MM (2006) Targeting multidrug resistance in cancer. Nat Rev Drug Discov 5:219–234
46. Hamann PR, Hinman LM, Beyer CF, Greenberger LM, Lin C, Lindh D, Menendez AT, Wallace R, Durr FE, Upeslacis J (2005) An anti-MUC1 antibody-calicheamicin conjugate for treatment of solid tumors. Choice of linker and overcoming drug resistance. Bioconjug Chem 16:346–353
47. Matsui H, Takeshita A, Naito K, Shinjo K, Shigeno K, Maekawa M, Yamakawa Y, Tanimoto M, Kobayashi M, Ohnishi K, Ohno R (2002) Reduced effect of gemtuzumab ozogamicin (CMA-676) on P-glycoprotein and/or CD34-positive leukemia cells and its restoration by multidrug resistance modifiers. Leukemia 16:813–819
48. Walter RB, Raden BW, Hong TC, Flowers DA, Bernstein ID, Linenberger ML (2003) Multidrug resistance protein attenuates gemtuzumab ozogamicin-induced cytotoxicity in acute myeloid leukemia cells. Blood 102:1466–1473
49. Toppmeyer DL, Slapak CA, Croop J, Kufe DW (1994) Role of P-glycoprotein in dolastatin 10 resistance. Biochem Pharmacol 48:609–612
50. Butryn RK, Smith KS, Adams EG, Abraham I, Stackpole J, Sampson KE, Bhuyan BK (1994) V79 Chinese hamster lung cells resistant to the bis-alkylator bizelesin are multidrug-resistant. Cancer Chemother Pharmacol 34:44–50
51. Zsido TJ, Beerman TA, Meegan RL, Woynarowski JM, Baker RM (1992) Resistance of CHO cells expressing P-glycoprotein to cyclopropylpyrroloindole (CPI) alkylating agents. Biochem Pharmacol 43:1817–1822
52. Tang R, Cohen S, Perrot JY, Faussat AM, Zuany-Amorim C, Marjanovic Z, Morjani H, Fava F, Corre E, Legrand O, Marie JP (2009) P-gp activity is a critical resistance factor against AVE9633 and DM4 cytotoxicity in leukaemia cell lines, but not a major mechanism of chemoresistance in cells from acute myeloid leukaemia patients. BMC Cancer 9:199
53. Loo TW, Clarke DM (2005) Recent progress in understanding the mechanism of P-glycoprotein-mediated drug efflux. J Membr Biol 206:173–185
54. Kovtun Y, Jones G, Audette C, Mayo M, Leece B, Zhao R, Clancy L, Sun X, Chari R, Singh R (2010) 235. Negatively-charged sulfonate group in linker improves potency of antibody–maytansinoid conjugates against multidrug-resistant cancer cells. 22nd EORTC-NCI-AACR symposium on molecular targets and cancer therapeutics, Berlin, Germany
55. Qin A, Watermill J, Mastico RA, Lutz RJ, O'Keeffe J, Zildjian S, Mita AC, Phan AT, Tolcher AW (2008) The pharmacokinetics and pharmacodynamics of IMGN242 (huC242-DM4) in patients with CanAg-expressing solid tumors. ASCO Meet Abstr 26:3066

56. Tolcher AW, Ochoa L, Hammond LA, Patnaik A, Edwards T, Takimoto C, Smith L, de Bono J, Schwartz G, Mays T, Jonak ZL, Johnson R, DeWitte M, Martino H, Audette C, Maes K, Chari RV, Lambert JM, Rowinsky EK (2003) Cantuzumab mertansine, a maytansinoid immunoconjugate directed to the CanAg antigen: a phase I, pharmacokinetic, and biologic correlative study. J Clin Oncol 21:211–222
57. Xie H, Audette C, Hoffee M, Lambert JM, Blattler WA (2004) Pharmacokinetics and biodistribution of the antitumor immunoconjugate, cantuzumab mertansine (huC242-DM1), and its two components in mice. J Pharmacol Exp Ther 308:1073–1082
58. Younes A, Gordon L, Kim S, Romaguera J, Copeland AR, de Castro Farial S, Kwak L, Fayad L, Hagemeister F, Fanale M, Lambert J, Bagulho T, Morariu-Zamfir R (2009) Phase I multidose escalation study of the anti-CD19 maytansinoid immunoconjugate SAR3419 administered by intravenous (IV) infusion every 3 weeks to patients with relapsed/refractory B-Cell non-Hodgkin's lymphoma (NHL). ASH Annu Meet Abstr 114:585
59. Lapusan S, Vidriales MB, Thomas X, de Botton S, Vekhoff A, Tang R, Dumontet C, Morariu-Zamfir R, Lambert JM, Ozoux ML, Poncelet P, San Miguel JF, Legrand O, Deangelo DJ, Giles FJ, Marie JP (2012) Phase I studies of AVE9633, an anti-CD33 antibody-maytansinoid conjugate, in adult patients with relapsed/refractory acute myeloid leukemia. Invest New Drugs 30(3):1121–1131
60. Thompson DS, Patnaik A, Bendell JC, Papadopoulos K, Infante JR, Mastico RA, Johnson D, Qin A, O'Leary JJ, Tolcher AW (2010) A phase I dose-escalation study of IMGN388 in patients with solid tumors. ASCO Meet Abstr 28:3058
61. Lambert JM (2010) Antibody-maytansinoid conjugates: a new strategy for the treatment of cancer. Drugs of the future 35:471–480

Part IV
Antibody-Drug Conjugates for Hematologic Malignancies

Chapter 8
Antibody–Drug Conjugates for the Treatment of B-Cell Malignancies

Andrew G. Polson

Malignancies of B-cell origin constitute a diverse set of neoplasms that vary in B-cell subtype of origin and underlying genetic drivers. In addition, they vary widely in clinical outcome. Follicular non-Hodgkin's lymphoma (FL) or chronic lymphocytic leukemia (CLL), are indolent and incurable diseases with a median survival of 8–10 years whereas the more aggressive diseases such as Diffuse large B-cell lymphoma (DLBCL) and Mantle cell lymphoma (MCL) can have a median survival of 6 months if left untreated. DLBCL is the most common type of NHL accounting for approximately 30–40% of all NHL diagnosis followed by follicular lymphoma (20–25% of NHL diagnosis) and MCL (6–10% NHL diagnosis). B-cell chronic lymphocytic leukemia (B-CLL) is the most common of the chronic leukemias in adults with approximately 15,000 new cases per year in the United States [1]. These diseases are quite diverse; however, most of them are treated with the anti-CD20 chimeric monoclonal antibody rituximab (Rituxan®, MabThera®) in combination with cytotoxic chemotherapy. Although durable responses can be achieved in some patients, approximately half of patients with aggressive NHL will ultimately experience progressive or relapsed disease. In addition, indolent B-cell malignancies remain incurable despite longer durations of response with current therapies. Thus, there is still a need for treatments that can significantly extend disease-free and overall survival in these patients, with at least acceptable if not superior safety profiles.

The development of antibody–drug conjugates (ADCs) for the treatment of B-cell malignancies provides a unique opportunity to fill these unmet medical needs. NHL is responsive to chemotherapy, unconjugated antibody therapies, and radioimmunoconjugate therapies, suggesting that these tumors are accessible by antibody-based therapies and would be responsive to cytotoxics delivered by an ADC. Furthermore,

A.G. Polson (✉)
Genentech Research and Early Development, 1 DNA Way,
South San Francisco, CA 94080, USA
e-mail: polson@gene.com

G.L. Phillips (ed.), *Antibody-Drug Conjugates and Immunotoxins: From Pre-Clinical Development to Therapeutic Applications*, Cancer Drug Discovery and Development,
DOI 10.1007/978-1-4614-5456-4_8,

rituximab (chimeric IgG1 anti-CD20) depletes normal B cells and has a generally acceptable safety profile in humans, suggesting that expression of an ADC target on normal B cells that results in depletion of normal B cells will not result in unacceptable toxicities [2]. There are a number of potential ADC targets that are B-lineage markers whose expression is restricted to the B-cell compartment and are also expressed on non-Hodgkin's lymphoma NHL including CD19, CD20, CD21, CD22, and CD79. Additional targets that have a wider expression pattern that extends beyond B cells but could also be good ADCs targets for NHL include CD70, CD72, and CD180. The expression pattern and biology of these targets as well as the properties of the linker-drugs being explored bring a diverse and promising collection of ADCs for the treatment of B-cell malignancies.

ADCs for the Treatment of NHL Currently in Clinical Trials

There are three ADCs in clinical trials designed only to treat B-cell malignancies inotuzumab ozogamicin (IO, CMC-544), SAR3419, and DCDT2980S. IO and DCDT2980S both target the CD22 antigen and SAR3419 targets CD19. CD22 is a member of the SIGLEC family of proteins and binds to α2,6 linked sialic acid residues; it functions as a negative regulator of B-cell antigen receptor signaling [3]. CD22 expression is restricted to the B-cell lineage. During B-cell development, CD22 is first detected at the pre-B-cell stage, is expressed through the development of mature B cells, and is decreased during differentiation into plasma cells [4]. CD22 is expressed in the vast majority of NHLs. Similar levels of CD22 expression are observed in DLBCL, FL, and marginal zone lymphomas. CD22 expression is slightly higher in hairy cell leukemia compared to other tumor types and normal B lymphocytes and is comparatively lower in CLL [5].

Inotuzumab ozogamicin (IO, CMC-544) is a human IgG4 monoclonal antibody to CD22 conjugated via an acid-labile hydrazone linker to a cytotoxic DNA damaging agent calicheamicin [6, 7]. This is the same linker-drug used in gemtuzumab ozogamicin (Mylotarg), which was the first approved ADC for the treatment of acute myeloid leukemia. IO has been tested in several Phase 1 clinical trials for the treatment of NHL as a single agent, in combination with rituximab [8–10] and in combination with rituximab, vincristine, and cyclophosphamide and prednisone (R-CVP) [11]. In a Phase 1 open-label dose escalation study in heavily pretreated (≥2 prior therapies) FL and DLBCL patients ($n=79$), the maximum tolerated dose (MTD) of single-agent IO was 1.8 mg/m^2 dosed every 4 weeks. The dose-limiting toxicities (DLTs) were thrombocytopenia and neutropenia. IO also demonstrated antitumor activity in relapsed and refractory FL and DLBCL patients with an ORR of 68 and 15%, and median progression free survival (PFS) of 10.4 months and 1.6 months, respectively. Results from a Phase 1b expansion in combination with rituximab (375 mg/m^2) showed that in a similar population of patients enrolled into the single-agent Phase I study, the MTD remained 1.8 mg/m^2 and tolerability was unaffected by the addition of rituximab. The PFS at 1 year was 80% in follicular patients

($n=41$) and was 56% in relapsed DLBCL patients. The overall response rate (ORR) in both these populations was 80% [8, 12]. Also, when used as an early line of therapy, the combination of rituximab and IO potentially adds efficacy without changing safety [8]. Based on these results, IO is being studied in a phase III trial in patients with relapsed/refractory DLBCL who are not candidates for high-dose chemotherapy with stem cell rescue. This study is comparing IO in combination with rituximab vs. physician's choice of rituximab plus bendamustine or rituximab plus gemcitabine (ClinicalTrials.gov identifier NCT01232556).

In addition to combinations with rituximab, IO has been studied in combination with immunochemotherapy regimens. In combination with R-CVP (rituximab 375 mg/m^2, vincristine 1.4 mg/m^2, and cyclophosphamide 750 mg/m^2 all given on day 1, and prednisone 40 mg/m^2 given on days 1 through 5 on a 3-week cycle) in patients with relapsed/refractory NHL the MTD of IO was 0.8 mg/m^2, which is lower than the MTD of single-agent IO or IO when combined with rituximab only. The DLTs were acute hepatitis, thrombocytopenia, and neutropenia requiring support with G-CSF. Preliminary efficacy data from the dose–escalation portion of the study ($n=15$ evaluable patients) showed an ORR of 87% (33% with complete response; 53% with partial response). In patients with FL, which constituted the majority of the evaluable study patient population, the ORR was 100% (45% with complete response) [11]. IO in combination with other agents for the treatment of NHL and Acute lymphoblastic leukemia (ALL) continues to be studied in ongoing Phase I and Phase II clinical trials.

The second ADC targeted to CD22 is DCDT2980S. DCDT2980S is an anti-CD22-humanized IgG1 conjugated to the potent tubulin-destabilizing agent monomethyl auristatin E (MMAE) via antibody cysteines residues by a maleimidocaproyl–valine–citrulline-*p*-aminobenzyloxycarbonyl (MC-vc-PAB) linker that is designed to be cleaved by cathepsins. This is the same linker-drug that is used in the recently approved anti-CD30 ADC brentuximab vedotin (SGN-35) that has shown excellent efficacy and safety in the treatment of relapsed/refractory Hodgkin lymphoma (see Chap. 10). The promising results with the MC-vc-PAB-MMAE ADC in Hodgkin's lymphoma and with IO (anti-CD22 ADC) are encouraging for the clinical possibilities for DCDT2980S. DCDT2980S is currently in Phase I testing both as a single agent and in combination with rituximab (ClinicalTrials.gov identifier NCT01209130).

The third ADC in clinical trials for the treatment of NHL is SAR3419, which consists of a humanized anti-CD19 antibody and with a linker cleavable by disulfide reduction (SPDB) attached to the maytansinoid DM4 through lysine residues [13]. CD19 is a member of the Ig superfamily of proteins. It is expressed on all mature B cells, exists in the B-cell membrane in a complex with CD21, CD81 and CD225, and complexes with the B-cell receptor (BCR) to lower the threshold for antigen receptor stimulation and regulate B-cell receptor signaling. CD19, like CD22, is expressed only in the B-cell lineage starting at the pre-B-cell stage and not expressed in plasma cells. CD19 is also expressed in the vast majority of NHLs [14, 15]. There have been two Phase I trials of SAR3419 in relapsed and refractory NHL testing every 3-week and weekly dose schedules. These studies established the MTD of

160 mg/m^2 dosed every 3 weeks and 55 mg/m^2 dosed weekly. In both cases DLT was reversible ocular toxicity, with affected patients experiencing some level of blurred vision or vision impairment; the incidence and frequency was lower with the weekly schedule. The efficacy also appears to be better in the weekly schedule with a 33% ORR compared to 17% for every 3 week dosing although as patient in the dose escalation are included so a direct comparison of efficacy should be treated with caution [16]. SAR3419 is currently being tested in phase 2 trials as a single agent and in combination with rituximab. Additional information about SAR3419 is detailed in Chap. 10.

The combination of any of the aforementioned ADCs with rituximab would seem very promising for several reasons. Rituximab is generally well tolerated and can be combined safely with and enhance the efficacy of chemotherapy. Evidence supporting this is the demonstration that, the combination of rituximab and IO was just as tolerated as IO at maximum single-agent doses and the combination did not lead to unacceptable toxicity while potentially resulting in enhanced antitumor activity [8]. Another reason that the combination of these ADCs with rituximab is of interest is that the expression patterns of CD20, CD19, and CD22 on normal B cells are overlapping. Consequently, the depletion of normal B cells with rituximab treatment could potentially remove the antigen sink and increase the exposure of the tumor to the ADC. If this increase in exposure does not decrease the tolerability of the ADCs, as seems to be the case with IO plus rituximab, this would provide an additional rationale to expect an increase in efficacy of these ADCs in combination with rituximab.

Another indication currently under study for the use of anti-CD19 and anti-CD22 ADCs is in B-cell acute lymphoblastic leukemia (B-ALL). In adults who are treated with intensive chemotherapy long-term survival is approximately 40%; however, the treatments are poorly tolerated and the majority of patients are not cured. CD19 is expressed on greater than 99% of B-ALL and CD22 is expressed on 93% of B-ALL [17]. B-ALL remains a major unmet medical need—despite the incorporation of aggressive induction and consolidation chemotherapy, the majority of adults with B-ALL will ultimately have disease relapse and die of their disease. Patterns of CD19 and CD22 expression in B-ALL have not surprisingly led to the investigation of IO and SAR3419 in clinical trials for adult B-ALL. IO was tested in relapsed/refractory ALL dosed every 3 weeks at 1.8 mg/m^2 and the major side effects were thrombocytopenia and hepatic toxicity as observed in the NHL trials. The ORR was 57% ($n=49$) with 18% CRs [18]. Based on the data with SAR3419 in NHL described above, SAR3419 is currently being tested in a Phase II trial for the treatment of relapsed/refractory ALL (ClinicalTrials.gov Identifier NCT01440179).

In addition to the three ADCs in clinical development specifically targeting B-cell malignancies, two ADCs targeting CD70 (SGN-75 and MDX-1203), which is expressed in both hematologic and solid tumors, are in clinical development. CD70 is a TNF family member and the ligand of CD27 and is transiently expressed on normal activated B and T cells [19]. CD70 is expressed in ~70% of NHL [20] as well as solid tumors including renal cell, thymic, and nasopharyngeal carcinomas ([21] and references there in), and in glioblastomas and astrocytomas [22].

The restricted expression pattern of CD70 in normal tissue and its prevalence in a variety of tumors make it a promising target for ADCs. SGN-75 consists of the antibody anti-CD70 (h1F6) conjugated via a noncleavable maleimidocaproyl linker (MC) to monomethyl auristatin F (MC-MMAF) [21]. MMAF is less permeable to the cell but more potent than MMAE and requires internalization of the ADC for activity. The resulting lysosomal degradation of the antibody results in the generation of the active catabolite cysteine-MC-MMAF inside tumor cells [23]. SGN-75 is being evaluated in Phase I clinical trial for CD70-positive relapsed and refractory Non-Hodgkin Lymphoma and metastatic renal cell carcinoma.

MDX-1203 is an anti-CD70 ADC using a derivative of the DNA alkylating agent duocarmycin (described below) is also in early Phase 1 clinical development (ClinicalTrials.gov Identifier NCT00944905). MDX-1203 consists of a human anti-CD70 antibody to which duocarmycin (MED-2460) is conjugated via a cleavable peptide-based linker [24]. The duocarmycins are a derivative of the antibiotic CC-1065, a DNA alkylating agent. Like the other drugs used in the ADC format, the duocarmycins are highly potent cytotoxic agents with a narrow therapeutic window when administered as free agents. For example, the duocarmycin KW-2189 was tested for the treatment of solid tumors in early clinical trials [25]. However, KW-2189 did not demonstrate efficacy at tolerated doses as systemic chemotherapy. With MDX-1203, however, activity of the duocarmycin derivative is dependent on two events, cleavage of the linker by lysosomal proteases and activation by carboxyesterases that remove a protecting carbamate [24]. The active drug then causes alkylation of the -3 position of adenine in the DNA. This mechanism of action ensures that the internalization and conversion to active drug will be highly specific to tumor cells whereas normal tissues will be minimally exposed to active drug, thus theoretically providing an additional level of safety without compromising efficacy.

While still preliminary, the data reported to date of ADCs in the treatment of B-cell malignancies and their combinability with existing therapies offer the potential to further provide better outcomes for patients.

Preclinical ADCs for the Treatment of B-Cell Malignancies

Three other ADCs using different drug-linker technologies are being studied targeting CD19 or CD22. The first, anti-CD19(hBU12)-MC-MMAF (SGN-CD19A) [26], consists of an anti-CD19-directed antibody (hBU12) conjugated to the MC-MMAF linker-drug used in SGN-75. The second ADC, MDX-1206, targets CD19 and is conjugated to the same duocarmycin DNA alkylating agent as in the anti-CD70 ADC MDX-1203. MDX-1206 has been shown to have significant activity in preclinical models of NHL, and appears to have a well-tolerated profile with a significant therapeutic index based on pilot results obtained in cynomolgus monkeys [27].

The third reported ADC to these two targets is the anti-CD22 ADC Epratuzumab-SN-38 [28]. Epratuzumab is a humanized anti-CD22 antibody (unconjugated) that is currently in clinical trials for the treatment of B-cell malignancies

[29] and lupus [30]. The drug, SN-38, is the active metabolite of the topoisomerase I inhibitor irinotecan. SN-38 is attached to the antibody through cysteines and contains a short polyethylene glycol segment and a lysine that increase solubility. Once internalized into the cell, the drug is mostly likely released through a pH-sensitive benzyl carbonate bond to SN-38's lactone ring [28]. The linker appears to be relatively labile in vitro as control conjugates and Epratuzumab-SN-38 were equally effective in vitro suggesting efficient release of free drug. Furthermore, anti-CD20 antibody-SN38 ADCs, which do not internalize upon binding, were also effective in vivo. In xenograft studies, Epratuzumab-SN-38 was more efficacious than non-anti-CD22-directed control conjugates, suggesting that this type of linker could be the optimal choice to use with targeted delivery of SN-38, which itself is less potent that the other drugs used in the ADCs discussed in this chapter, to CD22-positive tumor cells. This suggests that the combination of a cytotoxic drug that is reasonably well tolerated combined with a linker that readily facilitates its release as free drug could be an alternate approach to ADC design. This contrasts with the other ADCs described in this chapter, which emphasize the combination of highly stable linkers and highly potent cytotoxic drugs. Epratuzumab-SN-38 has not been tested in the clinic. Given the other ADCs that targeted CD22, it would be interesting to see the comparisons of safety and tolerability with these different linker–cytotoxic combinations.

In addition to the targets for the treatment of NHL by ADCs that are currently in clinical trials, B-cell surface proteins CD20, CD21, CD72, CD180, CD79a, and CD79b have all shown efficacy as ADC targets for NHL [31–33]. CD20 differs from the other targets listed in that it is very poorly internalized upon antibody binding and is therefore less suited as an ADC target. Still, an unconjugated anti-CD20 (rituximab) is an effective therapy for NHL and CLL either as a single agent or in combination with standard chemotherapy. Additionally, anti-CD20 ADCs were shown to be more effective than comparable unconjugated anti-CD20 antibodies with three different linker-drugs [31–33]. An ADC that could engage the effector function of the antibody component resulting in potential enhancement of ADC-mediated cell killing is an attractive concept, and this approach has proven to be clinically viable with T-DM1 in HER2+ breast cancer [34]. However, as discussed above, any ADC to other NHL targets could be combined with an anti-CD20 antibody with maximal exposure to both therapies and probably little increase in toxicity, thus diminishing the rationale for an anti-CD20 ADC.

A promising ADC target for the treatment of B-cell malignancies is the signaling component of the B-cell receptor CD79. CD79 is a heterodimer (CD79a/CD79b) and, similar to CD20 and CD22, it is expressed only on pre-B-cells, mature B cells, and the majority of NHLs and CLLs from both treated and untreated patients. Additionally, most likely due to its function in class II antigen presentation, antibodies that bind CD79 rapidly internalize to the lysosomal compartment. ADCs targeting CD79b were shown to be very efficacious in preclinical models with both cleavable (SPP-DM1 and MC-vc-PAB-MMAE) and uncleavable linkers [35–37] presumably due to exploitation of this unique and efficient intercellular trafficking mechanism. The safety of targeting CD79b was tested preclinically with a surrogate antibody recognizing the cynomolgus monkey CD79b protein with binding properties similar to that of an antibody recognizing the human CD79b that had preclinical efficacy as an ADC. Both the ADC and unconjugated antibody were shown to be well tolerated in cynomolgus monkeys [35]. Based on preclinical data, CD79b has the potential of being a highly effective ADC target, and drug conjugates targeting this receptor could have significant clinical potential.

Conclusions

The rich pipeline of ADCs in the clinic and in preclinical development has great potential to change the way B-cell malignancies are treated and to improve patient outcome for these unmet medical needs. It also presents an opportunity to better understand the key parameters that make for a safe and effective ADC. Appropriate analysis of the tumors in the clinical trials could help us understand what makes a tumor sensitive or resistant to the ADC. In the three cases where the in vitro sensitivity of NHL cells lines to the ADC was compared to the sensitivity to free drug and the levels of surface receptor, little correlation of ADC sensitivity and surface receptor or free drug sensitivity was found [5, 26, 36]. These data suggest that, although sensitivity to the free drug and the surface receptors may play a role in tumor response to an ADC, neither one of these factors would be the main driver of response. It would be interesting to see if this observation plays out in the clinic. There have been three ADCs described that use the MC-vc-PAB-MMAE linker-drug but have different targets (anti-CD22, anti-CD19 and anti-CD79b [26, 36]). One (DCDT2980S, anti-CD22-MC-vc-PAB-MMAE) is in clinical testing, if one of the other two were tested in the clinic this could allow us to understand how target and antibody affect the properties of the ADC. Does the target effect influence which indication the ADC is most effective in? How much does the target characteristics affect the efficacy of the ADC? Further, there are two ADCs with the same target in the clinic, IO and DCDT2980S. Preclinical data suggest that IO is more potent, both tolerated and effective at very low doses, compared to DCDT2980S and the drugs used have different mechanisms of action. If both are effective this would indicate that there are many paths to effective ADC development and that ADCs have great potential as a technology to treat B-cell malignancies and cancer cancers in general.

References

1. Jemal A, Siegel R, Ward E, Hao Y, Xu J, Thun M (2009) Cancer statistics, 2009. CA Cancer J Clin 59(4):225–249
2. Solal-Celigny P (2006) Safety of rituximab maintenance therapy in follicular lymphomas. Leuk Res 30(Suppl 1):S16–S21
3. Billadeau DD, Leibson PJ (2002) ITAMs versus ITIMs: striking a balance during cell regulation. J Clin Invest 109(2):161–168

4. Tedder TF, Tuscano J, Sato S, Kehrl JH (1997) CD22, a B lymphocyte-specific adhesion molecule that regulates antigen receptor signaling. Annu Rev Immunol 15:481–504
5. Polson AG, Williams M, Gray AM et al (2010) Anti-CD22-MCC-DM1: an antibody-drug conjugate with a stable linker for the treatment of non-Hodgkin's lymphoma. Leukemia 24(9):1566–1573
6. DiJoseph JF, Armellino DC, Boghaert ER et al (2004) Antibody-targeted chemotherapy with CMC-544: a CD22-targeted immunoconjugate of calicheamicin for the treatment of B-lymphoid malignancies. Blood 103(5):1807–1814
7. Zein N, Poncin M, Nilakantan R, Ellestad GA (1989) Calicheamicin gamma 1I and DNA: molecular recognition process responsible for site-specificity. Science 244(4905):697–699
8. Dang N, Smith M, Offner F et al (2009) Anti-CD22 immunoconjugate inotuzumab ozogamicin (CMC-544)+rituximab: clinical activity including survival in patients with recurrent/refractory follicular or 'aggressive' lymphoma. Blood (ASH Annual Meeting Abstracts) 114(22):Abstract 584
9. Fayad L, Patel H, Verhoef G et al (2008) Safety and clinical activity of the anti-CD22 immunoconjugate inotuzumab ozogamicin (CMC-544) in combination with rituximab in follicular lymphoma or diffuse large B-cell lymphoma: preliminary report of a phase 1/2 study. ASH Annu Meet Abstr 112(11):266
10. Ogura M, Tobinai K, Hatake K et al (2010) Phase I study of inotuzumab ozogamicin (CMC-544) in Japanese patients with follicular lymphoma pretreated with rituximab-based therapy. Cancer Sci 101(8):1840–1545
11. Ogura M, Uchida T, MacDonald DA et al (2011) An open-label, Phase I Study of R-CVP in combination with inotuzumab ozogamicin in patients with relapsed/refractory CD22-positive B-cell non-Hodgkin lymphoma. ASH Annu Meet Abstr 118(21%U http://abstracts.hematologylibrary.org/cgi/content/abstract/ashmtg;118/21/3715 %8 November 18, 2011):3715
12. Advani A, Coiffier B, Czuczman MS et al (2010) Safety, pharmacokinetics, and preliminary clinical activity of inotuzumab ozogamicin, a novel immunoconjugate for the treatment of B-cell non-Hodgkin's lymphoma: results of a phase I study. J Clin Oncol 28(12):2085–2093
13. Younes A, Gordon L, Kim S et al (2009) Phase I multi-dose escalation study of the anti-CD19 maytansinoid immunoconjugate SAR3419 administered by intravenous (IV) infusion every 3 weeks to patients with relapsed/refractory B-cell non-Hodgkin's lymphoma (NHL). ASH Annu Meet Abstr 114(22):585
14. Barclay AN, Brown M, Law SKA, McKinght AJ, Tomlinson MG, Anton van der Merwe P (1997) The leucocyte antigen facts book. Academic, San Diego, CA
15. Olejniczak SH, Stewart CC, Donohue K, Czuczman MS (2006) A quantitative exploration of surface antigen expression in common B-cell malignancies using flow cytometry. Immunol Invest 35(1):93–114
16. Coiffier B, Ribrag V, Dupuis J et al (2011) Phase I/II study of the anti-CD19 maytansinoid immunoconjugate SAR3419 administered weekly to patients (pts) with relapsed/refractory B-cell non-Hodgkin lymphoma (NHL). ASCO Meet Abstr 29(Suppl 15):8017
17. Raponi S, Stefania De Propris M, Intoppa S et al (2011) Flow cytometric study of potential target antigens (CD19, CD20, CD22, CD33) for antibody-based immunotherapy in acute lymphoblastic leukemia: analysis of 552 cases. Leuk Lymphoma 52(6):1098–1107
18. O'Brien S, Thomas DA, Ohanian M et al (2011) Inotuzumab Ozogamycin (I0), a CD22 monoclonal antibody conjugated to calecheamicin, is active in refractory-relapse acute lymphocytic leukemia (R-R ALL). ASH Annu Meet Abstr 118(21):875
19. Arens R, Schepers K, Nolte MA et al (2004) Tumor rejection induced by CD70-mediated quantitative and qualitative effects on effector CD8+ T cell formation. J Exp Med 199(11):1595–1605
20. Lens SM, Drillenburg P, den Drijver BF et al (1999) Aberrant expression and reverse signalling of CD70 on malignant B cells. Br J Haematol 106(2):491–503
21. Oflazoglu E, Stone IJ, Gordon K et al (2008) Potent anticarcinoma activity of the humanized anti-CD70 antibody h1f6 conjugated to the tubulin inhibitor auristatin via an uncleavable linker. Clin Cancer Res 14(19):6171–6180

22. Wischhusen J, Jung G, Radovanovic I et al (2002) Identification of CD70-mediated apoptosis of immune effector cells as a novel immune escape pathway of human glioblastoma. Cancer Res 62(9):2592–2599
23. Alley SC, Benjamin DR, Jeffrey SC et al (2008) Contribution of linker stability to the activities of anticancer immunoconjugates. Bioconjug Chem 19(3):759–765
24. Derwin D, Passmore D, Sung J et al (2010) Activation of antibody drug conjugate MDX-1203 by human carboxylesterase. Meeting of the American Association for Cancer Research
25. Alberts SR, Erlichman C, Reid JM et al (1998) Phase I study of the duocarmycin semisynthetic derivative KW-2189 given daily for five days every six weeks. Clin Cancer Res 4(9):2111–2117
26. Gerber H-P, Kung-Sutherland M, Stone I et al (2009) Potent antitumor activity of the anti-CD19 auristatin antibody drug conjugate hBU12-vcMMAE against rituximab-sensitive and -resistant lymphomas. Blood 113(18):4352–4361
27. Rao C, Pan C, Vangipuram R et al (2010) Efficacy and toxicity of an anti-CD19 antibody drug conjugate. Annual Meeting of the American Association for Cancer Research, Washington, DC, p. 2452
28. Sharkey RM, Govindan SV, Cardillo TM, Goldenberg DM (2012) Epratuzumab-SN-38: a new antibody-drug conjugate for the therapy of hematologic malignancies. Mol Cancer Ther 11(1):224–234
29. Leonard JP, Goldenberg DM (2007) Preclinical and clinical evaluation of epratuzumab (anti-CD22 IgG) in B-cell malignancies. Oncogene 26(25):3704–3713
30. Traczewski P, Rudnicka L (2011) Treatment of systemic lupus erythematosus with epratuzumab. Br J Clin Pharmacol 71(2):175–182
31. Dijoseph JF, Dougher MM, Armellino DC et al (2007) CD20-specific antibody-targeted chemotherapy of non-Hodgkin's B-cell lymphoma using calicheamicin-conjugated rituximab. Cancer Immunol Immunother 56(7):1107–1117
32. Law C-L, Cerveny CG, Gordon KA et al (2004) Efficient elimination of B-lineage lymphomas by anti-CD20-auristatin conjugates. Clin Cancer Res 10(23):7842–7851
33. Polson AG, Calemine-Fenaux J, Chan P et al (2009) Antibody-drug conjugates for the treatment of non-Hodgkin's lymphoma: target and linker-drug selection. Cancer Res 69(3):2358–2364
34. Krop IE, Beeram M, Modi S et al (2010) Phase I study of trastuzumab-DM1, an HER2 antibody-drug conjugate, given every 3 weeks to patients with HER2-positive metastatic breast cancer. J Clin Oncol 28(16):2698–2704
35. Zheng B, Fuji RN, Elkins K et al (2009) In vivo effects of targeting CD79b with antibodies and antibody-drug conjugates. Mol Cancer Ther 8(10):2937–2946
36. Dornan D, Bennett F, Chen Y et al (2009) Therapeutic potential of an anti-CD79b antibody-drug conjugate, anti-CD79b-vc-MMAE, for the treatment of non-Hodgkin lymphoma. Blood 114(13):2721–2729
37. Polson AG, Yu SF, Elkins K et al (2007) Antibody-drug conjugates targeted to CD79 for the treatment of non-Hodgkin lymphoma. Blood 110(2):616–623

Chapter 9
Targeting CD19 with SAR3419, an anti-CD19-Maytansinoid Conjugate for the Treatment of B Cell Malignancies

John M. Lambert, Veronique Blanc, Nathalie Le Bail, and Anne Bousseau

Introduction

CD19 is a 95 kDa type 1 transmembrane gylcoprotein that is a member of the immunoglobulin superfamily of cell surface proteins [1]. It contains two extracellular immunoglobulin-like domains and an extensive cytoplasmic domain. Expression of CD19 is highly restricted to cells of B-lineage, appearing on the cell surface of early B progenitor cells in the bone marrow, and continuing to be expressed during all stages of differentiation during of B cell ontogeny, until terminal differentiation into the final plasma cell when expression of CD19 is lost [1–5].

On the B cell surface, CD19 associates with CD21, CD81, and CD225 to form the B cell co-receptor complex [6]. The complex assembles with the B cell receptor (BCR) to modulate signal transduction triggered by the BCR [7, 8]. Upon activation, the cytoplasmic domain of CD19 becomes phosphorylated, which causes recruitment of src-family kinases and PI3 kinase to the plasma membrane and activation of pathways that increase intracellular calcium levels, resulting in a decrease in the threshold for antigen receptor signaling [9]. Mutations in CD19 are associated clinically with antibody-deficiency syndromes [10], while CD19-deficient mice have significantly reduced germinal center formation [4]. These observations attest to the critical role of CD19 in regulation of B cell development, activation, and differentiation [2, 5, 9].

J.M. Lambert (✉)
ImmunoGen, Inc., 830 Winter Street, Waltham, MA 02451, USA
e-mail: john.lambert@immunogen.com

V. Blanc • N. Le Bail • A. Bousseau
Sanofi Oncology, Vitry sur Seine, France
e-mails: Veronique.blanc@sanofi.com; Nathalie.lebail@sanofi.com; Anne.bousseau@sanofi.com

G.L. Phillips (ed.), *Antibody-Drug Conjugates and Immunotoxins: From Pre-Clinical Development to Therapeutic Applications*, Cancer Drug Discovery and Development,
DOI 10.1007/978-1-4614-5456-4_9,

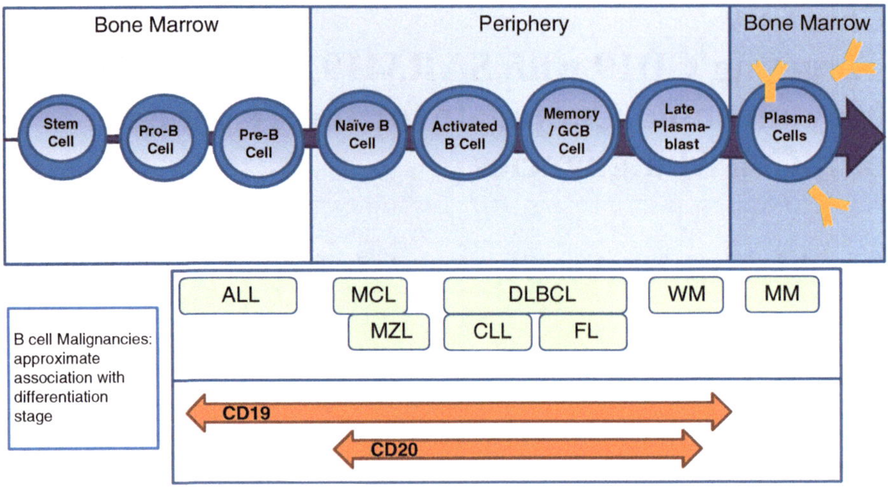

Fig. 9.1 Schematic representation of B cell ontogeny. A simplified cartoon of B lineage differentiation to show the approximate expression pattern of CD19, compared with that of CD20, during differentiation, based on published information [2, 64]. The approximate positions of B cell malignancies associated with different B lineage differentiation stages are also indicated

CD19 expression is maintained in B-lineage cells that have undergone malignant transformation, including all subtypes of B cell lymphoma from indolent phenotypes such as follicular lymphoma to aggressive phenotypes such as diffuse large B cell lymphoma (DLBCL), as well as B cell chronic lymphocytic leukemia and non-T acute lymphoblastic leukemia [3, 11]. Since CD19 is expressed on the earliest recognizable B-lineage cells and persists throughout B cell maturation until the final plasma cell, it is an exquisitely selective target that covers a wider range of B lymphoid malignancies than CD20, the target for rituximab (Fig. 9.1).

Anti-CD19 Antibodies as Therapeutics for B Cell Malignancies

Many approaches to exploit anti-CD19 monoclonal antibodies to treat B cell malignancies have been explored since the 1980s. However, as yet there is no approved anti-CD19 antibody therapeutic. Recent innovations in antibody engineering have yielded a number of promising new approaches to enhancing the potency of "naked" anti-CD19-targeting antibodies that are undergoing current evaluation in clinical trials [12–15]. Unlike rituximab, such antibodies display little direct ability to induce apoptosis or inhibit B cell proliferation, their antitumor activity being principally via mediation of antibody-dependent cellular cytotoxicity (ADCC). Antibodies such as MEDI-55 and MOR-208 that are currently undergoing clinical testing have been engineered for enhanced ADCC by enhancing the affinity of IgG1 antibodies for the FcγRIII, either by glycoengineering approaches [13] or by amino acid substitution in the Fc domain of the antibodies [14].

Bispecific antibodies are another approach to antibody engineering that can exploit the specificity of anti-CD19 antibodies for cancer treatment. By coupling an anti-CD19 binding domain of an antibody to an antibody-binding domain selective for a target on a T cell or an NK cell, one can attract cytotoxic immune effector cells to bind to and kill malignant B cells [16, 17]. The most advanced of these compounds, blinatumomab, is a bi-specific molecule with an anti-CD19 single chain variable antibody domain (scFv) fused to an anti-CD3 scFv which targets T cells to CD19-positive cells; it has shown activity in early clinical trials [16, 18].

Development of Anti-CD19 Immunoconjugates

Another approach to enhancing the potency of anti-CD19 antibodies for treatment of B cell malignancies is by conjugation of such antibodies to a cytotoxic moiety for antibody-directed delivery to CD19-expressing cancer cells. Early efforts to exploit the specificity of antibodies to CD19 for therapeutic intervention in B cell malignancies via conjugation to a cytotoxic moiety focused on delivery of potent protein toxins [19–22]. Such antibody–protein toxin conjugates, or immunotoxins, generated from murine monoclonal anti-CD19 antibodies, were developed with different highly potent plant-derived protein toxins including ricin, in the form of ricin A chain or blocked ricin [19–21, 23, 24], and single chain ribosome-inactivating proteins such as gelonin [25], pokeweed activated protein [22], and saporin [26]. The anti-CD19 immunotoxin that received the most extensive evaluation in clinical testing was a blocked ricin conjugate, anti-B4-bR [20, 27–36]. Early phase I clinical trials showed one complete remission, two partial remissions, and several transient biological responses [20]. However subsequent phase I and phase II trials showed no obvious activity [27–34], and a phase III trial in the setting of minimal residual disease post-autologous bone marrow transplant (BMT) failed to support a role for anti-B4-bR as consolidation therapy after BMT [35]. Among the factors that may have limited efficacy was that the majority of patients developed anti-mouse Ig and anti-ricin antibodies that precluded treatment beyond two 7-day cycles of treatment, despite the fact that these patients were significantly immunocompromised from their B cell disease and prior therapies [29, 35].

Early attempts at developing ADCs by conjugating small molecular weight payloads to murine monoclonal anti-CD19 antibodies utilized cytotoxic effector molecules such as idarubicin [37] and the tyrosine kinase inhibitor, genistein [38]. However, the clinical effectiveness of such compounds was limited by development of human anti-mouse Ig antibodies [39] and by the relatively poor potency of the payloads [40, 41]. From the early work with immunotoxins and immunoconjugates, it became apparent that successful development of ADCs would require non-immunogenic antibodies to allow multiple dosing, as well as payloads of greater cytotoxic potency [40–42]. These innovations led to the development of an anti-CD19 ADC which

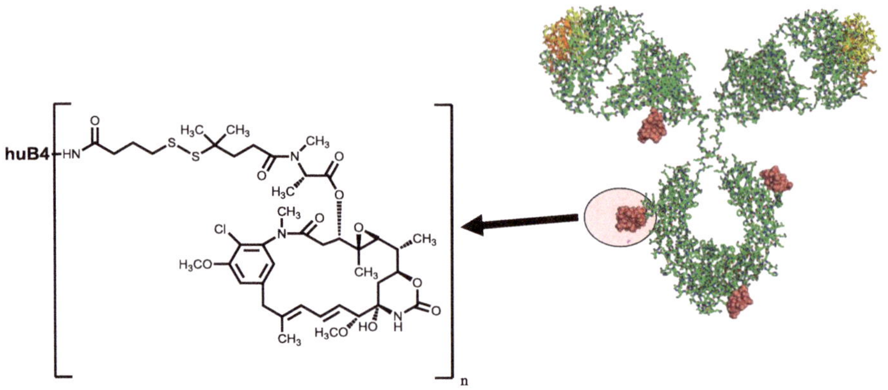

Fig. 9.2 Structure of SAR3419. A model of an IgG1 antibody conjugated to four molecules of maytansinoid (*salmon-colored* space-filling structures) to illustrate the general structure of an antibody–maytansinoid conjugate. Residues of the complementarity-determining region of the heavy chain and light chain of the antibody model are colored *orange* and *yellow*, respectively. The chemical structure of DM4 linked via the SPDB linker to an amino group of a lysine amino acid residue is shown. SAR3419 contains an average of 3.5 molecules of DM4 per molecule of antibody, with a binomial distribution of DM4 loading, as shown for other maytansinoid ADCs [65]

utilized a potent maytansinoid payload and a humanized antibody. This compound, SAR3419, overcomes many of the limitations of the earlier CD19-targeting immunotoxins and immunoconjugates. The structure, mechanism of action, as well as preclinical evaluation and early clinical development are the focus of this chapter.

SAR3419: Structure and Mechanism of Action

SAR3419 is composed of a humanized monoclonal IgG1 antibody (huB4) attached to the highly potent cytotoxic agent, the maytansinoid *N*2′-deacetyl-*N*2′-(4-mercapto-4-methyl-1-oxopentyl)maytansine, also known as DM4 [42–44], through reaction with the disulfide-containing linker, *N*-succinimidyl-4-(2-pyridyldithio) butyrate (SPDB). Figure 9.2 shows a schematic representation of the structure of SAR3419 and also shows the chemical structure of its DM4-linker moiety.

The Anti-CD19 Antibody Component of SAR3419

The murine monoclonal antibody, anti-B4, from which huB4 is derived was developed at the Dana-Farber Cancer Institute (Boston, MA) by Nadler and colleagues using human chronic lymphocytic leukemia cells as the immunogen [45]. The anti-B4 antibody binds specifically to CD19 with high affinity, with an apparent dissociation constant of about 2 to 3×10^{-10} M measured under nonequilibrium conditions, while that measured under conditions where full equilibrium was reached resulted in an estimated value of 8×10^{-12} M [46]. The murine antibody was humanized by the method of immunoglobulin variable domain resurfacing [47, 48]. The humanized antibody, huB4, is indistinguishable from the murine anti-B4 antibody in its binding properties measured in a variety of assay formats [47, 48].

The Cytotoxic "Payload" Component of SAR3419

Maytansine, the first compound of a class of benzoansamacrolide antibiotics called maytansinoids [43, 49], is a highly cytotoxic natural product that binds to tubulin and inhibits microtubule assembly, resulting in arrest of cells at mitosis and, ultimately, in cell death [50]. Maytansinoids bind to tubulin at a similar site as the *Vinca* alkaloids, although many maytansinoids are 100–1,000-fold more cytotoxic towards cell lines in vitro than vincristine or vinblastine [41, 43]. Maytansine was extensively tested clinically, and while some responses were documented, development was ultimately discontinued for the lack of a therapeutic window [51].

Although maytansine was not effective in clinical trials, its very high cytotoxic potency made it an attractive candidate as a payload for an ADC approach [40–42]. A series of new maytansinoids bearing a thiol or disulfide substituent were synthesized and several of these were found to be similar in potency to maytansine itself in vitro [43], with EC_{50} values in the picomolar range on many cancer cell lines. The hindered thiol-containing maytansinoid DM4 was selected as the payload component for SAR3419 (see Fig. 9.2).

The Linker Component of SAR3419 and Conjugation

The huB4 antibody was modified by the SPDB linker; the *N*-hydroxysuccinimide ester group reacts with amino groups of lysine amino acid residues in the antibody forming stable amide bonds that introduce pyridyldithio groups into the antibody. These provide the sites of attachment for DM4 to the antibody through the linker via thiol-disulfide exchange reactions to form a hindered disulfide-containing linkage. The SPDB linker/DM4 combination was selected to "arm" the huB4 antibody to create SAR3419 based on its superior activity as assessed in vivo compared with a number of other combinations of linker and maytansinoid in studies analogous to those described by Kellogg and colleagues [42, 52]. The linker reaction is controlled so that SAR3419 contains an average of about 3.5 maytansinoid molecules per antibody molecule. The overall molecular weight of SAR3419 is about 150,000; its DM4 content is about 1.8% by weight.

Mechanism of Action of SAR3419

SAR3419 displays potent in vitro cytotoxicity towards CD19-positive lymphoma cell lines, with EC_{50} values in the nanomolar to subnanomolar range [44, 53]. Within 24 h of exposure of cells to SAR3419, the majority of cells were arrested at the G2/M phase of the cell cycle, followed by increased apoptotic cell death from 24 to 48 h [44], as expected upon delivery of a tubulin-acting agent into cells. Experiments with SAR3419 in which the DM4 moiety was radiolabeled [54, 55], provided further insight into the mechanism of action. The conjugate binds to CD19 on the cell surface, is internalized, presumably via endocytosis and is routed into the lysosomal degradation pathway where the huB4 antibody moiety is completely degraded to its constituent amino acids, thus yielding lysine–SPDB–DM4 as the initial maytansinoid metabolite within cells [55]. Over several hours, likely in the reducing environment of the cytoplasm of the cell, the disulfide in the lysine–SPDB–DM4 metabolite is subject to further cleavage by thiol-disulfide exchange reactions to release the free thiol, DM4. Erickson and colleagues have shown that intracellular DM4 is readily methylated in cancer cells by an endogenous *S*-methyl-transferase to form *S*-methyl-DM4 [54]. This final metabolite of SAR3419 processing in CD19-positive cells has potency similar to that of maytansine itself when evaluated for cytotoxic potency in vitro on different tumor cell lines [43, 56, 57].

The huB4 component of SAR3419 induces ADCC, an activity that was conserved following conjugation to DM4 [44]. Neither the naked antibody, nor its conjugate, shows any complement-dependent cytotoxicity [44]. The "naked" huB4 antibody has not been shown to exhibit any direct antiproliferative or pro-apoptotic activity on cell lines in vitro prior to its conjugation with maytansinoids [44, 53].

Activity of SAR3419 in Preclinical Models

SAR3419 has shown efficacy in several different models of lymphoma, including Burkitt's lymphoma (Namalwa, Ramos, and Raji cell lines) and DLBCL (RL, WSU-DLCL2, and WSU-FSCCL models) implanted into SCID mice as either subcutaneous or intravenous (systemic) models [53, 58]. The high level of activity in preclinical models is exemplified in Fig. 9.3, which shows a dose–response study of the antitumor activity of SAR3419 in the Ramos subcutaneous lymphoma xenograft model. A *single* dose of 7 mg/kg (antibody dose) of the conjugate produced complete regressions in 100% of the mice, while at higher doses the majority (at 13 mg/kg) or all (at 27 mg/kg) of mice remained tumor free for at least 100 days postinoculation. All doses were well tolerated as evidenced by no loss in body weight. A nonbinding control conjugate showed no activity up to 13 mg/kg and only minimal activity at the highest dose tested. In several models, it was established that unconjugated DM4, at doses equivalent to the doses of SAR3419 that result in complete regressions, showed no significant antitumor activity, indicating that conjugation of

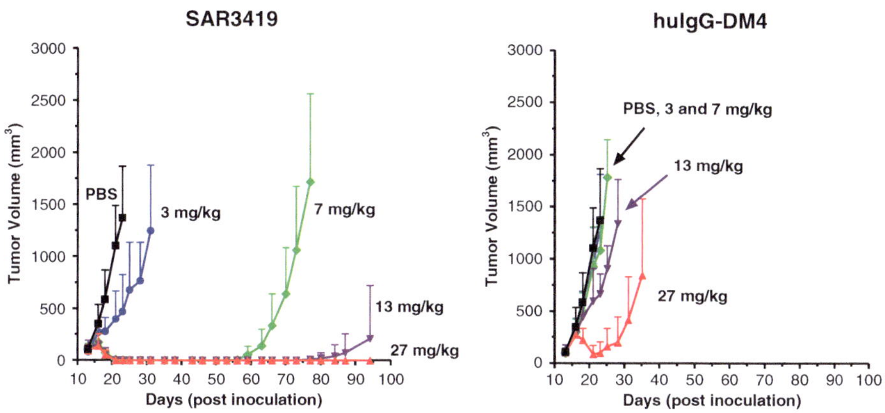

Fig. 9.3 Specificity of dose-dependent activity of SAR3419 against established CD19-positive Ramos tumor xenografts in SCID mice. SCID mice were inoculated subcutaneously with Ramos B lymphoma cells. Groups of mice (6 per group) were treated with a *single* intravenous injection of either SAR3419 (*left panel*) or a nonbinding control conjugate (huIgG-DM4) (*right panel*), at the doses indicated (given as mg of antibody in the conjugate), when the xenografts were approximately 100 mm^3 in size. One group received vehicle (*PBS*) which is plotted in both graphs of mean tumor volume of each group versus day postinoculation

DM4 to the anti-CD19 antibody was critical for delivery of sufficient maytansinoid to the tumor in vivo to induce tumor shrinkage [44, 53, 58]. Large doses, 30–50 mg/kg, of the "naked" huB4 antibody were completely inactive [44, 53]. The antitumor activity of a 10 mg/kg dose of SAR3419 can be completely blocked by coadministration with an excess (50 mg/kg) of "naked" huB4 antibody, demonstrating that the antitumor activity of in vivo is mediated by its binding to CD19 on the tumor cell surface [44, 58]. The preclinical results provide a strong rationale for the development of SAR3419 for clinical use, the activity of the immunoconjugate comparing very favorably with rituximab or with standard chemotherapeutic treatments in a variety of xenograft models [44, 53, 58].

Early Clinical Development of SAR3419

SAR3419 has been evaluated clinically in two phase I dose escalation studies exploring two different schedules of administration, every 3 weeks [59, 60] and weekly [61], in patients with refractory/relapsed B cell non-Hodgkin's lymphoma expressing CD19.

The trial of administration of SAR3419 once every 3 weeks for up to six cycles showed that the maximum tolerated dose (MTD) was 160 mg/m^2 (~4.3 mg/kg), a dose-level subsequently used to treat an expanded cohort of 16 patients [44, 59, 60]. Of the 35 response-evaluable patients who completed at least two cycles of treatment, tumor shrinkage was reported in twenty-six patients (74%), with six objective responses including complete responses (CR) [59, 60]. Notably, seven of 15 patients with rituximab-refractory disease showed tumor shrinkage, with one objective response. Tumor shrinkage was seen in a variety of lymphoma subtypes including follicular lymphoma and marginal zone lymphoma [44, 60]. The dose-limiting toxicity (DLT) at doses >200 mg/m^2 was reversible ocular toxicity that did not preclude continued dosing at 208 mg/m^2 with dose delays of 1–2 weeks, with no other clinically significant grade 3 or 4 toxicities reported [59, 60]. The reversible ocular toxicity, typically in the second cycle or beyond, was blurred vision associated with observed microcystic corneal deposits, very similar in nature to the reported reversible DLTs observed for the phase I studies with albumin-bound paclitaxel that were found to be manageable at the dosing regimen used for its phase III trial [62, 63]. As with other antibody–maytansinoid conjugates, there was no clinically significant myelosuppression (38 patients evaluable for safety), suggesting that SAR3419 may be readily combined with conventional chemotherapy regimens [42, 44, 59]. The half-life of SAR3419 in these patients was estimated to be about 1 week with dose-proportional pharmacokinetics and low clearance of about 0.5 L/d/m^2 [44, 59, 60], giving SAR3419 the greatest reported exposure at MTD of any ADC yet reported. These early results from a phase I trial demonstrated promising activity and tolerability, especially considering the wide dose range (10–270 mg/m^2), the heavy pretreatment of these patients (28% had prior stem cell transplant), and the mixed histology of those enrolled [59, 60].

A second study with a schedule of weekly dosing for 8 weeks, with the possibility of a further 4 weeks if warranted for clinical benefit, established an MTD of 55 mg/m^2 (about 1.5 mg/kg/week) [61]. The dose intensity reached was similar to that of the 3-week dosing schedule. Pharmacokinetic analysis showed a half-life of 8–9 days, with accumulation noted until a steady state C_{max} was reached after about 4 cycles [61]. A total of 21 patients received the 55 mg/m^2 dose, from a total of 44 patients treated at doses ranging from 10 to 70 mg/m^2 per week. Of 40 patients receiving doses of ≥14 mg/m^2 per week, 12 (30%) achieved an objective response including 6 with CR/CRu [44, 61]. The response rate at the MTD was 33% (7/21), with responses seen in both follicular lymphoma and DLBCL [61]. SAR3419 was well tolerated on this dosing schedule, with a median number of doses delivered per patient of eight overall, and a median relative dose intensity of 0.96 at the MTD, with investigators commenting on the noteworthy lack of clinically significant myelosuppression [61]. While reversible ocular toxicity was reported on this dosing regimen, it was with a late onset (mainly post cycle 7 or 8) and the incidence and severity of the observations was markedly reduced relative to the 3-week schedule [44, 61]. A modified schedule consisting of four weekly doses of 55 mg/m^2 followed by four biweekly doses, based on pharmacokinetic simulations and pharmacodynamic observations, was ongoing at the time of data cutoff, to evaluate an approach to reduce even further the incidence of this toxicity [44, 61]. While these results are not yet reported, the sponsor has initiated three phase II trials in the latter half of 2011, evaluating SAR3419 as a single agent in DLBCL and in ALL, as well as in combination with rituximab in DLBCL (http://www.clinicaltrials.gov).

Summary

For nearly 15 years, rituximab has had a profound positive impact in treatment of non-Hodgkin's lymphoma. However, a significant number of patients ultimately relapse, and, in the effort to improve therapy, several strategies are being explored in clinical and discovery research for targeting B cell lymphomas using monoclonal antibodies directed to B cell antigens. CD19 is the target that was exploited in developing SAR3419, an ADC designed to deliver the potent tubulin poison, the maytansinoid DM4, to malignant B cells. The highly restricted expression of CD19 for B cells has the potential to allow effective treatment of B cell malignancies with SAR3419, without toxicity to other hematologic non-B cell compartments.

The preliminary clinical activity shown by SAR3419 in two phase I clinical trials is encouraging for its future development [44, 59–61]. In a heavily pretreated phase I patient population, there were objective responses seen in both follicular lymphoma and DLBCL, including complete responses. There was a low incidence of clinically significant hematological toxicity, and the reversible ocular toxicity that defined the DLT on the 3-week schedule appeared to be manageable on an alternative dosing regimen. The potential of SAR3419 is now being evaluated in a multi-trial phase II program which started in the second half of 2011. It will include a robust assessment of activity in patients with relapsed DLBCL, a patient population where responses were seen in the phase I trials and where there is a clear unmet medical need.

References

1. Tedder TF, Issacs CM (1989) Isolation of cDNAs encoding the CD19 antigen of human and mouse B lymphocytes. A new member of the immunoglobulin superfamily. J Immunol 143:712–717
2. Uckun FM (1990) Regulation of human B-cell ontogeny. Blood 76:1908–1923
3. Scheuermann RH, Racila E (1995) CD19 antigen in leukemia and lymphoma diagnosis and immunotherapy. Leuk Lymphoma 18:385–397
4. Sato S, Steeber DA, Jansen PJ, Tedder TF (1997) CD19 expression levels regulate B lymphocyte development: human CD19 restores normal function in mice lacking endogenous CD19. J Immunol 158:4662–4669
5. Sato S, Steeber DA, Tedder TF (1995) The CD19 signal transduction molecule is a response regulator of B-lymphocyte differentiation. Proc Natl Acad Sci USA 92:11558–11562
6. Bradbury LE, Kansas GS, Levy S, Evans RL, Tedder TF (1992) The CD19/CD21 signal transducing complex of human B lymphocytes includes the target of antiproliferative antibody-1 and Leu-13 molecules. J Immunol 149:2841–2850
7. Pesando JM, Bouchard LS, McMaster BE (1989) CD19 is functionally and physically associated with surface immunoglobulin. J Exp Med 170:2159–2164
8. Carter RH, Tuveson DA, Park DJ, Rhee SG, Fearon DT (1991) The CD19 complex of B lymphocytes. Activation of phospholipase C by a protein tyrosine kinase-dependent pathway that can be enhanced by the membrane IgM complex. J Immunol 147:3663–3671
9. Carter RH, Fearon DT (1992) CD19: lowering the threshold for antigen receptor stimulation of B lymphocytes. Science 256:105–107
10. van Zelm MC, Reisli I, van der Burg M, Castaño D, van Noesel CJ, van Tol MJ et al (2006) An antibody-deficiency syndrome due to mutations in the CD19 gene. N Engl J Med 354:1901–1912

11. Anderson KC, Bates MP, Slaughenhoupt BL, Pinkus GS, Schlossman SF, Nadler LM (1984) Expression of human B-cell associated antigens on leukemias and lymphomas: a model of human B-cell differentiation. Blood 63:1424–1433
12. Yazawa N, Hamaguchi Y, Poe JC, Tedder TF (2005) Immunotherapy using unconjugated CD19 monoclonal antibodies in animal models for B lymphocyte malignancies and autoimmune disease. Proc Natl Acad Sci USA 102:15178–15183
13. Herbst R, Wang Y, Gallagher S, Mittereder N, Kuta E, Damschroder M et al (2010) B-cell depletion in vitro and in vivo with an afucosylated anti-CD19 antibody. J Pharmacol Exp Ther 335:213–222
14. Horton HM, Bernett MJ, Pong E, Peipp M, Karki S, Chu SY et al (2008) Potent in vitro and in vivo activity of an Fc-engineered anti-CD19 monoclonal antibody against lymphoma and leukemia. Cancer Res 68:8049–8057
15. Awan FT, Lapalombella R, Trotta R, Butchar JP, Yu B, Benson DM Jr et al (2010) CD19 targeting of chronic lymphocytic leukemia with a novel Fc-domain-engineered monoclonal antibody. Blood 115:1204–1213
16. Nagorsen D, Baeuerle PA (2011) Immunomodulatory therapy of cancer with T cell-engaging BiTE antibody blinatumomab. Exp Cell Res 317:1255–1260
17. Kipriyanov SM, Cochlovius B, Schäfer HJ, Moldenhauer G, Bähre A, Le Gall F et al (2002) Synergistic antitumor effect of bispecific CD19 x CD3 and CD19 x CD16 diabodies in a preclinical model of non-Hodgkin's lymphoma. J Immunol 169:137–144
18. Bargou R, Leo E, Zugmaier G, Klinger M, Goebeler M, Knop S et al (2008) Tumor regression in cancer patients by very low doses of a T cell-engaging antibody. Science 321:974–977
19. Lambert JM, Goldmacher VS, Collinson AR, Nadler LM, Blättler WA (1991) An immunotoxin prepared with blocked ricin: a natural plant toxin adapted for therapeutic use. Cancer Res 51:6236–6242
20. Grossbard ML, Freedman AS, Ritz J, Coral F, Goldmacher VS, Eliseo L et al (1992) Serotherapy of B-cell neoplasms with anti-B4-blocked ricin: a phase I trial of daily bolus infusion. Blood 79:576–585
21. Grossbard ML, Press OW, Appelbaum FR, Bernstein ID, Nadler LM (1992) Monoclonal antibody-based therapies of leukemia and lymphoma. Blood 80:863–878
22. Uckun FM, Manivel C, Arthur D, Chelstrom LM, Finnegan D, Tuel-Ahlgren L et al (1992) In vivo efficacy of B43 (anti-CD19)-pokeweed antiviral protein immunotoxin against human pre-B cell acute lymphoblastic leukemia in mice with severe combined immunodeficiency. Blood 79:2201–2214
23. Ghetie MA, May RD, Till M, Uhr JW, Ghetie V, Knowles PP et al (1988) Evaluation of ricin A chain-containing immunotoxins directed against CD19 and CD22 antigens on normal and malignant human B-cells as potential reagents for in vivo therapy. Cancer Res 48:2610–2617
24. Messmann RA, Vitetta ES, Headlee D, Senderowicz AM, Figg WD, Schindler J et al (2000) A phase I study of combination therapy with immunotoxins IgG-HD37-defucosylated ricin A chain (dgA) and IgG-RFB4-dgA (Combotox) in patients with refractory CD19(+), CD22(+) B cell lymphoma. Clin Cancer Res 6:1302–1313
25. Goldmacher VS, Scott CF, Lambert JM, McIntyre GD, Blättler WA, Collinson AR et al (1989) Cytotoxicity of gelonin and its conjugates with antibodies is determined by the extent of their endocytosis. J Cell Physiol 141:222–234
26. Flavell DJ, Flavell SU, Boehm DA, Emery L, Noss A, Ling NR et al (1995) Preclinical studies with the anti-CD19-saporin immunotoxin BU12-SAPORIN for the treatment of human-B-cell tumours. Br J Cancer 72(6):1373–1379
27. Grossbard ML, Lambert JM, Goldmacher VS, Spector NL, Kinsella J, Eliseo L et al (1993) Anti-B4-blocked ricin: a phase I trial of 7-day continuous infusion in patients with B-cell neoplasms. J Clin Oncol 11:726–737
28. Grossbard ML, Gribben JG, Freedman AS, Lambert JM, Kinsella J, Rabinowe SN et al (1993) Adjuvant immunotoxin therapy with anti-B4-blocked ricin after autologous bone marrow transplantation for patients with B-cell non-Hodgkin's lymphoma. Blood 81:2263–2271
29. Grossbard ML, Multani PS, Freedman AS, O'Day S, Gribben JG, Rhuda C et al (1999) A phase II study of adjuvant therapy with anti-B4-blocked ricin after autologous bone marrow

transplantation for patients with relapsed B-cell non-Hodgkin's lymphoma. Clin Cancer Res 5:2392–2398
30. Longo DL, Duffey PL, Gribben JG, Jaffe ES, Curti BD, Gause BL et al (2000) Combination chemotherapy followed by an immunotoxin (anti-B4-blocked ricin) in patients with indolent lymphoma: results of a phase II study. Cancer J 6:146–150
31. Scadden DT, Schenkein DP, Bernstein Z, Luskey B, Doweiko J, Tulpule A, Levine AM (1998) Immunotoxin combined with chemotherapy for patients with AIDS-related non-Hodgkin's lymphoma. Cancer 83:2580–2587
32. Dinndorf P, Krailo M, Liu-Mares W, Frierdich S, Sondel P, Reaman G (2001) Phase I trial of anti-B4-blocked ricin in pediatric patients with leukemia and lymphoma. J Immunother 24:511–516
33. Szatrowski TP, Dodge RK, Reynolds C, Westbrook CA, Frankel SR, Sklar J et al (2003) Lineage specific treatment of adult patients with acute lymphoblastic leukemia in first remission with anti-B4-blocked ricin or high-dose cytarabine: Cancer and Leukemia Group B Study 9311. Cancer 97:1471–1480
34. Tsimberidou AM, Giles FJ, Kantarjian HM, Keating MJ, O'Brien SM (2003) Anti-B4-blocked ricin post chemotherapy in patients with chronic lymphocytic leukemia—long-term follow-up of a monoclonal antibody-based approach to residual disease. Leuk Lymphoma 44:1719–1725
35. Furman RR, Grossbard ML, Johnson JL, Pecora AL, Cassileth PA, Jung SH et al (2011) A phase III study of anti-B4-blocked ricin as adjuvant therapy post-autologous bone marrow transplant: CALGB 9254. Leuk Lymphoma 52:587–596
36. Roy DC, Perreault C, Bélanger R, Gyger M, Le Houillier C, Blättler WA et al (1995) Elimination of B-lineage leukemia and lymphoma cells from bone marrow grafts using anti-B4-blocked-ricin immunotoxin. J Clin Immunol 15:51–57
37. Rowland AJ, Pietersz GA, McKenzie IF (1993) Preclinical investigation of the antitumour effects of anti-CD19-idarubicin immunoconjugates. Cancer Immunol Immunother 37:195–202
38. Uckun FM, Evans WE, Forsyth CJ, Waddick KG, Ahlgren LT, Chelstrom LM et al (1995) Biotherapy of B-cell precursor leukemia by targeting genistein to CD19-associated tyrosine kinases. Science 267:886–891
39. Uckun FM, Messinger Y, Chen CL, O'Neill K, Myers DE, Goldman F et al (1999) Treatment of therapy-refractory B-lineage acute lymphoblastic leukemia with an apoptosis-inducing CD19-directed tyrosine kinase inhibitor. Clin Cancer Res 5:3906–3913
40. Chari RVJ (1998) Targeted delivery of chemotherapeutics: tumor-activated prodrug therapy. Adv Drug Delivery Rev 31:89–105
41. Lambert JM (2005) Drug-conjugated monoclonal antibodies for the treatment of cancer. Curr Opin Pharmacol 5:543–549
42. Lambert JM (2010) Antibody-maytansinoid conjugates: a new strategy for the treatment of cancer. Drugs Fut 35:471–480
43. Widdison WC, Wilhelm SD, Cavanagh EE, Whiteman KR, Leece BA, Kovtun Y et al (2006) Semisynthetic maytansine analogues for the targeted treatment of cancer. J Med Chem 49:4392–4408
44. Blanc V, Bousseau A, Caron A, Carrez C, Lutz RJ, Lambert JM (2011) SAR3419: an anti-CD19-maytansinoid immunoconjugate for the treatment of B-cell malignancies. Clin Cancer Res 17:6448–6458
45. Nadler LM, Anderson KC, Marti G, Bates M, Park E, Daley JF, Schlossman SF (1983) B4, a human B lymphocyte-associated antigen expressed on normal, mitogen activated, and malignant B lymphocytes. J Immunol 131:244–250
46. Vater CA, Reid K, Bartle LM, Goldmacher VS (1995) Characterization of antibody binding to cell surface antigens using a plasma membrane-bound plate assay. Anal Biochem 224:39–50
47. Roguska MA, Pedersen JT, Keddy CA, Henry AH, Searle SJ, Lambert JM et al (1994) Humanization of murine monoclonal antibodies through variable domain resurfacing. Proc Natl Acad Sci USA 91:969–973
48. Roguska MA, Pedersen JT, Henry AH, Searle SMJ, Roja CM, Avery B et al (1996) A comparison of two murine monoclonal antibodies humanized by CDR-grafting and variable domain resurfacing. Protein Eng 9:895–904, Erratum: Protein Eng. 1997; 10:181

49. Kupchan SM, Komoda Y, Court WA, Thomas GT, Smith RM, Karim A et al (1972) Maytansine, a novel antileukemic ansa macrolide from *Maytenus ovatus*. J Am Chem Soc 94:1354–1356
50. Remillard S, Rebhun LI, Howie GA, Kupchan SM (1975) Antimitotic activity of the potent tumor inhibitor maytansine. Science 189:1002–1005
51. Issell BF, Crooke ST (1978) Maytansine. Cancer Treat Rev 5:199–207
52. Kellogg BA, Garrett L, Kovtun Y, Lai KC, Leece B, Miller M et al (2011) Disulfide-linked antibody-maytansinoid conjugates: optimization of *in vivo* activity by varying the steric hindrance at carbon atoms adjacent to the disulfide linkage. Bioconjug Chem 22:717–727
53. Lutz RJ, Zuany-Amorim C, Vrignaud P, Mayo MF, Guerif S, Xie H et al (2006) Preclinical evaluation of SAR3419 (huB4-DM4), an anti-CD19-maytansinoid immunoconjugate, for the treatment of B-cell lymphoma. Proc Am Assoc Cancer Res 47 (Abstract 3731)
54. Erickson HK, Park PU, Widdison WC, Kovtun YV, Garrett LM, Hoffman K et al (2006) Antibody-maytansinoid conjugates are activated in targeted cancer cells by lysosomal degradation and linker-dependent intracellular processing. Cancer Res 66:4426–4433
55. Erickson HK, Provenzano CA, Mayo MF, Widdison WC, Audette C, Leece B et al (2009) Target-cell processing of the anti-CD19 antibody maytansinoid conjugate SAR3419 in preclinical models. Proc Am Assoc Cancer Res (Abstr 5473)
56. Lopus M, Oroudjev E, Wilson L, Wilhelm S, Widdison W, Chari R et al (2010) Maytansine and cellular metabolites of antibody-maytansinoid conjugates strongly suppress microtubule dynamics by binding to microtubules. Mol Cancer Ther 9:2689–2699
57. Erickson HK, Widdison WC, Mayo MF, Whiteman K, Audette C, Wilhelm SD et al (2010) Tumor delivery and *in vivo* processing of disulfide-linked and thioether linked antibody-maytansinoid conjugates. Bioconjug Chem 21:84–92
58. Al Katib AM, Aboukameel A, Mohammad R, Bissery M-C, Zuany-Amorim C (2009) Superior antitumor activity of SAR3419 to rituximab in xenograft models for non-Hodgkin's lymphoma. Clin Cancer Res 15:4038–4045
59. Younes A, Gordon L, Kim S, Romaguera J, Copeland AR, de Castro Farial S et al (2009) Phase I multi-dose escalation study of the anti-CD19 maytansinoid immunoconjugate SAR3419 administered by intravenous (IV) infusion every 3 weeks to patients with relapsed/refractory B-Cell non-Hodgkin's lymphoma (NHL). ASH annual meeting abstracts. Blood 114 (Abstr 585)
60. Younes A, Kim S, Romaguera J, Copeland A, de Castro Farial S, Kwak LW et al (2012) Phase I multi-dose escalation study of the anti-CD19 maytansinoid immunoconjugate SAR3419 administered by intravenous infusion every 3 weeks to patients with relapsed/refractory B-cell lymphoma. J Clin Oncol 30(22):2776–2782
61. Coiffier B, Ribrag V, Dupuis J, Tilly H, Haioun C, Morschhauseret F et al (2011) Phase I/II study of the anti-CD19 maytansinoid immunoconjugate SAR3419 administered weekly to patients with relapsed/refractory B-cell non-Hodgkin's lymphoma (NHL). J Clin Oncol 29(Suppl):Abstr 8017
62. Ibrahim NK, Desai N, Legha S, Soon-Shiong P, Theriault RL, Rivera E et al (2002) Phase I and pharmacokinetic study of ABI-007, a Cremophor-free, protein stabilized, nanoparticle formulation of paclitaxel. Clin Cancer Res 8:1038–1044
63. Gradishar WJ, Tjulandin S, Davidson N, Shaw H, Desai N, Bhar P et al (2005) Phase III of nanoparticle albumin-bound paclitaxel compared with polyethylated castor-oil-based paclitaxel in women with metastatic breast cancer. J Clin Oncol 23:7794–7803
64. Janeway CA, Travers P, Walport M, Shlomchik M (2004) Immunobiology, the Immune System in Health and Disease. 6th Edition, Churchill Livingstone
65. Lazar AC, Wang L, Blättler WA, Amphlett GA, Lambert LM, Zhang W (2005) Analysis of the composition of immunoconjugates using size-exclusion chromatography coupled to mass spectrometry. Rapid Commun Mass Spectrom 19:1806–1814

Chapter 10
Brentuximab Vedotin (SGN-35) for CD30-Positive Malignancies

Andres Forero, Christos Vaklavas, and Albert F. LoBuglio

Introduction

Although the prognosis of patients with Hodgkin's lymphoma (HL) and anaplastic large cell lymphoma (ALCL) has improved over the past decade, there are still subpopulations of these patients with a poor prognosis including HL patients with chemotherapy-refractory disease, HL patients who fail or relapse with high-dose chemotherapy with autologous stem cell rescue and who have less than a 50% overall survival at 10 years [1], HL patients who receive alternate salvage chemotherapy [2–5], and elderly patients with HL who often cannot tolerate aggressive combination therapy. Similarly, patients with relapsed or refractory systemic ALCL (approximately 40–65% of adult patients) have few effective salvage therapies [6, 7]. Thus, there is an unmet medical need for these patients, and the effort is ongoing to develop novel therapeutic strategies.

Unlabeled monoclonal antibodies are the most widely used type of targeted biological therapy as evidenced by the number of such drugs approved for oncologic indications since 1995 [8]. These antibodies are effective against tumor cells through induction of apoptosis, antibody-dependent cellular cytotoxicity, and/or complement-dependent cytotoxicity. However, these antibody therapeutics are seldom curative, encouraging numerous approaches to enhance efficacy [9–11]. One of the strategies to enhance the antitumor activity of monoclonal antibodies is the use of antibody–drug conjugates or ADCs [12, 13]. HL and ALCL express cell membrane CD30 as a potential antibody target.

A. Forero (✉) • C. Vaklavas • A.F. LoBuglio
Comprehensive Cancer Center, University of Alabama at Birmingham NP 2510, 1720 2nd Avenue South Birmingham, Alabama 35294-3300, USA
e-mail: aforero@uab.edu

G.L. Phillips (ed.), *Antibody-Drug Conjugates and Immunotoxins: From Pre-Clinical Development to Therapeutic Applications*, Cancer Drug Discovery and Development, DOI 10.1007/978-1-4614-5456-4_10,

ADCs comprise a human or "humanized" monoclonal antibody conjugated to a cytotoxic drug via a chemical linker [14]. The therapeutic concept of ADCs is to use the antibody as a vehicle to deliver a cytotoxic drug or toxin directly to a tumor cell by means of binding to a target cell surface antigen. ADCs are "prodrugs" requiring intracellular drug release for activation. They have significant potential for enhancing the antitumor activity of antibodies especially in patients with malignant cells resistant to apoptosis induction and/or patients who lack an adequate immune system; in addition, ADCs have the potential of reducing the systemic toxicity of the conjugated drugs. The clinical potential of ADCs has been greatly enhanced by improved choices of targets, more potent drugs in conjunction with linkers of improved stability, and greatly expanded knowledge of ADC tumor cell biology and pharmacology [15–18]. This review will summarize data on brentuximab vedotin (SGN-35), an anti-CD30 ADC for the treatment of HL and ALCL.

CD30 Antigen

CD30, also known as TNFRSF8, is a member of the TNF-receptor (TNF-R) superfamily of proteins that was originally identified as a surface marker for the malignant Reed–Sternberg cells of Hodgkin disease [19]. It is a transmembrane glycoprotein receptor of 120 kDa and is normally found on the surface of mitogen-activated, but not resting, T and B cells, and decidual cells [20–22]. In addition, CD30 has also been detected on a variety of cell types of hematopoietic origin. The CD30 antigen has a very low expression on normal cells but is found on the Reed–Sternberg (RS) cell of HL, on tumor cells of ALCL, and some T cell lymphoproliferative disorders. It is also expressed in embryonal carcinoma but not in seminoma.

While the function of CD30 has not been clearly defined, CD30 has been implicated in both cell death and proliferation [23, 24]. Two studies have shown that monoclonal antibodies directed against CD30 were able to inhibit the growth of HL cells in severe combined immunodeficiency mice in the absence of immune effector cells, suggesting a direct effect of CD30 on tumor cells (apoptosis-inducing characteristics) [24, 25]. Structurally, CD30 does not possess the death domains found in CD95/Fas and TNF receptor 1; the CD30 cytoplasmic tail, however, binds to TNFR-associated factor (TRAF) family members; CD30 has been shown to activate nuclear factor κB (NF-κB), extracellular-regulated kinase (ERK), Jun N-terminal kinase (JNK), and p38 [26–28]. The utility of CD30 as a diagnostic marker for HL and ALCL, its limited expression profile, and its apoptosis-inducing characteristics have led to the investigation of this antigen as a target for monoclonal antibody therapy in patients with CD30-positive hematological malignancies.

Brentuximab Vedotin (SGN-35)

Brentuximab vedotin is an antibody–drug conjugate consisting of the chimeric monoclonal antibody cAC10 and the small molecule anti-tubulin agent monomethylauristatin E (MMAE).

cAC10, also known as SGN30, is an antagonist chimeric monoclonal antibody constructed from the variable region of the anti-CD30 murine antibody AC10 and the human gamma 1 heavy chain and kappa light chain constant regions [24]. SGN-30 has specificity for CD30 that is unique from other anti-CD30 antibodies with antitumor activity in both HL and ALCL cell lines in disseminated and localized xenograft models [24]. It has shown cytotoxic synergism with different chemotherapy agents in vitro including bleomycin, etoposide, and cytarabine [29]. MMAE is a small synthetic analog of the natural product dolastatin 10, binds to tubulin, and inhibits tubulin polymerization. It appears to have little or no immunogenicity. Brentuximab vedotin is produced by the conjugation of MMAE to cAC10. The points of attachment are cysteines produced by mild reduction of the interchain disulfides of the antibody, and the linker consists of a thiol-reactive maleimide, a caproyl spacer, the dipeptide valine–citrulline, and *p*-aminobenzyloxycarbonyl, a self-immolative fragmenting group (Fig. 10.1). The overall average drug-to-antibody mole ratio (MR) is approximately 4. The calculated molecular mass (monoisotopic) for the nominal form of brentuximab vedotin is approximately 153 kDa.

Brentuximab vedotin is proposed to have a multistep mechanism of action that is initiated by binding to the cell surface marker CD30 followed by internalization and trafficking to lysosomes where MMAE is released through proteolytic degradation of the drug linker (Fig. 10.2) [30]. Binding of released MMAE to tubulin disrupts the microtubule network, leading to G2/M phase cell cycle arrest and apoptosis [31].

Preclinical Studies of Brentuximab vedotin (SGN-35)

The ability of brentuximab vedotin to selectively kill CD30-positive cell lines was assessed with human CD30-positive Karpas 299 (anaplastic large cell lymphoma) and L540cy (Hodgkin's lymphoma) cell lines and the CD30-negative WSU-NHL cell line. Brentuximab vedotin was cytotoxic to CD30-positive lines (IC_{50}s of 0.031 and 0.089 nM), but was not effective against the CD30-negative cell line (IC_{50} >6.75 nM). All three cell lines were similarly sensitive to MMAE, suggesting that the lack of sensitivity by WSU-NHL is not attributable to drug resistance.

The in vivo efficacy of brentuximab vedotin was examined in CD30-positive xenograft models; Karpas 299 [32, 33] and L540cy [34] cells were implanted either subcutaneously to model solid tumors or intravenously to model disseminated disease. In the subcutaneous model a dose-dependent delay in tumor growth was observed in the brentuximab vedotin treated groups. When administered separately or together, cAC10 or MMAE did not show tumor growth inhibition compared with

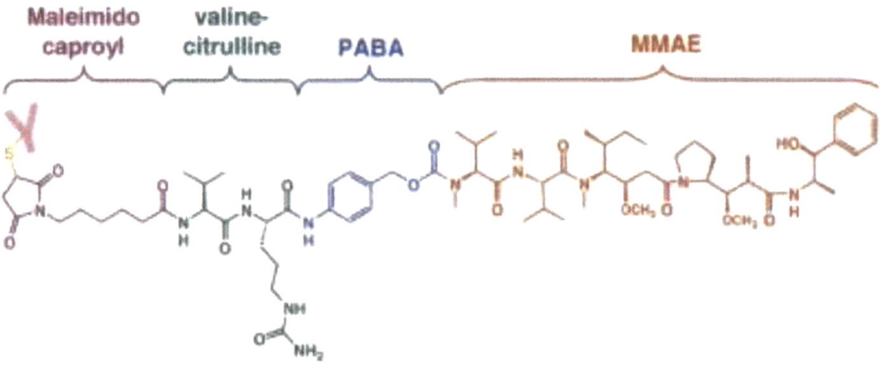

Fig. 10.1 Structure of brentuximab vedotin. Brentuximab vedotin consists of the chimeric mAb cAC10, a linker (consists of a thiol-reactive maleimide, a caproyl spacer, the dipeptide valine–citrulline, and *p*-aminobenzyloxycarbonyl) and the small molecule anti-tubulin agent monomethylauristatin E. Image provided by Seattle Genetics

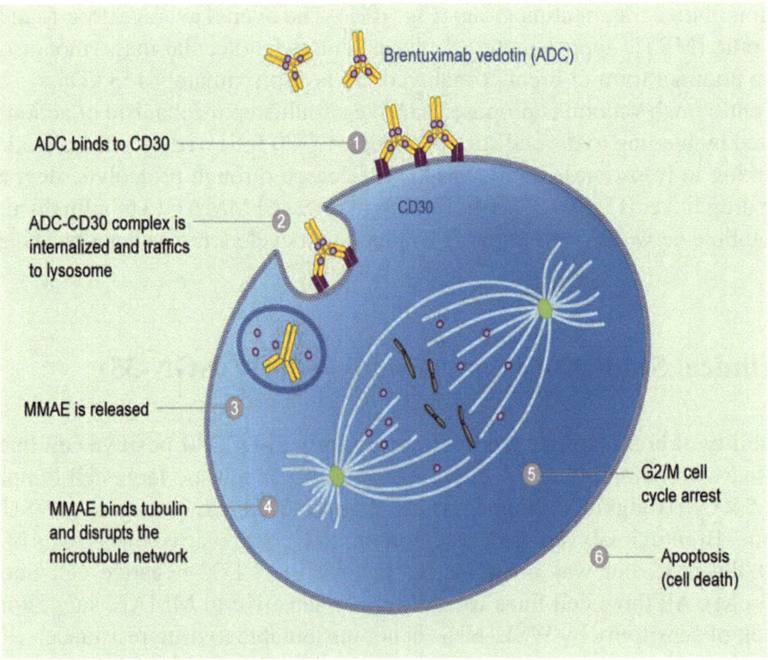

Fig. 10.2 Brentuximab vedotin mechanism of action. The cytotoxin MMAE is released from the antibody–drug conjugate intracellularly via lysosomal protease cleavage at the valine–citrulline dipeptide. Image provided by Seattle Genetics

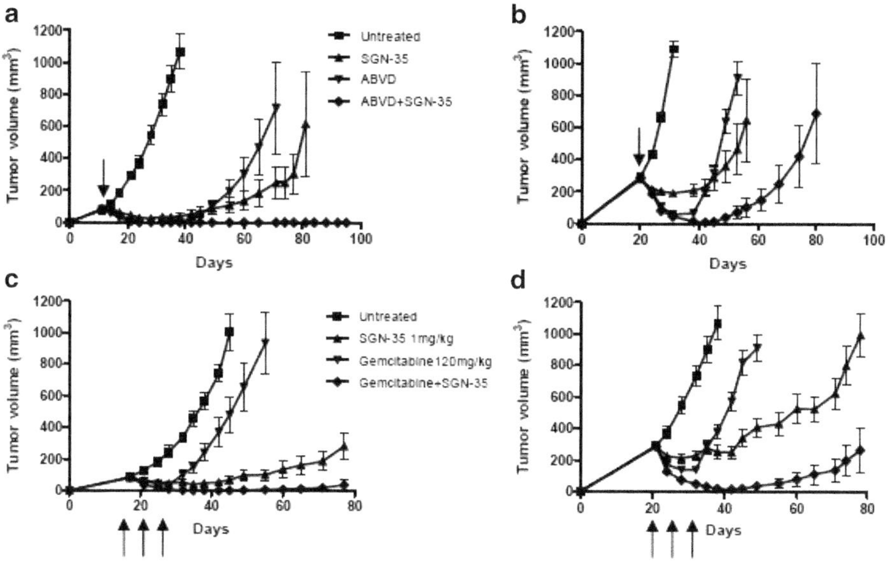

Fig. 10.3 In vivo activity of brentuximab vedotin in combination with chemotherapy agents. SCID mice were implanted with L540cy HL cells in the right flank. Groups of mice (5–10/group) were untreated or received brentuximab vedotin (SGN-35), gemcitabine, or brentuximab vedotin + gemcitabine (IP) when tumor size averaged approximately 100 mm3 (*panel* **c**) or 300 mm3 (*panel* **d**). The dosing schedule (q4dx3) is indicated by *arrows*. *Bars* represent standard deviation. SCID mice were implanted with L540cy HL cells in the right flank. Groups of mice (5–10/group) were untreated or received brentuximab vedotin (SGN-35) (1 mg/kg, q4dx3, i.p.) and/or ABVD: (adriamycin (0.75 mg/kg, q4dx3, i.v.), bleomycin (6 μg/kg, q4dx3, i.p.), vinblastine (0.01 mg/kg, q4dx3, i.p.), and dacarbazine (15 mg/kg, q3dx4, i.p.)) when tumor sized averaged approximately 100 mm^3 (*panel* **a**) or 300 mm^3 (*panel* **b**). The start of the dosing schedule is indicated by *arrows*. *Bars* represent standard deviation. Figure provided by Seattle Genetics

the untreated mice. This demonstrates that the ADC is more active than an admixture of the antibody and drug. In the disseminated models [33], a dose-dependent improvement of survival was observed in mice treated with brentuximab vedotin. A dose equivalent mixture of cAC10 and MMAE was much less effective than brentuximab vedotin.

The efficacy of combination therapy with brentuximab vedotin and chemotherapy has been studied in a subcutaneous SCID mouse model with the L540cy HL cell line. As seen in Fig. 10.3a, the combination of brentuximab vedotin and ABVD produced 9/9 durable complete regressions, while individually, the tumor regressions were significant but not durable. Even larger tumors (300 mm^3) responded well to the combination therapy (Fig. 10.3b) including 5/10 animals with durable complete regressions. Similar studies with the combination of brentuximab vedotin and gemcitabine (Fig. 10.3c, d) demonstrated a similar pattern of superior efficacy of the combination as compared to either single agent regimen particularly in large tumor size model (Fig. 10.3d).

The toxicity profile of brentuximab vedotin has been assessed in rats and monkeys. In both species, the dose-limiting toxicity was characterized by hypocellularity of the bone marrow and lymphoid depletion of the thymus. Histopathologic lesions were also observed in the spleen in monkeys and in the liver and testes in rats. In addition, decreases in peripheral blood counts were observed in both species, and elevations in liver enzymes were seen in rats only. The most significant toxicity was neutropenia, which in monkeys resulted in secondary bacterial infections leading to early deaths at the 6 mg/kg dose. Toxicity was dose-dependent, with a no-observable-adverse-effect level of 0.5 mg/kg in rats and 1 mg/kg in monkeys. Reversibility of toxicity was demonstrated for all of the findings (SGN-35 Investigator's Brochure).

Phase I Studies with Brentuximab Vedotin (SGN-35)

The first phase 1 study using brentuximab vedotin was an open-label, multicenter, dose-escalation trial at a dose range of 0.1–3.6 mg/kg every 3 weeks to 45 patients with relapsed or refractory CD30-positive hematologic malignancies [35]. Forty-two patients with Hodgkin's lymphoma, 2 patients with systemic anaplastic lymphoma, and 1 patient with CD30 angioimmunoblastic T cell lymphoma were enrolled. Patients had relapsed or refractory disease to multiple systemic therapies with a median of three previous chemotherapy regimens (range, 1–7) and 33 patients (73%) had failed high-dose chemotherapy with autologous stem cell rescue previously. The maximal tolerated dose was exceeded at 3.6 mg/kg and the dose selected for further studies was 1.8 mg/kg every 3 weeks since it was better tolerated than an intermediate dose of 2.7 mg/kg [35].

The majority of the adverse events observed with brentuximab vedotin were grade 1 or 2, including fatigue, pyrexia, diarrhea, nausea, neutropenia, and peripheral neuropathy. Peripheral neuropathy was reported in 16 patients, was typically sensory (grade 1 or 2), and the median time to onset was 9 weeks (range, 3–24). Peripheral neuropathy was generally reversible, although three patients discontinued treatment due to this side effect. Only one patient had a grade 3 peripheral neuropathy (2.7 mg/kg cohort) which returned to grade 1 within 4 months. Nine out of the 27 serious adverse events reported in the study were considered by the investigators to be related with brentuximab vedotin and those events occurred in five patients. The only laboratory abnormality seen in more than ten patients was grade 3 lymphopenia. Only two patients developed antibodies against brentuximab vedotin: one in the 0.1 mg/kg dose cohort and one in the 1.2 mg/kg dose cohort; both were low titer and both patients had stable disease [35]. Thus, brentuximab vedotin was shown to be well tolerated.

Although not the primary objective of the study, 17/42 patients enrolled had objective responses, 11 complete remissions, and 6 partial responses (Table 10.1). Nine of 11 complete responders had previously failed high-dose chemotherapy with stem cell rescue. Ten of 11 complete responders were among the 24 patients treated at

Table 10.1 Brentuximab vedotin phase I trial—every 3-week schedule best clinical responses

	Dose (mg/kg)								
Response	0.1 (*N*=3)	0.2 (*N*=4)	0.4 (*N*=3)	0.6 (*N*=3)	0.8 (*N*=3)	1.2 (*N*=4)	1.8 (*N*=12)	2.7 (*N*=12)	3.6 (*N*=1)
Complete remission	0	0	0	0	0	1	4	6	0
Partial remission	0	0	0	2	0	1	2	1	0
Stable disease	2	0	2	1	2	2	5	5	0
Progressive disease	1	4	1	0	1	0	1	0	0
Not evaluated	0	0	0	0	0	0	0	0	1

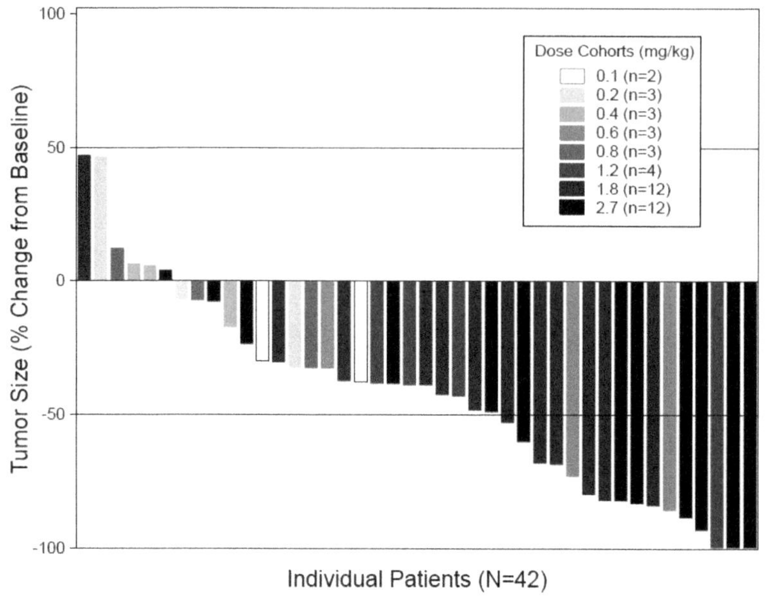

Fig. 10.4 Brentuximab vedotin Phase I trial maximum reduction in target lesion size. Change in target lesion data are presented for 42 patients enrolled in the 8 different dose cohorts of the Phase I trial evaluating the administration of brentuximab vedotin intravenously every 3 weeks. Figure provided by Seattle Genetics

1.8 mg/kg or 2.7 mg/kg doses. The median duration of response for the 17 patients with an objective response was 17.3 months. As can be seen in the waterfall diagram (Fig. 10.4), tumor regressions were observed in 36 of the 42 evaluated patients [35]. This represented a remarkable degree of antitumor efficacy for a phase I clinical trial.

The second phase 1 study using brentuximab vedotin on a weekly schedule was an open-label, multicenter, dose-escalation trial using doses of 0.4–1.4 mg/kg (3 weeks on and 1 week off) in 44 patients with relapsed or refractory CD30-positive hematologic malignancies [36]. Thirty-eight patients had Hodgkin lymphoma, five patients had systemic anaplastic large cell lymphoma, and one patient had peripheral T cell lymphoma. As in the every 3-week phase I trial, all patients were heavily pretreated with a median of 3 prior to chemotherapy regimens (range 1–8); 62% had previously failed high-dose chemotherapy with stem cell rescue; 45% had been resistant to their prior treatment regimen.

Dose-limiting toxicities included grade 3 diarrhea, grade 3 vomiting, and grade 4 hyperglycemia. The maximum tolerated dose was exceeded at 1.4 mg/kg; at this level, 2 of the 6 patients enrolled experienced dose-limiting toxicities (hyperglycemia and diarrhea). Subsequently, the 1.0 mg/kg and 1.2 mg/kg cohorts were both expanded to include 12 patients each. At the 1.2 mg/kg dose cohort no dose-limiting toxicities were seen; thus, this dose was considered the highest dose that did not cause unacceptable adverse effects [36].

The most common treatment-related adverse events were peripheral neuropathy, nausea, fatigue, diarrhea, and neutropenia; most were grade 1 or 2 in severity.

Table 10.2 Brentuximab vedotin phase I trial—weekly schedule best clinical responses

	Dose (mg/kg)					
Response	0.4 (*N*=4)	0.6 (*N*=4)	0.8 (*N*=6)	1.0 (*N*=11)	1.2 (*N*=9)	1.4 (*N*=5)
Complete remission	0	0	4	5	2	2
Partial remission	0	2	0	3	2	2
Stable disease	4	1	1	2	4	1
Progressive disease	0	1	1	1	1	0

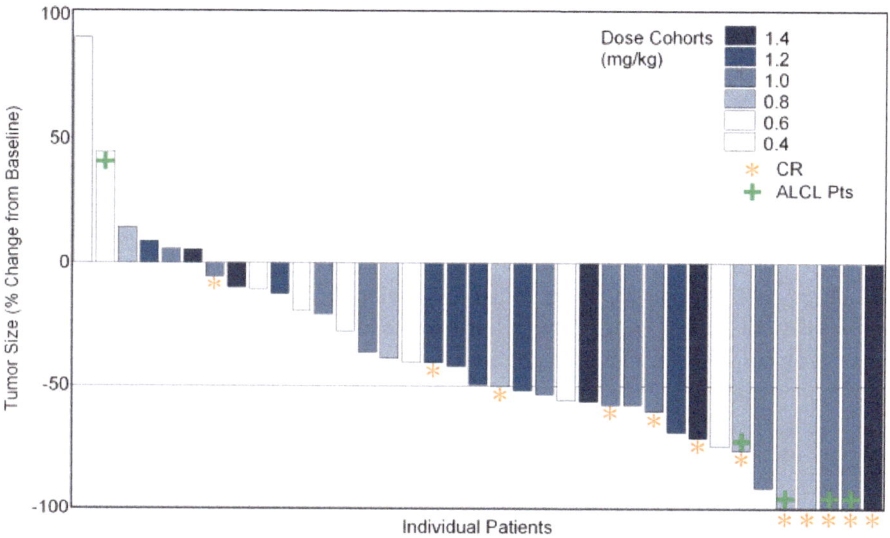

Fig. 10.5 Brentuximab vedotin phase I trial maximum reduction in target lesion size. Change in target lesion data are presented for 37 patients enrolled in the 6 different dose cohorts of the phase I trial evaluating the administration of brentuximab vedotin intravenously weekly. Image provided by Seattle Genetics

Twenty four of the 44 patients enrolled had some degree of peripheral neuropathy (generally sensory) which was observed more frequently with this schedule compared with the every 3-week schedule. The laboratory abnormalities seen in more than 8 patients were grade 3 lymphopenia and grade 2 hypophosphatemia [36].

Twenty two of 39 evaluable patients had objective responses (56%) including 13 (33%) with complete remissions (Table 10.2). The median duration of response at the time of the poster presentation in December 2009 was at least 16 weeks (range, 0.1+ to 34+). As can be seen in the waterfall diagram (Fig. 10.5), tumor regressions were observed in 84% of the patients [36]. Thus, weekly brentuximab vedotin showed antitumor activity against CD30-positive malignancies similar to the every 3-week regimen with an increase in toxicity.

Table 10.3 Cycle I pharmacokinetics for brentuximab vedotin for the 1.8 mg/kg dose level with the every 3-week schedule

Parameter	Brentuximab vedotin (N=12)	MMAE (N=12)	Serum total antibody (N=12)
AUC0-21 day (μg/ml)	76.7	36.1	169
Cmax (μg/ml)	32.0	4.97	36.6
Tmax (day)	0.089 (0.084–0.254)	2.09 (1.08–3.93	0.132 (0.084–1.10)
$T_{½}$ (day)	4.43	3.60	–
Cl (L/day)	1.76	–	–

In both phase I studies, retreatment with brentuximab vedotin was allowed if patients had stable disease (with reduced tumor volume) or better to initial treatment. They received doses of 1 mg/kg weekly or 1.8 mg/kg every 3 weeks, depending on which study they participated [37]. A total of 8 patients received 11 retreatment experiences and included 7 patients with HL and 7/8 who had previously failed high-dose chemotherapy with stem cell rescue [37]. Among the retreatment experiences, there were 2 complete remissions, 5 partial remissions, 3 stable diseases, and 1 progressive disease. The toxicity profile on retreatment was similar to the experiences in the original phase I trials.

Pharmacokinetic parameters for individual patients were determined in both phase I studies using concentrations of brentuximab vedotin antibody–drug conjugate, plasma MMAE, and serum total antibody.

In both trials, serum levels were dose proportional. The terminal half-life for the ADC was 4–6 days and for MMAE was 3–4 days. Pharmacokinetic parameters for the 1.8 mg/kg every 3-week schedule are presented in Table 10.3 [35].

Pivotal Studies of Brentuximab Vedotin

In consultation with the FDA, pivotal trials were undertaken in HL and a second one in systemic ALCL using the 1.8 mg/kg every 3-week dose and schedule.

The primary objective of the study in patients with Hodgkin's lymphoma was overall objective response rate as assessed by an independent review facility according to the Revised Response Criteria for Malignant Lymphoma [38] in patients with relapsed or refractory disease following high-dose chemotherapy with autologous stem cell rescue. The safety and pharmacokinetics of brentuximab vedotin, duration of response, progression-free survival, and overall survival were also evaluated. An Independent Data Monitoring Committee (IDMC) had oversight of the safety of the patients on a periodic basis.

A total of 102 patients with relapsed or refractory HL were treated at 26 study centers inside and outside the United States. Brentuximab vedotin was administered intravenously at 1.8 mg/kg every 3 weeks. The median age of the patients was 31 years (range 15–77) and approximately half of the patients were female (53%). The patients had an Eastern Cooperative Oncology Group (ECOG) performance status at baseline of 0 or 1 and were heavily pretreated with a median number of prior chemotherapy regimens of 3.5 (range 1–13). More than 70% of the patients had primary refractory disease, defined as failure to achieve a complete remission or progression within 3 months of completing frontline therapy. In addition, 39% of patients were refractory to the most recent salvage therapy excluding high-dose chemotherapy with stem cell rescue. The median duration of brentuximab vedotin treatment on this study was 27 weeks (range 3–54) and the median number of cycles was 9 (range 1–16).

By the time of the pivotal trial publication [39], the objective response rate was 72% (34% CR and 38% PR) per investigator assessment. Of the 35 patients who had B symptoms at baseline, 29 (83%) experienced resolution of these symptoms. The median time to B symptom resolution was 3 weeks (range <1–16 weeks). Ninety seven of 102 patients (95%) had tumor size reductions. The median progression-free survival was 5.6 months and the median duration of response for those patients in CR was 20.5 month.

The most common treatment-related adverse events (seen in more than 15% of the patients) of any grade were peripheral sensory neuropathy (43%), fatigue (40%), nausea (35%), neutropenia (19%), diarrhea (18%), pyrexia (16%), and vomiting (22%); most events were grade 1 or 2 and reversible. Grade 3 treatment-related adverse events reported in more than 1 patient were neutropenia (14%), peripheral sensory neuropathy (5%), thrombocytopenia and hyperglycemia (3% each), and fatigue (2%). Grade 4 treatment-related events were neutropenia (4%), thrombocytopenia, abdominal pain, and pulmonary embolism (1% each). No related grade 5 events were observed. 18 patients discontinued treatment due to an adverse event.

The antitumor activity of brentuximab vedotin in patients with relapsed or refractory systemic ALCL was also assessed in a second pivotal trial. Brentuximab vedotin was administered intravenously at 1.8 mg/kg every 3 weeks. The primary objective of the study was overall objective response rate as assessed by an independent review facility according to the Revised Response Criteria for Malignant Lymphoma [38] in patients with relapsed or refractory disease. The safety and pharmacokinetics of brentuximab vedotin, duration of response, progression-free survival, and overall survival were also evaluated. An Independent Data Monitoring Committee (IDMC) had oversight of the safety of the patients on a periodic basis.

A total of 58 patients with relapsed or refractory anaplastic large cell non-Hodgkin's lymphoma were treated at 25 study centers inside and outside the United States. By the time of the pivotal trial publication [40], the median age of those patients was 52 years (range 14–76) and 25 patients were female. Ninety eight percent of the patients had an Eastern Cooperative Oncology Group (ECOG) performance status at baseline of 0 or 1, and 72% of the patients were ALK-negative. Patients were heavily pretreated with a median number of prior chemotherapy regimens of 2 (range 1–6); 26% of the patients had previously failed high-dose chemotherapy with stem cell rescue. Sixty-two percent of the 58 patients presented had primary refractory disease, defined as failure to achieve a complete remission or progression within 3 months of completing frontline therapy. In addition, 50% of patients were refractory to their most recent salvage therapy.

The objective response rate for the 58 patients treated was 86% (57% CR and 29% PR) per investigator assessment. Interestingly, the responses seen in ALK-positive and negative patients were similar. The median time to objective response was 5.9 weeks (range 4.3–14), the duration of objective response was 12.6 months, and the median duration of CR was 13.2 months. B symptoms resolved in 9 of the 10 patients who had these symptoms at baseline. Ninety-seven percent of the patients had reductions in tumor size.

The most common treatment-related adverse events of any grade (seen in more than 10% of the patients) for those 58 patients treated were peripheral sensory neuropathy (41%), nausea (40%), fatigue (38%), pyrexia (34%), diarrhea (29%), neutropenia (21%), dyspnea (17%), and insomnia (16%); most events were grade 1 or 2 and reversible. Grade 3/4 treatment-related adverse events reported in more than 1 patient were neutropenia (21%), thrombocytopenia (14%), peripheral sensory neuropathy (12%), and diarrhea (3%). No related grade 5 events were observed. Seven patients discontinued treatment due to an adverse event.

Summary

Brentuximab vedotin, an antibody–drug conjugate, represents a unique strategy for target-based immunotherapy using a monoclonal antibody to deliver MMAE, an anti-tubulin agent intracellularly. The striking activity demonstrated in animal models with CD30-positive hematological malignancies was also observed in clinical trials using brentuximab vedotin in patients with relapsed and/or refractory CD30-positive Hodgkin's lymphoma and anaplastic large cell lymphoma. Brentuximab vedotin has been well tolerated at the recommended dose of 1.8 mg/kg every three weeks with peripheral neuropathy as the main reversible side effect. The data from the pivotal trials were presented to the FDA and brentuximab vedotin was approved in 2011. Clinical trials using the combination of brentuximab vedotin and chemotherapy as well as trials using maintenance brentuximab vedotin in patients with high risk disease after high-dose chemotherapy with stem cell rescue have been initiated.

References

1. Moskowitz CH, Kewalramani T, Nimer SD, Gonzalez M, Zelenetz AD, Yahalom J (2004) Effectiveness of high dose chemoradiotherapy and autologous stem cell transplantation for patients with biopsy-proven primary refractory Hodgkin's disease. Br J Haematol 124(5):645–652
2. Longo DL, Duffey PL, Young RC, Hubbard SM, Ihde DC, Glatstein E, Phares JC, Jaffe ES, Urba WJ, DeVita VT Jr (1992) Conventional-dose salvage combination chemotherapy in

patients relapsing with Hodgkin's disease after combination chemotherapy: the low probability for cure. J Clin Oncol 10(2):210–218
3. Schmitz N, Haverkamp H, Josting A, Diehl V, Pfistner B, Carella AM, Haenel M, Boissevain F, Bokemeyer C, Goldstone AH (2005) Long term follow up in relapsed Hodgkin's disease: updated results of the HD-R1 study comparing conventional chemotherapy to high-dose chemotherapy with autologous haemopoetic stem cell transplantation of the German Hodgkin Study Group and the Working Party Lymphoma of the European Group for Blood and Marrow Transplantation. J Clin Oncol 23(16s):Abstract 6508
4. Schmitz N, Pfistner B, Sextro M, Sieber M, Carella AM, Haenel M, Boissevain F, Zschaber R, Müller P, Kirchner H, Lohri A, Decker S, Koch B, Hasenclever D, Goldstone AH, Diehl V, German Hodgkin's Lymphoma Study Group, Lymphoma Working Party of the European Group for Blood and Marrow Transplantation (2002) Aggressive conventional chemotherapy compared with high-dose chemotherapy with autologous haemopoietic stem-cell transplantation for relapsed chemosensitive Hodgkin's disease: a randomised trial. Lancet 359(9323):2065–2071
5. Linch DC, Winfield D, Goldstone AH, Moir D, Hancock B, McMillan A, Chopra R, Milligan D, Hudson GV (1993) Dose intensification with autologous bone-marrow transplantation in relapsed and resistant Hodgkin's disease: results of a BNLI randomised trial. Lancet 341(8852):1051–1054
6. Pileri S, Bocchia M, Baroni CD, Martelli M, Falini B, Sabattini E, Gherlinzoni F, Amadori S, Poggi S, Mazza P et al (1994) Anaplastic large cell lymphoma (CD30+/Ki-1+): results of a prospective clinico-pathological study of 69 cases. Br J Haematol 86(3):513–523
7. Pileri SA, Piccaluga A, Poggi S, Sabattini E, Piccaluga PP, De Vivo A, Falini B, Stein H (1995) Anaplastic large cell lymphoma: update of findings. Leuk Lymphoma 18(1–2):17–25
8. Reichert JM, Valge-Archer VE (2007) Development trends for monoclonal antibody cancer therapeutics. Nat Rev Drug Discov 6(5):349–356
9. Carter PJ (2006) Potent antibody therapeutics by design. Nat Rev Immunol 6(5):343–357
10. Schrama D, Reisfeld RA, Becker JC (2006) Antibody targeted drugs as cancer therapeutics. Nat Rev Drug Discov 5(2):147–159
11. Weiner LM (2007) Building better magic bullets—improving unconjugated monoclonal antibody therapy for cancer. Nat Rev Cancer 7(9):701–706
12. Carter PJ, Senter PD (2008) Antibody-drug conjugates for cancer therapy. Cancer J 14(3):154–169
13. Teicher BA (2009) Antibody-drug conjugate targets. Curr Cancer Drug Targets 9(8):982–1004
14. Lambert JM (2005) Drug-conjugated monoclonal antibodies for the treatment of cancer. Curr Opin Pharmacol 5(5):543–549
15. Carter P, Smith L, Ryan M (2004) Identification and validation of cell surface antigens for antibody targeting in oncology. Endocr Relat Cancer 11(4):659–687
16. Wu AM, Senter PD (2005) Arming antibodies: prospects and challenges for immunoconjugates. Nat Biotechnol 23(9):1137–1146
17. Xie H, Blättler WA (2006) In vivo behaviour of antibody-drug conjugates for the targeted treatment of cancer. Expert Opin Biol Ther 6(3):281–291
18. Kovtun YV, Goldmacher VS (2007) Cell killing by antibody-drug conjugates. Cancer Lett 255(2):232–240
19. Dürkop H, Latza U, Hummel M, Eitelbach F, Seed B, Stein H (1992) Molecular cloning and expression of a new member of the nerve growth factor receptor family that is characteristic for Hodgkin's disease. Cell 68(3):421–427
20. Horie R, Watanabe T (1998) CD30: expression and function in health and disease. Semin Immunol 10(6):457–470
21. Dürkop H, Foss HD, Eitelbach F, Anagnostopoulos I, Latza U, Pileri S, Stein H (2000) Expression of the CD30 antigen in non-lymphoid tissues and cells. J Pathol 190(5):613–618

22. Pera MF, Bennett W, Cerretti DP (1997) Expression of CD30 and CD30 ligand in cultured cell lines from human germ-cell tumors. Lab Invest 76(4):497–504
23. Muta H, Boise LH, Fang L, Podack ER (2000) CD30 signals integrate expression of cytotoxic effector molecules, lymphocyte trafficking signals, and signals for proliferation and apoptosis. J Immunol 165(9):5105–5111
24. Wahl AF, Klussman K, Thompson JD, Chen JH, Francisco LV, Risdon G, Chace DF, Siegall CB, Francisco JA (2002) The anti-CD30 monoclonal antibody SGN-30 promotes growth arrest and DNA fragmentation in vitro and affects antitumor activity in models of Hodgkin's disease. Cancer Res 62(13):3736–3742
25. Borchmann P, Treml JF, Hansen H, Gottstein C, Schnell R, Staak O, Zhang HF, Davis T, Keler T, Diehl V, Graziano RF, Engert A (2003) The human anti-CD30 antibody 5F11 shows in vitro and in vivo activity against malignant lymphoma. Blood 102(10):3737–3742
26. Duckett CS, Gedrich RW, Gilfillan MC, Thompson CB (1997) Induction of nuclear factor kappaB by the CD30 receptor is mediated by TRAF1 and TRAF2. Mol Cell Biol 17(3):1535–1542
27. Harlin H, Podack E, Boothby M, Alegre ML (2002) TCR-independent CD30 signaling selectively induces IL-13 production via a TNF receptor-associated factor/p38 mitogen-activated protein kinase-dependent mechanism. J Immunol 169(5):2451–2459
28. Zheng B, Fiumara P, Li YV, Georgakis G, Snell V, Younes M, Vauthey JN, Carbone A, Younes A (2003) MEK/ERK pathway is aberrantly active in Hodgkin disease: a signaling pathway shared by CD30, CD40, and RANK that regulates cell proliferation and survival. Blood 102(3):1019–1027
29. Cerveny CG, Law CL, McCormick RS, Lenox JS, Hamblett KJ, Westendorf LE, Yamane AK, Petroziello JM, Francisco JA, Wahl AF (2005) Signaling via the anti-CD30 mAb SGN-30 sensitizes Hodgkin's disease cells to conventional chemotherapeutics. Leukemia 19(9): 1648–1655
30. Sutherland MS, Sanderson RJ, Gordon KA, Andreyka J, Cerveny CG, Yu C, Lewis TS, Meyer DL, Zabinski RF, Doronina SO, Senter PD, Law CL, Wahl AF (2006) Lysosomal trafficking and cysteine protease metabolism confer target-specific cytotoxicity by peptide-linked anti-CD30-auristatin conjugates. J Biol Chem 281(15):10540–10547
31. Francisco JA, Cerveny CG, Meyer DL, Mixan BJ, Klussman K, Chace DF, Rejniak SX, Gordon KA, DeBlanc R, Toki BE, Law CL, Doronina SO, Siegall CB, Senter PD, Wahl AF (2003) cAC10-vcMMAE, an anti-CD30-monomethyl auristatin E conjugate with potent and selective antitumor activity. Blood 102(4):1458–1465
32. Fischer P, Nacheva E, Mason DY, Sherrington PD, Hoyle C, Hayhoe FG, Karpas A (1988) A Ki-1 (CD30)-positive human cell line (Karpas 299) established from a high-grade non-Hodgkin's lymphoma, showing a 2;5 translocation and rearrangement of the T-cell receptor beta-chain gene. Blood 72(1):234–240
33. Tian ZG, Longo DL, Funakoshi S, Asai O, Ferris DK, Widmer M, Murphy WJ (1995) In vivo antitumor effects of unconjugated CD30 monoclonal antibodies on human anaplastic large-cell lymphoma xenografts. Cancer Res 55(22):5335–5341
34. Kapp U, Wolf J, von Kalle C, Tawadros S, Röttgen A, Engert A, Fonatsch C, Stein H, Diehl V (1992) Preliminary report: growth of Hodgkin's lymphoma derived cells in immune compromised mice. Ann Oncol 3(Suppl 4):21–23
35. Younes A, Bartlett NL, Leonard JP, Kennedy DA, Lynch CM, Sievers EL, Forero-Torres A (2010) Brentuximab vedotin (SGN-35) for relapsed CD30-positive lymphomas. N Engl J Med 363(19):1812–1821
36. Fanale M, Bartlett NL, Forero-Torres A, Rosenblatt J, Horning SJ, Franklin AR, Lynch CM, Sievers EL, Kennedy DA (2009) The antibody-drug conjugate Brentuximab Vedotin (SGN-35) induced multiple objective responses in patients with relapsed or refractory CD30-positive lymphomas in a phase 1 weekly dosing study. ASH 2009 annual meeting (Abstract #2731)
37. Bartlett N, Grove LE, Kennedy DA, Sievers EL, Forero-Torres A (2010) Objective responses with Brentuximab Vedotin (SGN-35) retreatment in CD30-positive hematologic malignancies: a case series. J Clin Oncol 28:15s (Abstract #8062)

38. Cheson BD, Pfistner B, Juweid ME et al (2007) Revised Response Criteria for Malignant Lymphoma. J Clin Oncol 25:579
39. Younes A, Gopal AK, Smith SE, Ansell SM, Rosenblatt JD, Savage KJ, Ramchandren R, Bartlett NL, Cheson BD, de Vos S, Forero-Torres A, Moskowitz CH, Connors JM, Engert A, Larsen EK, Kennedy DA, Sievers EL, Chen R (2012) Results of a pivotal phase II study of brentuximab vedotin for patients with relapsed or refractory Hodgkin's lymphoma. J Clin Oncol 30(18):2183–2189
40. Pro B, Advani R, Brice P, Bartlett NL, Rosenblatt JD, Illidge T, Matous J, Ramchandren R, Fanale M, Connors JM, Yang Y, Sievers EL, Kennedy DA, Shustov A (2012) Brentuximab vedotin (SGN-35) in patients with relapsed or refractory systemic anaplastic large-cell lymphoma: results of a phase II study. J Clin Oncol 30(18):2190–2196

Part V
Antibody-Drug Conjugates for Solid Tumors

Chapter 11
Trastuzumab Emtansine (T-DM1) for the Treatment of HER2-Positive Cancer with a Focus on Breast Cancer

Hope S. Rugo, Ian E. Krop, and Yu-Waye Chu

Introduction

Overexpression of human epidermal growth factor receptor type 2 (HER2; *neu*; ErbB2) is an important histopathologic feature in a variety of human solid tumors. HER2 is a member of the type I receptor tyrosine kinase family that also includes epidermal growth factor receptor (EGFR, HER1, ErbB1), HER3 (ErbB3), and HER4 (ErbB4). HER2 serves as a coreceptor in the dimerization and subsequent activation of the other members of the HER receptors, notably HER3, which forms the major oncologic unit in a subset of breast cancer. HER2 overexpression occurs in 15–20% of all breast cancers and is associated with poor prognosis without treatment [1, 2]. Biologically, HER2 overexpression has been shown to have important functions in malignant transformation and/or progression of tumors and is associated with decreased response to endocrine therapy. Although HER2 overexpression has been most extensively studied in the context of breast cancer, it has also been observed in other cancers including gastric, ovarian, and pancreatic cancer [3].

Given the importance of HER2 overexpression in tumor initiation and progression and its pattern of overexpression that is restricted predominantly to tumor versus normal tissue, HER2 has been intensely investigated as a target for anticancer therapies. The humanized anti-HER2 monoclonal antibody trastuzumab (Herceptin™),

H.S. Rugo (✉)
H.S.R., University of California San Francisco, Helen Diller Family Comprehensive Cancer Center, San Francisco, CA, USA
e-mail: hrugo@medicine.ucsf.edu

I.E. Krop
I.E.K., Dana Farber Cancer Institute, Boston, MA, USA

Y.-W. Chu
Y-W.C., Exploratory Clinical Development, Genentech, Inc., South San Francisco, CA, USA

G.L. Phillips (ed.), *Antibody-Drug Conjugates and Immunotoxins: From Pre-Clinical Development to Therapeutic Applications*, Cancer Drug Discovery and Development, DOI 10.1007/978-1-4614-5456-4_11,

in combination with chemotherapy, prolongs survival of patients with HER2-overexpressing (HER2-positive [HER2+]) breast cancer in the metastatic (MBC) and adjuvant settings [4–7], which has led to its adoption as a standard of care. More recently, trastuzumab in combination with chemotherapy was shown to prolong survival in patients with HER2-positive metastatic gastric cancer, which led to its approval for this indication as well.

In addition to trastuzumab, the oral dual tyrosine kinase inhibitor lapatinib (Tykerb™/Tyverb™), which binds to the ATP-binding pocket of the EGFR and HER2 kinase domains and prevents activation of the downstream signaling cascade, has been approved as single-agent therapy or in combination with capecitabine for the treatment of patients with HER2-positive breast cancers previously treated with trastuzumab [8]. Lapatinib was also recently approved in combination with the aromatase inhibitor letrozole for postmenopausal hormone receptor-positive, HER2-positive MBC [9]. Similar to trastuzumab, lapatinib is being investigated in other HER2-positive tumors, including HER2-positive gastric cancer [10]. Together with the clinical experience of trastuzumab, these results demonstrate the importance of HER2 as an important target for anticancer therapy.

Progression free survival (PFS) following treatment with trastuzumab combined with taxane based chemotherapy is only about one year (references 4, 6 from chapter), and can be extended to about 18 months with the addition of pertuzumab, a novel HER2 targeted antibody approved by the U.S.FDA in June of 2012 as first-line therapy for HER2 positive advanced breast cancer in combination with trastuzumab and docetaxel [46]. However, despite the gains in clinical benefit of trastuzumab and lapatinib in the treatment of HER2-positive breast cancer, the majority of patients with HER2+ MBC eventually develop progressive disease [11]. Consequently, the development of additional therapeutic options for patients whose tumors progress following initial HER2-directed therapy is warranted. This chapter will describe the clinical experience to date of the antibody–drug conjugate (ADC) trastuzumab emtansine (T-DM1) as a novel therapeutic option in the treatment of HER2-positive tumors focusing on the treatment of metastatic breast cancer.

Trastuzumab Emtansine

Structure

T-DM1 (Fig. 11.1) is a novel anti-HER2 ADC in development for the treatment of patients with HER2+ breast cancer [12]. T-DM1 combines the HER2-targeting properties of trastuzumab with intracellular delivery of DM1, a highly potent derivative of the antimicrotubule agent maytansine [13–15]. The conjugation of DM1 to trastuzumab results in a range of DM1 to antibody ratios with the average being 3.5 molecules of DM1 conjugated to every one molecule of trastuzumab. DM1 binds to tubulin at the same binding site as the vinca alkaloids but inhibits microtubule assembly with a potency 20–100 times that of vincristine or vinblastine [13]. Similar to the vinca alkaloids, DM1 causes apoptosis through inhibition of microtubule

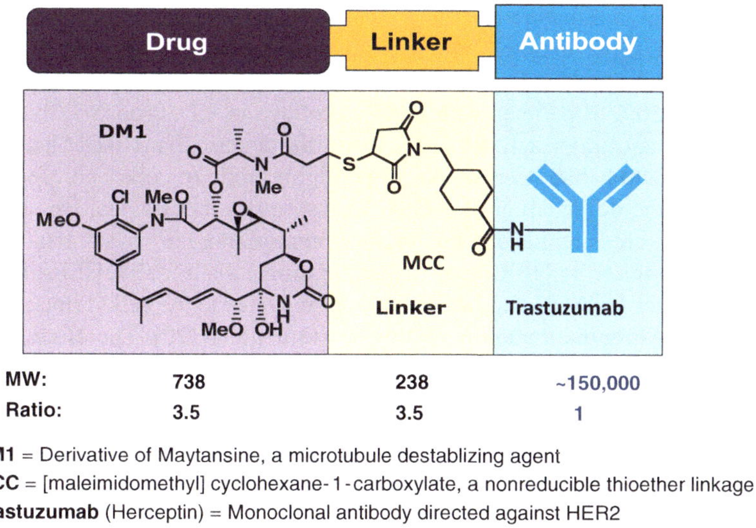

Fig. 11.1 Schematic representation of trastuzumab emtansine

assembly, which in turn leads to G2-M cell cycle arrest. The parent molecule of DM1, maytansine, was studied as a potential chemotherapeutic agent by the National Cancer Institute in phase II studies in over 35 tumor types. Of over 800 patients treated with single-agent maytansine, objective responses were observed in only about 20 patients. Dose-limiting toxicities (DLT) were established in the range of 1–2 mg/m^2 with toxicities including neurotoxicity, gastrointestinal toxicity, weakness, nausea, vomiting, and diarrhea. Because of the narrow therapeutic window afforded by maytansine, its development as a potential agent for clinical use was suspended [14].

There are several features of T-DM1 that make it a suitable candidate to be successful as an ADC. First, trastuzumab and DM1 are covalently linked via a non-reducible thioether linker (*N*-maleimidomethyl)cyclohexane-1-carboxylate (MCC). The stability of MCC, compared with disulfide linkers, was shown to strongly contribute to T-DM1's favorable activity and toxicity profiles in preclinical testing [16, 17] and in clinical studies resulted in systemic levels of DM1 that were more than 50-fold lower by molar equivalents (see below). Thus, despite the narrow therapeutic window previously established by maytansine, when DM1 is administered as a component of an ADC, its exposure to HER2+ tumors is maximized while exposure of normal tissue is minimized, resulting in expansion of the therapeutic window. Second, T-DM1 appears to retain trastuzumab's antitumor properties, including flagging HER2+ tumor cells for destruction by antibody-dependent cellular cytotoxicity, as well as inhibiting HER2 shedding and HER2-dependent PI3K/AKT signaling [16–18]. The additional anticancer property provided by the parent antibody trastuzumab, on top of the targeted delivery of a cytotoxic agent, is a feature that distinguishes T-DM1 among other ADCs currently in development. For example, the unconjugated antibody that is the backbone of the ADC brentuximab vedotin (SGN-35), which resulted in durable objective responses in 50% of patients with relapsed/refractory CD30-positive lymphomas, had minimal antitumor activity [19]. Third, the predominant T-DM1 metabolite, lysine-MCC-DM1, has been shown to be highly toxic to cells upon intracellular release with the degradation of T-DM1 in lysosomes, but its positive charge precludes it from crossing plasma membranes, minimizing the "bystander" cytotoxic effects on neighboring HER2 non-overexpressing cells. Finally, HER2 itself is an attractive target for ADCs in that it passively recycles to the cell surface and is not subject to downregulation upon binding to trastuzumab [20]. Therefore, the availability of HER2 as a T-DM1 target is retained with repeated dosing.

Preclinical Studies

Results of preclinical studies in vitro and in vivo have provided strong evidence supporting a broad therapeutic window for T-DM1. A key finding in these initial studies was the importance of linker stability in defining the efficacy, pharmacokinetics, and safety profile of trastuzumab-DM1 conjugates. Earlier generation ADCs utilized disulfide-based linkers where deconjugation of the drug from the antibody was achieved by intracellular reduction. However, the observation that reductive cleavage of drug linked to the antibody by disulfide-based linkers is extremely inefficient [21] led to evaluation of different linker types. Compared to reducible disulfide linkers, conjugation of DM1 to trastuzumab via the non-reducible thioether linker MCC resulted in increased antitumor efficacy, increased serum ADC concentrations over time, minimized release of DM1 into the circulation, and less toxic effects in short-term single-dose toxicity studies in rats as measured by changes in body weight over time [17]. Based on these initial observations, trastuzumab-MCC-DM1 was further studied in preclinical testing.

In murine xenograft models of HER2-overexpressing trastuzumab-resistant tumors, specifically the tumor-derived cell line BT-474 EEI and Fo5 tumor transplant model (derived from transgenic mice where HER2 expression is driven by the mouse mammary tumor virus promoter), treatment with T-DM1 resulted in reduction in tumor volume in a dose-dependent manner. In contrast, treatment of the Fo5 xenograft model with unconjugated trastuzumab or free DM1 did not result in reduction of tumor volume [17]. In addition to trastuzumab-resistant cell lines and tumor xenografts, T-DM1 exhibited antitumor effects against cell lines and tumor xenografts that were resistant to lapatinib. In addition to the aforementioned antitumor activity in the Fo5 tumor transplant model, where treatment with lapatinib did not inhibit tumor growth, T-DM1 exhibited robust antitumor activity against tumors derived from the MCF7-neo/HER2 cell line, which are trastuzumab resistant due to an activating mutation (E545K) in PIK3CA. Together, these results support the premise that T-DM1 can have an effect on tumors that have developed potential resistance to trastuzumab and lapatinib [18].

Preclinical safety findings following T-DM1 treatment suggested that T-DM1 had a favorable safety and tolerability profile. In rats, where there is no cross-reactivity of T-DM1 against rat HER2 protein, treatment with T-DM1 resulted in transient liver enzyme elevations and mild reversible thrombocytopenia [17]. Similar results were observed in studies of cynomolgus monkeys where there exists cross-reactivity of T-DM1 to HER2 and included reversible increases in hepatic transaminases, dose-dependent irreversible axonal degeneration, and modest reversible decreases in platelet counts; however, platelet counts typically remained within normal limits [12]. Studies of radiolabeled T-DM1 in rats demonstrated that the primary route of elimination was via the hepatobiliary route [22].

Given the promising preclinical results of T-DM1 and the potential to develop a novel class of HER2-directed agents, clinical testing of T-DM1 was initiated in patients in HER2-positive breast cancer. A listing of clinical studies of T-DM1 is summarized in Table 11.1. In addition to studies of single-agent T-DM1, combinations of T-DM1 with systemic chemotherapy and the HER2-directed monoclonal antibody pertuzumab are being studied [23, 24]. Results of clinical studies that attest to the efficacy and safety of T-DM1 are highlighted in the following sections.

Phase I Study in HER2-Positive Metastatic Breast Cancer

A phase I dose-escalation study evaluated T-DM1 administered intravenously in patients with HER2+ MBC that had progressed on trastuzumab-based therapy [12]. The purpose of this study was to determine the maximally tolerated dose using two dosing schedules, every 3 weeks and weekly. For the every-3-week (q3w) schedule, the range of doses tested was 0.3 mg/kg to 4.8 mg/kg. A total of 24 patients were enrolled in this portion of the study. For the weekly schedule, a total of 28 patients were enrolled. The range of doses tested at the weekly schedule was 1.2–2.9 mg/kg. Enrolled patients had received a median of four prior chemotherapeutic agents for MBC in addition to progressing on prior trastuzumab therapy. Patients were assessed for safety and pharmacokinetics with exploratory assessments of efficacy.

For the q3w schedule, the maximum tolerated dose (MTD) of T-DM1 was 3.6 mg/kg based on dose-limiting toxicity of grade 4 thrombocytopenia that was observed in two of three patients treated at 4.8 mg/kg. Exploratory efficacy results at the MTD were promising given a heavily pretreated patient population with demonstrated progression on prior trastuzumab. For the 15 patients treated at the MTD, the clinical benefit rate (CBR) (defined as the objective response rate plus stable disease for at least six months' duration) was 73%. Four of the nine patients (44%) with measurable disease had an objective response [12].

For the weekly schedule, based on an assessment of 19 patients, the MTD was 2.4 mg/kg due to toxicity that prevented on-schedule administration of the subsequent dose in two of three patients treated at the 2.9-mg/kg dose level. Among the

Table 11.1 Clinical studies of T-DM1 in HER2-positive breast cancer

Clinical study and reference	Phase	Clinical setting	Treatment regimen
TDM3569g [12, 25]	I	HER2-positive MBC following prior chemotherapy and progression on trastuzumab	T-DM1 0.3–4.8 mg/kg every 3 weeks; T-DM1 1.2 to 2.9 mg/kg weekly
TDM4258g [26]	II	HER-positive MBC following prior chemotherapy and progression on a HER2-directed agent	T-DM1 3.6 mg/kg every 3 weeks
TDM4374g [27]	II	HER-positive MBC following prior exposure to an antracycline, a taxane, capecitabine, trastuzumab, and lapatinib; two HER2-directed agents in the metastatic setting; progression on the last regimen	T-DM1 3.6 mg/kg every 3 weeks
TDM4450g/ BO21976 [36]	II	HER2-positive recurrent or progressive locally advanced or previously untreated MBC	T-DM1 3.6 mg/kg every 3 weeks versus trastuzumab 8 mg/kg loading dose then 6 mg/kg every 3 weeks, docetaxel 75 or 100 mg/m^2 every 3 weeks
TDM4688g	II	HER2-positive locally advanced or MBC following recurrence or progression on prior trastuzumab therapy	T-DM1 3.6 mg/kg every 3 weeks; for patients with early progression on single-agent T-DM1, pertuzumab 840-mg loading dose then 420 mg every 3 weeks is added
TDM4373g [23]	Ib/II	HER2-positive MBC following prior chemotherapy and HER2-directed therapy; includes patients treated in metastatic and in neoadjuvant/adjuvant settings	T-DM1 3.6 mg/kg every 3 weeks plus pertuzumab 840-mg loading dose then 420 mg every 3 weeks
TDM4652g [24]	Ib	HER2-positive MBC following prior trastuzumab	Starting T-DM1 dose 2.4 mg/kg every 3 weeks plus paclitaxel from 65 mg/m^2 weekly with dose adjustments based on safety; starting T-DM1 dose 2.0 mg/kg weekly plus paclitaxel 80 mg/m^2 weekly with dose adjustments based on safety

(continued)

Table 11.1 (continued)

Clinical study and reference	Phase	Clinical setting	Treatment regimen
BO22572	Ib	HER2-positive MBC or newly diagnosed locally advanced (stage III) breast cancer	MBC: starting T-DM1 dose 2.4 mg/kg every 3 weeks plus docetaxel dose escalation from 75 mg/m^2 every 3 weeks with dose adjustments based on safety; Locally advanced disease: starting T-DM1 dose 3.6 mg/kg every 3 weeks plus docetaxel 60 mg/m^2 every 3 weeks with dose adjustments based on safety
TDM4874g	II	HER2-positive early stage breast cancer	T-DM1 3.6 mg/kg every 3 weeks sequentially with neoadjuvant or adjuvant chemotherapy
TDM4370g	III	HER2-positive locally advanced or MBC previously treated with trastuzumab	T-DM1 3.6 mg/kg every 3 weeks versus lapatinib 1,250 mg/day day 1–21 and capecitabine 1,000 mg/m^2 day 1–14 every 3 weeks
BO22589/TDM4788g	III	HER2-positive progressive or recurrent locally advanced or previously untreated MBC	T-DM1 3.6 mg/kg every 3 weeks plus pertuzumab/pertuzumab placebo 840-mg loading dose then 420 mg every 3 weeks versus trastuzumab 8-mg/kg loading dose then 6 mg/kg every 3 weeks plus docetaxel 75 or 100 mg/m^2 every 3 weeks or trastuzumab 4 mg/kg loading dose then 2 mg/kg every week plus paclitaxel 80 mg/m^2 every week

15 patients across all dose levels who had evaluable measurable disease, eight (53%) had confirmed objective responses. Two of seven patients treated at the 2.4-mg/kg dose level had a partial response as their best response [25].

T-DM1's pharmacokinetic profile based on assessments following the first dose of 3.6 mg/kg was characterized by relatively slow clearance, a volume of distribution (60 ± 13.6 mL/kg) that approximates the physiologic blood volume, and a half-life of approximately 3.5 days. Notably, systemic DM1 exposure was low (average of ~5 ng/mL maximum plasma levels) compared to that of conjugated T-DM1, which had a C_{max} of 74.3 μg/mL [12]. For the 2.4-mg/kg weekly schedule, the peak T-DM1 serum concentration following cycle 1 dosing was lower (C_{max} 58.4 ± 13.8 μg/mL), but total exposure of T-DM1 over a 3-week period with this weekly schedule is expected to be approximately twofold higher than the exposure of T-DM1 when given at a dose of 3.6 mg/kg on a once-every-3-week schedule [25].

Based on these results, and because of the convenience of an every-3-week schedule for patients, the 3.6-mg/kg every-3-week dose schedule was selected for evaluation in subsequent phase II studies in patients with advanced HER2-positive breast cancer. However, the increased T-DM1 exposure provided by the weekly schedule does suggest that it may be worthwhile to evaluate this more dose-dense schedule in other disease settings, particularly as the exposure–efficacy relationships of T-DM1 become better characterized. On the other hand, the impact of a more intense dose schedule on safety and tolerability of T-DM1 is not known and will require additional investigation.

Phase II Studies in Advanced HER2-Positive Metastatic Breast Cancer

Two single-arm phase II studies of single-agent T-DM1 were conducted in patients with HER2-positive metastatic breast cancer (MBC) (Table 11.2). Study TDM4258g [26] was the first phase II study conducted with T-DM1 in patients with HER2-positive MBC after promising results were observed in the dose-escalation phase I study described in the previous section. Study TDM4374g [27] was subsequently initiated to assess the efficacy and safety of T-DM1 in patients with even more heavily pretreated disease. Both studies' primary endpoint was the objective response rate based on RECIST version 1.0 [28] as determined by independent radiologic review. Secondary endpoints included duration of response and progression-free survival (PFS) by independent radiologic review as well as objective response rate, duration of response, and PFS based on investigator assessment.

The demographic characteristics of patients enrolled in the two studies were similar (see Table 11.3). Most patients had an Eastern Cooperative Oncology Group (ECOG) performance status of 0 or 1. All patients' tumors were HER2 positive by local laboratory assessment, as evidenced by 3+ on IHC and/or HER2 gene amplification determined on fluorescence in situ hybridization (FISH), with the exception of one patient in study TDM4374g whose tumor, on clinical review, was determined to be HER2 2+ on IHC and FISH negative. At study entry, all patients in both studies had measurable disease as assessed by the investigator. In general, the patients enrolled in both studies had significant disease burden. The median time

Table 11.2 TDM4374g and TDM4258g study designs

	Study TDM4258g	Study TDM4374g
Stage and design	Multi-institutional, open-label, single-arm, phase II trial	Multi-institutional, open-label, single-arm, phase II trial
Number of patients enrolled	112	110
Patients	HER2-positive MBC: • At least one prior chemotherapy agent • Prior PD on HER2-directed regimen	HER2-positive MBC: • Prior exposure to an anthracycline, taxane, capecitabine, lapatinib, and trastuzumab • Two prior HER2-directed regimens in the metastatic setting • PD on last regimen received
Dose and schedule	T-DM1 at 3.6 mg/kg IV q3w for up to 1 year or until documented disease progression or unmanageable toxicity	T-DM1 at 3.6 mg/kg IV q3w until documented disease progression or unmanageable toxicity
Primary endpoint	ORR assessed by independent review	ORR assessed by independent review
Secondary endpoints	• DoR by IRF assessment • PFS by IRF assessment • ORR, DoR, and PFS by investigator assessment	• DoR by IRF assessment • PFS by IRF assessment • Clinical benefit rate by IRF assessment • ORR, DoR, PFS, and clinical benefit rate by investigator assessment
End of follow-up	30 days after last dose unless serious adverse event (90 days)	30 days after last dose unless serious adverse event (90 days)
First patient enrolled; last patient enrolled	20 July 2007; 31 July 2008	13 August 2008; 2 April 2009

from the diagnosis of metastatic breast cancer to treatment with TDM1 was 33.1 months in study TDM4258g and 41.4 months in study TDM4374g. The number and distribution of sites of metastatic disease were similar between the two studies, with the majority of patients having had disease involvement in three or more distinct sites, most frequently lung, liver, and bone.

Patients in both studies were heavily pretreated, having received a median of eight anticancer agents in all therapeutic settings, including the adjuvant and neoadjuvant settings. The two studies had different enrollment criteria for prior therapy before trial enrollment, resulting in variations in both the number of prior agents received for the treatment of locally advanced or metastatic disease as well as the duration of prior HER2-directed therapy received in the locally advanced or metastatic setting. Study TDM4258g required patients to have a history of disease

Table 11.3 Demographic and disease characteristics: enrolled patients in studies TDM4374g and TDM4258g

Characteristic	Study TDM4258g ($n = 112$)	Study TDM4374g ($n = 110$)
Median time since metastatic diagnosis, mo (range)	33.1 (2–258)	41.4 (1–149)
ECOG performance status		
0	60 (53.6%)	54 (49.1%)
1	43 (38.4%)	53 (48.2%)
2	8 (7.1%)	3 (2.7%)
3	1 (0.9%)	0
Number of distinct metastatic sites		
<3	28 (25%)	29 (26.4%)
≥3	84 (75%)	81 (73.6%)
Site of metastasis (occurring in 40% of patients)		
Local–regional	67 (59.8%)	70 (63.6%)
Lung	63 (56.3%)	69 (62.7%)
Bone	59 (52.7%)	57 (51.8%)
Liver	63 (56.3%)	49 (44.5%)
Median number of agents for metastatic disease (range)[a]	5.0 (1–17)	7.0 (3–17)
Median number of agents in all therapy settings (range)[a]	8.0 (2–19)	8.5 (5–19)
Prior trastuzumab		
Number of patients	112 (100%)	110 (100%)
Median duration of prior trastuzumab for treatment of locally advanced or metastatic breast cancer, mo (range)	17.6 (1–152)	19.7 (1.8–115.8)
Prior lapatinib		
Number of patients	67 (59.8%)	110 (100%)
Median duration of prior lapatinib for treatment of locally advanced or metastatic breast cancer, mo (range)	6.0 (1–24)	6.8 (0.2–23.3)

Source: Refs. [26, 27]

[a]Included all agents intended for the treatment of breast cancer except hormonal therapy and myeloablative therapy with stem cell transplant

progression during or within 60 days of completing one HER2-directed therapy and to have received at least one prior chemotherapy agent for MBC. Patients received a median of five agents in the locally advanced or metastatic setting.

Study TDM4374g was subsequently initiated to evaluate the efficacy of T-DM1 in a more strictly defined homogenous patient population and required eligible patients to have been treated with an anthracycline, trastuzumab, a taxane, lapatinib, and capecitabine, and to have been exposed to two HER2-directed agents in the metastatic setting. Patients must have also received at least two lines of therapy in the metastatic setting and progressed on the last regimen received. Consequently, all 110 patients enrolled on study TDM4374g had received trastuzumab, lapatinib, capecitabine, and an anthracycline prior to study enrollment, and all but one patient had previously received a taxane. The median number of agents received in the metastatic setting was seven in study TDM4374g.

As required, all patients in both studies TDM4374g and TDM4258g received trastuzumab prior to study enrollment. Additionally, all 110 patients enrolled in study TDM4374g, and 67 patients (59.8%) in study TDM4258g received lapatinib as a second HER2-directed agent. Because study TDM4258g was activated in July 2007, just after the approval of lapatinib in combination with capecitabine for HER2-positive metastatic breast cancer (March 2007), pretreatment with lapatinib was not required for enrollment in study TDM4258g. The median duration of treatment with trastuzumab and lapatinib was similar between the two studies.

Efficacy

Single-agent T-DM1 demonstrated antitumor efficacy in both studies. Among treated patients, 29 on study TMD4258g and 36 on study TDM4374g had an objective tumor response, all partial, by independent review, corresponding to an objective response rate (ORR) of 25.9% and 32.7%, respectively (Table 11.4). Based on investigator assessment, the ORR was 37.5% in study TDM4258g and 32.7% in study TDM4374g. CBR, defined as the proportion of patients with an objective response or with stable disease for at least 6 months' duration, was 39.3% and 48.2% by independent review and 44.6% and 46.4% by investigator assessment, in study TDM4258g and TDM4374g, respectively.

In study TDM4258g, among patients with prior lapatinib treatment ($n=67$), the ORR was 24.2% (95% CI, 14.5–36.0%) by independent radiologic review and 34.8% (95% CI, 23.5–46.8%) per investigator [26]. Together with the primary results of study TDM4374g, T-DM1 had demonstrable efficacy in tumors of patients who had previously received both approved HER2-directed therapies.

Responses to T-DM1 treatment in many cases were durable (Table 11.5). Based on investigator assessment, the median duration of response was similar in the two studies: 9.7 months in TDM4374g and 9.4 months in TDM4258g. The ranges of duration of objective response were also similar between the two studies. In both studies, the median duration of response based on independent radiologic assessment was not reached due to insufficient events.

PFS, defined as the time from the first day of treatment with T-DM1 to documented disease progression or death from any cause on study, whichever occurred first, is shown in Table 11.6. No notable differences were observed between the two studies, with the median PFS by IRF and investigator assessment being 6.9 and 5.5 months, respectively, in study TDM4374g and 4.6 months for both in study TDM4258g.

Table 11.4 Objective responses: treated patients in studies TDM4374g and TDM4258g

	Study TDM4258g[a]	Study TDM4374g[b]
Treated patients, *n*	112	110
IRF assessment		
Patients with objective response, *n* (%)	29 (25.9%)	38 (34.5%)
95% CI for ORR	(18.4%, 34.4%)	(26.1%, 43.9%)
Investigator assessment		
Patients with objective response, *n* (%)	42 (37.5%)	36 (32.7%)
95% CI for ORR	(28.6%, 46.6%)	(24.1%, 42.1%)

CI, confidence interval; CSR, clinical study report; IRF, independent review facility; ORR, objective response rate

[a]Approximately 12 months of follow-up after the last patient was enrolled

[b]Approximately 9 months of follow-up after the last patient was enrolled

Source: Refs. [26, 27]

Table 11.5 Duration of objective response: responding patients in studies TDM4374g and TDM4258g

	Study TDM4258g	Study TDM4374g
IRF assessment		
Duration of objective response (mo)		
Median	NR	7.2
(95% CI)	(6.2, NE)	(4.6, NE)
Investigator assessment		
Duration of objective response (mo)		
Median	9.4	9.7
(95% CI)	(7.0, NE)	(6.6, NE)

CI, confidence interval; CSR, clinical study report; IRF, independent review facility; NE, not estimable; NR, not reached

Source: Refs. [26, 27]

Table 11.6 Progression-free survival: treated patients in studies TDM4374g and TDM4258g

	Study TDM4258g ($n=112$)	Study TDM4374g ($n=110$)
IRF assessment		
Progression-free survival (mo)		
Median	4.6	6.9
(95% CI)	(3.9, 8.6)	(4.2, 8.4)
Investigator assessment		
Progression-free survival (mo)		
Median	4.6	5.5
(95% CI)	(4.0, 6.0)	(4.1, 7.5)

CI, confidence interval; CSR, clinical study report; IRF, independent review facility; NR, not reached

Source: Refs. [26, 27]

Exploratory HER2 Testing Analyses

The development of targeted therapies such as trastuzumab and lapatinib underscores the critical value of accurate testing in determining the presence and expression level of the intended target, that is, HER2. Currently, HER2 status is determined using IHC or FISH. Despite the availability of FDA-approved diagnostic kits to assess HER2 status, standardization of diagnostic procedures and reagents is still lacking, which may be a contributing factor to the estimation that 15–20% of HER2 status as assessed by local testing may not be concordant with testing performed in a high-volume central laboratory [29]. In an analysis of breast cancer specimens obtained from 2,600 patients comparing HER2 IHC and FISH results performed in local versus central laboratories, HER2 assessment by IHC and FISH performed at local laboratories had false-positive rates of 25% and 10%, respectively, and agreement rates (κ statistic) of 0.56 and 0.83, respectively [30]. The implication of the heterogeneity of HER2 testing methodologies is that some patients may be inappropriately selected to receive (or not to receive) HER2-directed therapy and that responses to HER2-directed therapy may be affected by discrepancies in HER2 testing.

In an exploratory analysis in the two phase II studies, tumor blocks or unstained slides from archival tumor tissue, where available, were reassessed for HER2 status using standardized methods for immunohistochemistry (IHC) and/or FISH by a central pathology laboratory.

In both studies, the discordance in HER2 results between local and central assessment was similar to what has been reported in published reports [29]. In study TDM4374g, 92 patients had data available from retrospective HER2 testing. Tumors from 77 patients were assessed to be HER2 positive, whereas tumors from 15 patients (16%) were assessed to be HER2 normal. Similarly, in study TDM4258g, 99 patients had data available from retrospective HER2 testing. Tumors from 78 patients were assessed to be HER2 positive, whereas tumors from 21 patients (21%) were assessed to be HER2 normal. Objective response rates in patients with centrally assessed HER2-positive and HER2-normal tumors as determined by the IRF in the two studies are shown in Table 11.7. In both studies, the objective response rate was modestly higher when the analysis was restricted to the centrally assessed HER2-positive patient population compared with that of the entire treated population. Furthermore, the objective response rates in patients with centrally assessed HER2-positive tumors in both studies were higher compared with those with centrally assessed HER2-normal tumors.

Further evidence for the specificity of T-DM1 against HER2-overexpressing disease is provided when assessing archival tumor tissue for HER2 expression as assessed by quantitative reverse-transcriptase polymerase chain reaction (qRT-PCR). Patients enrolled on either trial with retrospectively confirmed HER2+ disease were grouped according to HER2 expression levels (≥ or <median HER2 expression level in study TDM4258g) determined by qRT-PCR. Distributions and ranges of HER2 levels assessed by qRT-PCR (Fig. 11.2a, b) were consistent with the HER2 status assessed by IHC or FISH in that tumors determined to have normal

Table 11.7 Objective response by retrospectively assessed HER2 status per the IRF: treated patients in studies TDM4374g and TDM4258g

IRF assessment	Study TDM4374g	Study TDM4258g
All treated patients, *n*	110	112
Objective response rate	32.7%	25.9%
HER2-positive status, *n*	80	78
Objective response rate	41.3% (29.2%, 52.1%)	32.1% (21.9%, 43.4%)
HER2-normal status, *n*	15	21
Objective response rate	20.0% (5.7%, 44.9%)	4.8% (<1.0%, 21.8%)

CSR, clinical study report; IRF, independent review facility
Source: Refs. [26, 27]

levels of HER2 expression had lower levels of HER2 mRNA expression. Even within the group of patients with HER2-positive tumors, this data suggests that HER2 expression may have an effect on T-DM1 efficacy. With available data from 50 patients in study TDM4258g and 65 patients in study TDM4374g, ORR per IRF in patients with ≥median HER2 expression was 36% in study TDM4258g and 50% in study TDM4374g compared with ORR of 28% and 33.3% for patients whose tumors with <median HER2 expression (Fig. 11.2c). Additionally, in study TDM4258g, the median PFS of patients with tumors ≥ median HER2 expression was not reached compared to a median PFS of 4.2 months for patients with tumors having <median HER2 expression (Fig. 11.2c) [31].

Although these results are intriguing, a number of limitations in the analyses must be noted. First, the analyses were performed on archival specimens obtained at the time of initial diagnosis where technical differences in tissue preparation and extended storage times may affect the HER2 result from central retesting. Second, in most cases, central HER2 testing was performed on tumor tissue obtained at the time of initial diagnosis and not at the time of disease recurrence. Consequently, the impact of changes in HER2 expression between these two time points is not known. Prospective studies will be required to validate these findings and confirm whether HER2 expression is a predictive marker for response to T-DM1 and to further define RT-PCR-based cutoff values for HER2 expression that could reliably predict responsiveness to T-DM1. Nevertheless, these results support the specificity of T-DM1 against HER2-overexpressing tumors and reinforce the need for high-quality HER2 testing to ensure that targeted therapies like T-DM1 are provided to the appropriate patient population.

Safety

In the phase I and two phase II studies described above, there were a total of 237 patients treated with T-DM1 at the dose schedule of 3.6 mg/kg every 3 weeks. The nature and severity of adverse events that occurred during T-DM1 treatment in these

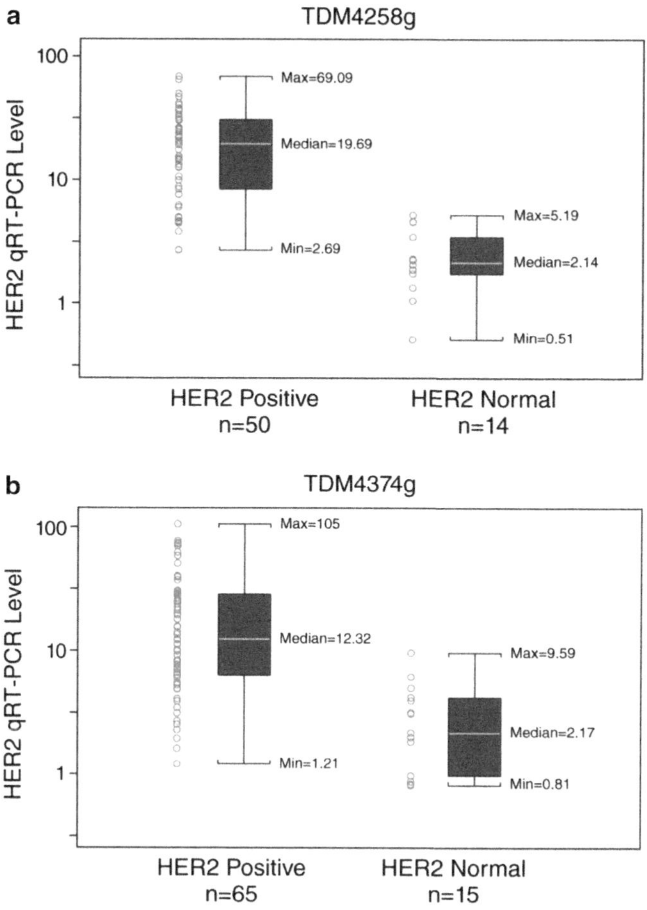

Fig. 11.2 Efficacy based on centrally assessed HER2 status and HER2 expression levels. Boxplots indicate levels of HER2 mRNA normalized to G6PDH mRNA expression, as assessed by qRT-PCR, for centrally assessed tumor samples that were found to be HER2 positive and HER2 normal in studies TDM4258g (**a**) and TDM4374g (**b**). The *upper* and *lower* limits within the *box* represent the 75th and 25th percentiles, respectively. *Open circles* represent HER2 expression levels from individual tumor samples. (**c**) Kaplan–Meier plot of PFS based on independent radiologic assessment for centrally confirmed HER2-normal patients and for HER2-positive patients based on expression of HER2 measured by qRT-PCR (≥median and <median levels) in study TDM4258g

patients are likely indicative of the safety and tolerability of T-DM1 in this population of patients with advanced MBC.

In study TDM4258g, treated patients received a median of seven doses of T-DM1 on study, with a median of 18.1 weeks duration of exposure. Twenty-one patients completed 1 year of study treatment, and 19 continued T-DM1 treatment as part of a separate extension study. In study TDM4374g, treated patients received a median of seven doses on study, with a median of 19.3 weeks duration of exposure. Most

Table 11.8 Adverse events that occurred in >20% of patients in TDM4258g or TDM4374g (all grades)

	TDM4258g			TDM4374g		
Adverse event	All grades (%)	Grade 1 or 2 (%)	Grade 3–4 (%)	All grades (%)	Grade 1 or 2 (%)	Grade 3–4 (%)
Fatigue	65.2	60.7	4.5	22.7	21.8	0.9
Nausea	50.9	50.0	0.9	37.3	36.4	0.9
Headache	40.2	40.2	0	21.8	21.8	0
Pyrexia	34.8	33.9	0.9	22.7	21.8	0.9
Epistaxis	35.7	33.9	1.8	22.7	21.8	0.9
Constipation	30.4	30.4	0	23.6	22.7	0.9
Cough	27.7	27.7	0	18.2	18.2	0
Diarrhea	25.9	25.9	0	12.7	12.7	0
Hypokalemia	24.1	15.2	8.9	20.9	20.0	0.9
Vomiting	24.1	23.2	0.9	16.4	16.4	0
Pain in extremity	22.3	22.3	0	13.6	12.8	1.8
Arthralgia	22.3	21.4	0.9	14.5	12.7	1.8
Anemia	20.5	17.9	2.7	20.0	18.2	1.8
Dyspnea	20.5	17.9	2.7	16.4	13.6	2.7
Thrombocytopenia	NR	NR	8.0	32.7	25.4	7.3
AST increased	NR	NR	NR	26.4	23.6	2.7
Decreased appetite	NR	NR	NR	20.9	20.0	0.9
Dry mouth	NR	NR	NR	20.0	20.0	0

Multiple occurrences of a specific AE for a patient were counted once at the highest NCI-CTCAE grade. Events are presented by MedDRA preferred terms
Source: Refs. [26, 27]

patients were able to receive T-DM1 until disease progression. Documented disease progression was listed as the reason for T-DM1 discontinuation in 81.2% of patients enrolled in study TDM4258g and 69.1% of patients enrolled in study TDM4374g. Four patients on study TDM4258g and seven patients in study TDM4374g discontinued T-DM1 treatment because of a documented adverse event.

The most common adverse events of any severity grade as measured by the NCI-CTCAE (version 3.0) for the two phase II studies are shown in Table 11.8. In general, the nature and severity of adverse events were consistent between the two studies. The vast majority of documented adverse events were grades 1–2 in severity. The most frequently observed grade 3–4 adverse events in study TDM4258g were hypokalemia (8.9%), thrombocytopenia (8.0%), and fatigue (4.5%); in study TDM4374g, the most frequently observed grade 3–4 adverse events were thrombocytopenia (7.3%), fatigue (4.5%), and cellulitis (3.6%). Regarding serious adverse events occurring in three or more patients, in study TDM4258g, cellulitis was reported in three patients, whereas in study TDM4374g, the most frequent serious adverse events were cellulitis in four patients and pyrexia and pneumonia each in three patients.

A total of three patients on the two phase II studies experienced adverse events leading to death including hepatic function abnormality, pneumonia, and interstitial lung disease. Four patients enrolled in study TDM4258g discontinued T-DM1 for the following reasons: concurrent thrombocytopenia and hepatotoxicity, thrombocytopenia, concurrent asthenia and failure to thrive, and secondary malignancy with onset retrospectively determined to occur prior to T-DM1 dosing. Seven patients enrolled in study TDM4374g discontinued T-DM1 for adverse events including abnormal hepatic function, spinal cord compression, fatigue, cholelithiasis/pancreatitis, dyspnea, atrial fibrillation, and thrombocytopenia.

Thrombocytopenia, defined as the DLT in the phase I study [12], was not associated with serious hemorrhage in either phase II study. Based on weekly laboratory evaluations of platelet count, thrombocytopenia was generally transient and noncumulative. Declines in platelet count were observed approximately 7 days after T-DM1 dose with sufficient recovery to allow subsequent T-DM1 dosing to take place on schedule. Clinically, thrombocytopenia was manifested primarily as a laboratory abnormality without significant bleeding events. Specifically, the most commonly reported hemorrhagic AE was grade 1–2 epistaxis in 34% and 21.8% of treated patients on studies TDM4258g and TDM4374g, respectively. Grade>2 thrombocytopenia was infrequent and, as described above, rarely led to discontinuation of T-DM1 treatment. Episodic platelet transfusions were also infrequent, and to date, there have been no documented instances where a patient required chronic platelet transfusions for recurrent thrombocytopenia.

The mechanism of action of thrombocytopenia resulting from T-DM1 treatment is not known and appears to be specific to the platelets and not other hematopoietic cell lines; anemia and leukopenia were less frequently observed than thrombocytopenia in each of the studies. Population PKPD (define) modeling from the phase I and phase II studies suggested that fluctuations in the platelet count with T-DM1 treatment resulted primarily from alterations in platelet production by megakaryocytes in the bone marrow [45]. This is consistent with the hypothesis that tubulin-dependent mechanisms related to pre-platelet release from mature megakaryocytes, rather than direct cytotoxic effects on megakaryocytes, are responsible for the thrombocytopenia associated with T-DM1. Moreover, based on covariate analysis to determine any baseline demographic or pathophysiologic characteristic could be used to predict a patient's platelet response to T-DM1 a priori, a baseline platelet count ≤200,000 μL^{-1} was the only factor that significantly contributed to an increased risk of developing grade 3–4 thrombocytopenia, suggesting that these patients' platelet counts should be carefully monitored.

Elevations in hepatic transaminases (aspartate aminotransferase [AST] and alanine aminotransferase [ALT]) were observed in the majority of patients enrolled in the two phase II studies. Similar to thrombocytopenia, elevations in AST and ALT were generally transient, reversible, and rarely resulted in discontinuation from T-DM1 treatment. However, grade 3 AST and ALT elevations were observed in 2.7% of patients in study TDM4374g and were associated with one patient death. The mechanism of action of T-DM1 associated hepatotoxicity is not known but has been observed with other maytansinoid ADCs [32].

Characterization of the cardiotoxicity profile of T-DM1 is of interest given the well-documented association of cardiotoxicity with trastuzumab treatment [33]. Despite the fact that many patients were previously treated with anthracyclines in addition to trastuzumab, no grade 3 LVEF declines or symptomatic congestive heart failure were observed in either phase II study, and no patients discontinued treatment due to cardiac toxicity. Two patients had LVEF declines to 40–45% on study TDM4258g; no patients on study TDM4374g had declines to ≤45%. It should be noted, however, that patients with a history of cardiac disease or LVEF < 50% by cardiac echocardiogram or MUGA at baseline were not eligible for study enrollment. An ongoing phase II study (TDM4874g, clinicaltrials.gov identifier NCT01196052) aims to assess cardiac adverse events in patients receiving T-DM1 following anthracycline-based therapy. Similarly, the effects of T-DM1 on potential QTc prolongation, which is qualitatively associated with the potentially fatal ventricular arrhythmia torsades de pointes, are being evaluated in another phase II study (TDM4688g, clinicaltrials.gov identifier NCT00943670).

Pharmacokinetics

Pharmacokinetic parameter values for T-DM1 from all PK-evaluable patients in study TDM4258g were consistent with those observed in the phase I study with added PK information following T-DM1 administration at cycle 4 (Fig. 11.3). T-DM1 C_{max} and area under curve (AUC) in cycles 1 and 4 were comparable, indicating no accumulation of T-DM1 with q3w dosing (Fig. 11.3B). As observed in the phase I study [12], total trastuzumab had a higher C_{max} and AUC and longer terminal half-life than T-DM1. While the reasons for the difference between T-DM1 and total trastuzumab PK are not definitively known, population PK modeling supports the presence of different routes of clearance of T-DM1 and trastuzumab as a potential

a Study TDM4258g: Pharmacokinetic Parameter Estimates following 3.6 mg/kg T-DM1 Administration Every Three Weeks

		Mean (SD)				
Cycle	Analyte	C_{max} (μg/mL)	AUC (μg•day/mL)	Terminal $t_{½}$ (day)	CL (mL/day/kg)	V_{ss} (mL/kg)
1	T-DM1	80.9 (20.7)	457 (129)	3.53 (0.7)	8.51 (2.7)	28.4 (12.9)
4	T-DM1	68.9 (21.8)	461 (136)	4.43 (1.7)	8.41 (4.3)	45.2 (43.0)

$AUC=AUC_{inf}$ (area under the concentration–time curve to infinity) for Cycle 1 and AUC_{last} (area under concentration curve to last sampling) for Cycle 4; CL=clearance; C_{max}=maximum plasma concentration; $t_{½}$=half-life; V_{ss}=volume of distribution at steady state.
Notes: n=101 for Cycle 1 and 61 for Cycle 4 for T-DM1. Pharmacokinetic parameters were not calculated for DM1 because measurable concentrations were observed only at the end of the infusion.

b

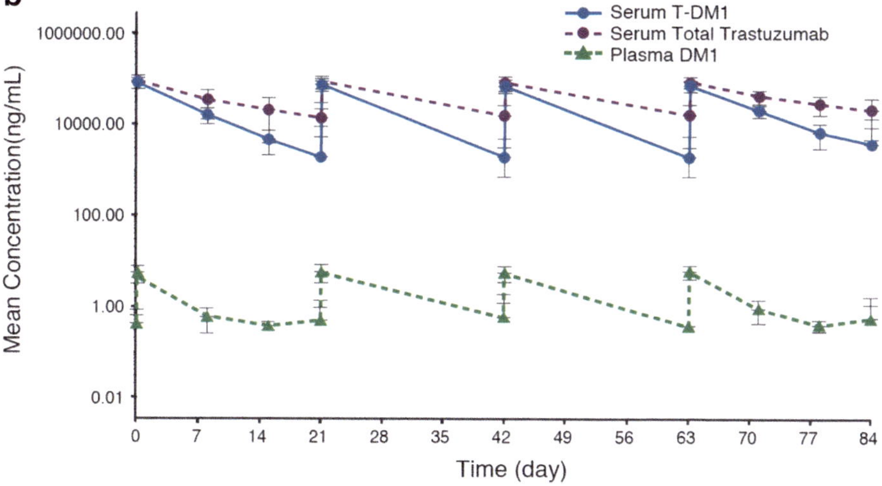

Fig. 11.3 Pharmacokinetics of T-DM1, total trastuzumab, and plasma DM1 in study TDM4258g. (**a**) Estimates of mean (and standard deviation) C_{max}, area under curve (*AUC*), terminal half-life, clearance, and volume of distribution at steady state (*V*ss) are shown for T-DM1 and total trastuzumab after cycle 1 and cycle 4 of T-DM1 treatment in PK-evaluable patients enrolled on study TDM4258g. The lower limit of quantitation for T-DM1 and trastuzumab by ELISA was 40 ng/mL. The lower limit of quantitation for DM1 was 0.74 ng/mL. (**b**) Mean concentration–time profiles for serum T-DM1, serum total trastuzumab, and plasma DM1 in study TDM4258g

determining factor. In this model, elimination of T-DM1 results from deconjugation of DM1 from trastuzumab (resulting in free trastuzumab) and proteolytic degradation; in contrast, elimination of trastuzumab would occur solely as a result of proteolytic degradation [34].

Important to the safety and tolerability profile of T-DM1, systemic exposure to DM1 was consistently very low; maximum DM1 levels averaged 5.35 ± 2.03 ng/mL in cycle 1. The highest observed concentration of DM1 was <17 ng/mL, and because DM1 was only measurable immediately following T-DM1 administration, no formal pharmacokinetic analysis of DM1 was possible. Moreover, repeated T-DM1 administration did not result in DM1 accumulation (Fig. 11.3B). Similar results were observed in study TDM4374g.

The appropriateness of the 3.6-mg/kg q3w dose schedule was further supported by a population PK analysis performed on 273 patients across the phase I and two phase II studies that was designed to identify clinical baseline covariates that could have an impact on T-DM1 pharmacokinetics. Based on this analysis, T-DM1 exposure was relatively consistent based on body weight dosing. Although there were statistically significant differences in interindividual variability associated with a number of covariates including body weight, serum albumin levels, tumor burden, and AST levels, the magnitude of these differences compared with typical parameter values was low (< 26% interindividual variability). As a result of the clinical and pharmacokinetic data, the 3.6-mg/kg q3w dose schedule has been adopted in most clinical trials of T-DM1 [35].

Forty-four percent of patients had measurable total serum trastuzumab (0.044–66.9 μg/mL) prior to receiving T-DM1, which was not unexpected since patients had received prior trastuzumab treatment and given trastuzumab's half-life of approximately 16 days when given on a typical q3w schedule to patients with HER2-positive breast cancer. Despite the presence of circulating trastuzumab, there was no impact on T-DM1 exposure.

With respect to immunogenicity, 7 of 108 evaluable patients in study TDM4258g developed anti-T-DM1 antibodies (ATA) with no obvious impact on pharmacokinetics (Table 11.9). The formation of ATA was not associated with significant clinical events [26].

Phase II Study of T-DM1 Compared to Docetaxel and Trastuzumab as First-Line Treatment in HER2-Positive Metastatic Breast Cancer

While the aforementioned single-arm phase II studies of T-DM1 in patients with advanced HER2-positive MBC showed strong evidence of antitumor efficacy combined with an apparently acceptable safety and tolerability profile, a clear demonstration of the clinical benefit with T-DM1 treatment would require a direct comparison with a standard regimen of trastuzumab combined with chemotherapy. To address this, a randomized open-label phase II study (TDM4450g; clinicaltrials.gov identifier: NCT00679341) was conducted to compare the efficacy and safety of single-agent T-DM1 administered at 3.6 mg/kg q3w with that of trastuzumab (8 mg/kg initial dose followed by 6 mg/kg q3w) and docetaxel (75 mg/m^2 or 100 mg/m^2 q3w) in patients with HER2-positive recurrent locally advanced breast cancer or previously untreated MBC. 137 patients were enrolled. Baseline demographic and disease characteristics between the two arms, including ECOG performance status, hormone receptor status, and prior therapies, were similar between the two arms. 27.1% and 17.9% of patients enrolled to the trastuzumab plus docetaxel arm and T-DM1 arm, respectively, received prior trastuzumab in the neoadjuvant and/or adjuvant settings.

Table 11.9 Impact of anti-therapeutic antibody on T-DM1 pharmacokinetics

		Mean (±SD)	
Patient population	Number of patients[a]	AUC_{inf} (μg day/mL)	C_{max} (μg/mL)
All PK-evaluable patients	101	457 (±129)	80.9 (±20.7)
Patients with positive ATA response[a]	7	409 (±149)	77.8 (±25.0)
Patients with negative ATA response	94	461 (±128)	81.2 (±20.5)

[a]Number of patients whose pretreatment (baseline) ATA response was negative but who had at least one positive confirmed ATA response after T-DM1 treatment

Primary efficacy and safety results based on a median of 6 months' duration of follow-up indicate that T-DM1 was superior in terms of the primary endpoint of the study, PFS. Based on investigator assessment, the median PFS in patients treated with T-DM1 was 14.2 months compared to 9.2 months among patients treated with trastuzumab and docetaxel (HR = 0.594; log-rank p value = 0.0353; Fig. 11.4a). Objective response rates were similar between the two treatment arms (58% for trastuzumab plus docetaxel versus 64.2% for T-DM1). However, more durable responses were observed in patients treated with T-DM1 (Fig. 11.4b). Moreover, the median duration of treatment was 10 months for T-DM1, 8.1 months for trastuzumab, and 5.5 months for docetaxel [36].

The safety profile of T-DM1 was also favorable compared to the combination of trastuzumab and docetaxel. Notably, the proportion of patients with reported grade ≥ 3 adverse events was 46.2% in the T-DM1 compared to 89.4% in the chemotherapy combination arm. Hematologic grade ≥ 3 adverse events commonly associated with docetaxel treatment, that is, neutropenia, leukopenia, and febrile neutropenia, were less frequently observed with T-DM1 (Table 11.10). In addition, alopecia, which is an event that has substantial psychosocial impact particularly on patients with advanced disease, was reported in only three patients treated with T-DM1 versus 44 patients treated with trastuzumab and docetaxel (Table 11.10). Beyond these specific adverse events, the spectrum of adverse events with T-DM1 treatment was consistent with those observed in the phase II studies in patients with more advanced HER2-positive MBC described earlier. Grade ≥ 3 thrombocytopenia was reported in 8.7% of patients (compared to 3.0% in the control arm); grade 3 elevations in AST and ALT each were observed in 8.7% of patients (compared to 0 in the control arm). Finally, based on regular echocardiogram/MUGA evaluations, T-DM1 was not associated with an increased of cardiotoxicity compared with trastuzumab and docetaxel [36].

Taken together, the preliminary results of study TDM4450g, which provide the first direct comparison with a trastuzumab-containing regimen, are strong evidence of an improved therapeutic window provided by T-DM1. The improvement in PFS with T-DM1 may result from a number of factors contributing to increased duration of T-DM1 treatment, including improved tolerability of T-DM1 over the combination of trastuzumab and docetaxel and the intrinsic antitumor potency of HER2-targeted delivery of DM1.

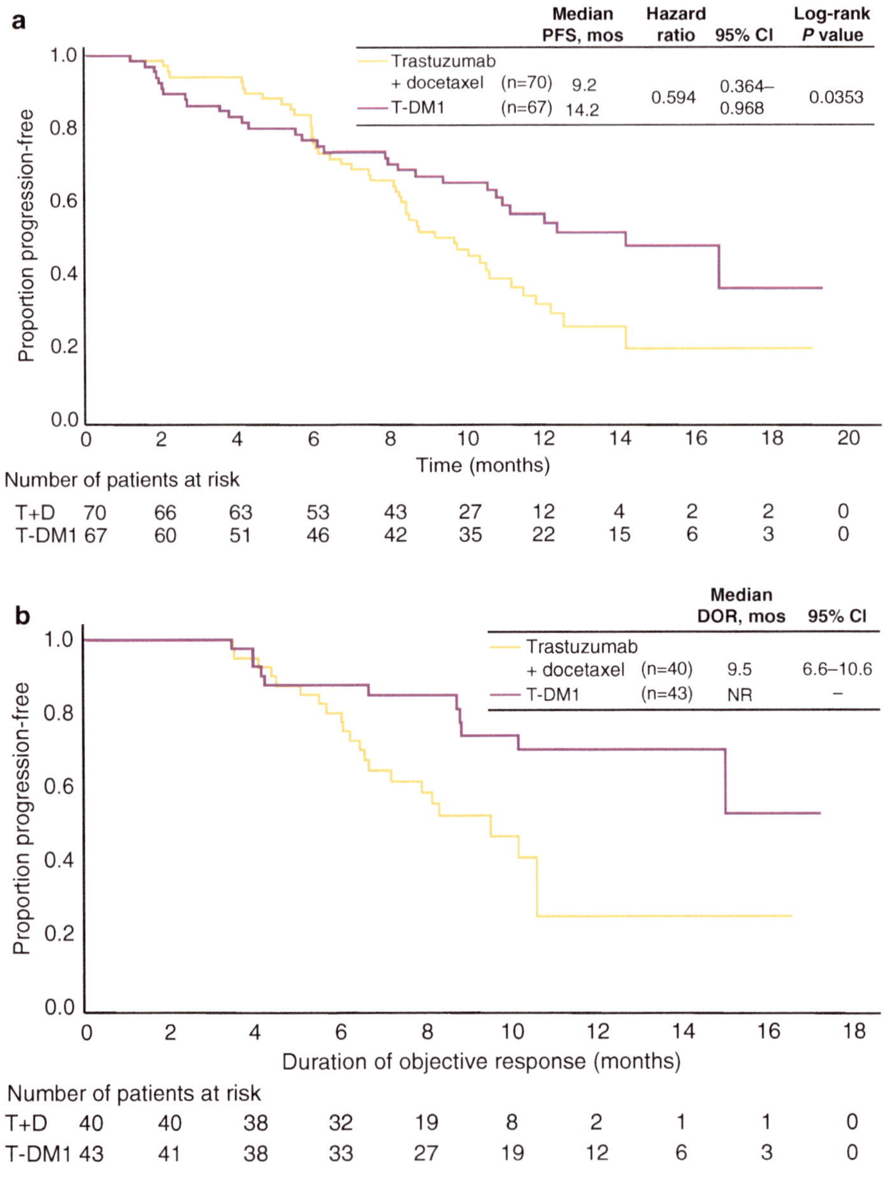

Fig. 11.4 Progression free survival (*PFS*) and duration of response in study TDM4450g. (**a**) Kaplan–Meier curves for PFS. Hazard ratio and log-rank *P* values were from stratified analysis. (**b**) Kaplan–Meier curves for duration of response. Note that the median duration of response for T-DM1 was not reached. *T+D* trastuzumab plus docetaxel; *CI* confidence interval; *NR* not reached

Table 11.10 Adverse events in study TDM4450; ≥30% (all grades) and/or ≥ 5% (grade ≥ 3) of patients in either treatment arm

	All grades, *n* (%)		Grade ≥ 3[a], *n* (%)	
	Trastuzumab + docetaxel (*n* = 66)[b]	T-DM1 (*n* = 69)[b,c]	Trastuzumab + docetaxel (*n* = 66)[b]	T-DM1 (*n* = 69)[b,c]
Non-hematologic adverse event				
Alopecia	44 (66.7)	3 (4.3)	[d]	[d]
Fatigue	30 (45.5)	34 (49.3)	3 (4.5)	3 (4.3)
Nausea	29 (43.9)	33 (47.8)	0	2 (2.9)
Diarrhea	30 (45.5)	11 (15.9)	2 (3.0)	0
Peripheral edema	29 (43.9)	7 (10.1)	3 (4.5)	0
Increased AST	4 (6.1)	27 (39.1)	0	6 (8.7)
Pyrexia	15 (22.7)	27 (39.1)	1 (1.5)	0
Headache	12 (18.2)	25 (36.2)	0	0
Back pain	20 (30.3)	18 (26.1)	3 (4.5)	1 (1.4)
Increased ALT	4 (6.1)	16 (23.2)	0	6 (8.7)
Pneumonia	1 (1.5)	6 (8.7)	0	4 (5.8)
Hematologic adverse event				
Neutropenia[e]	42 (63.6)	12 (17.4)	40 (60.6)	4 (5.8)
Febrile neutropenia	9 (13.6)	0	9 (13.6)	0
Thrombocytopenia[e]	4 (6.1)	21 (30.4)	2 (3.0)[f]	6 (8.7)[f]
Leukopenia[e]	18 (27.3)	6 (8.7)	17 (25.8)	0

[a]No adverse events listed were grade 5

[b]Two patients mistakenly received a dose of T-DM1 and were thus included in the T-DM1 arm for safety analyses

[c]Includes 3 patients who received at least 1 dose of trastuzumab alone or trastuzumab plus docetaxel

[d]National Cancer Institute Common Terminology Criteria for Adverse Events v.3 only categorizes alopecia as grade 1 or grade 2; there is no grade ≥3 for this AE

[e]Neutropenia includes events classified as MedDRA preferred terms neutropenia or neutrophil count decreased; thrombocytopenia includes events classified as MedDRA preferred terms thrombocytopenia, platelet count decreased, or heparin-induced thrombocytopenia; leukopenia includes events classified as MedDRA preferred terms leukopenia or white blood cell count decreased

[f]All of these events were grade 3

Phase III Studies

Results of the first phase III trial to demonstrate superiority of T-DM1compared with standard therapy were recently published in the New England Journal of Medicine [44]. EMILIA is a randomized, phase III study comparing T-DM1 (3.6 mg/kg every 3 weeks) to capecitabine and lapatinib in nearly 1000 patients with advanced breast cancer progressing on trastuzumab and a taxane (Fig. 11.5). The primary endpoint, PFS, was significantly longer in patients receiving T-DM1 compared with those treated with capecitabine and lapatinib (9.6 months vs. 6.4 months, $P < .0001$, Fig. 11.6a). With the exception of the 138 patients older than 65 years, this benefit was maintained across all subgroups. Treatment with T-DM1 also resulted in significantly improved overall response, and an almost doubling of median duration of response (Table 11.11). At a median follow-up of about 19 months, and after 331 deaths, overall survival was significantly longer in patients treated with T-DM1 compared to those treated with lapatinib and capecitabine, reaching the pre-specified study endpoint (30.9 versus 25.1 months respectively, HR 0.682, $P = .0006$, Fig. 11.6b). Final survival data is expected in 2014.

The EMILIA trial also reported less toxicity with T-DM1 compared to the control arm. Eighty-nine percent of patients in the lapatinib/capecitabine arm experienced grade ≥3 adverse events, compared with only 46% of patients in the T-DM1 arm; only 5.9% (29 patients) required treatment discontinuation due to toxicity in this arm compared with 10.7% (52 patients) treated with lapatinib and capecitabine (Table 11.12). Patients treated with lapatinib/capecitabine had a higher incidence of grade 3/4 diarrhea (20.7 versus 1.6%) and hand foot syndrome (16.4 versus 0%). In contrast, grade 3/4 thrombocytopenia was more common in patients treated with T-DM1 (12.8 versus 0.2%) but rarely led to hemorrhage. Transaminases were increased more frequently with T-DM1 as well, with grade 3/4 elevations occurring in less than 5% of study patients. Both thrombocytopenia and transaminase elevation responded to holding drug and dose reductions, when necessary.

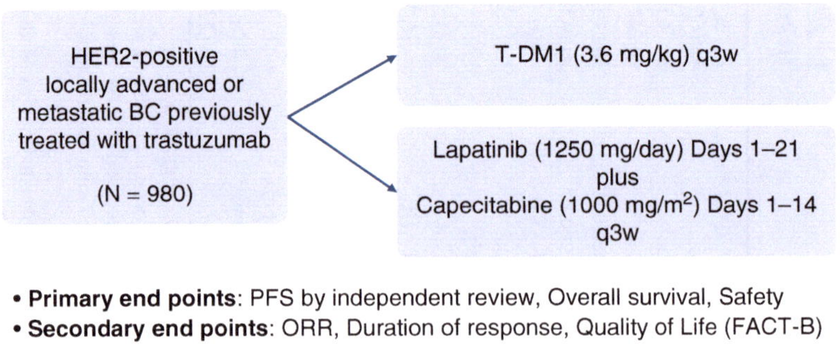

Fig. 11.5 Schema for the EMILIA study, a randomized open-label multi-institutional phase III study of single-agent T-DM1 versus the combination of lapatinib and capecitabine for the treatment of patients with HER2-positive locally advanced or metastatic breast cancer previously treated with trastuzumab

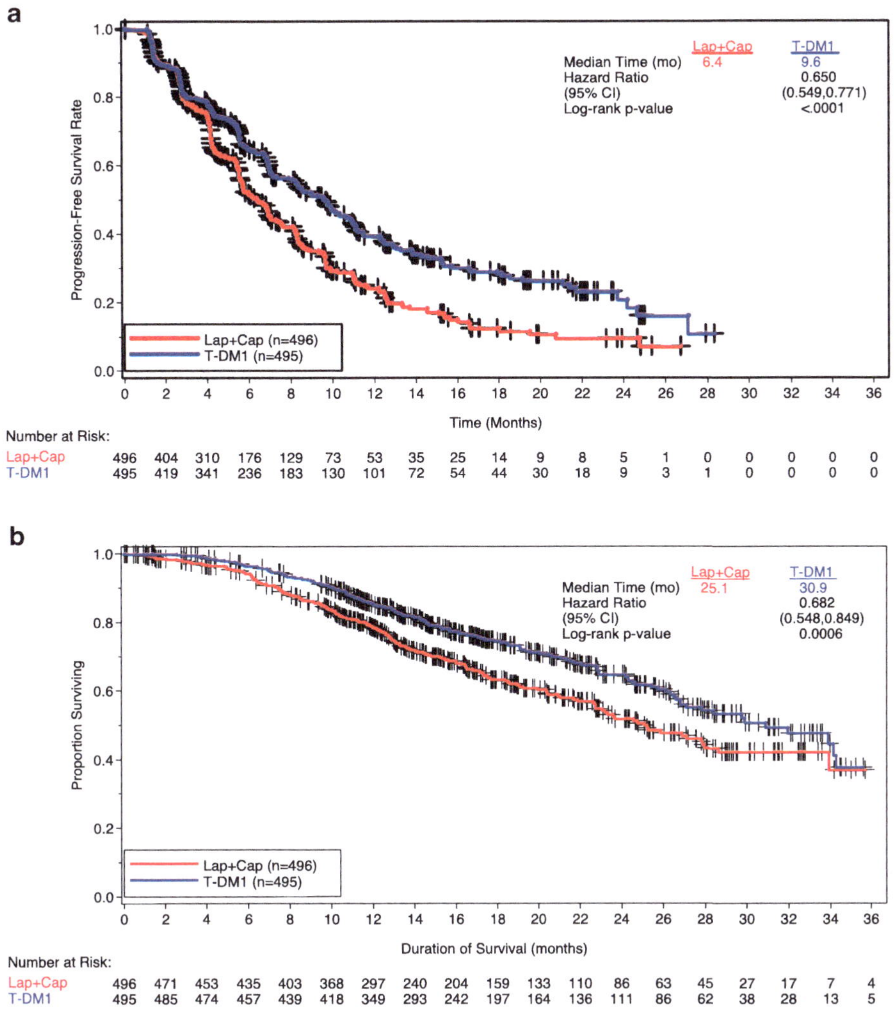

Fig. 11.6 Results of the EMILIA trial. (**a**) Progression free survival. (**b**) Overall survival at a median follow-up of about 19 months. Lap = lapatinib, Cap = capecitabine

Cardiotoxicity was not increased in the T-DM1 arm compared with the control arm (1.7% versus 1.6%, respectively). Patient-reported outcomes documented a significantly shorter time to symptom progression using the FACT Breast Trial Outcome Index in patients treated with capecitabine and lapatinib versus T-DM1 (4.6 versus 7.1 months, HR 0.8, $P = .012$). An application has been submitted to the FDA for T-DM1 based on this data, and approval is expected in 2013.

A second phase III trial, named MARIANNE (BO22589/TDM4788g Fig. 11.7a; clinicaltrials.gov identifier NCT01120184), is expected to report initial results in

Table 11.11 Overall response and duration of response in the EMILIA trial

Adverse Event	**Lapatinib Plus Capecitabine (n=488)**		**T-DM1 (n=490)**	
	All grades, n (%)	**Grade 3-4 n (%)**	**All grades, n (%)**	**Grade 3-4 n (%)**
Overall	477 (97.7)	278 (57.0)	470 (95.9)	200 (40.8)
Specific events				
Diarrhea	389 (79.7)	101 (20.7)	114 (23.3)	8 (1.6)
Palmar–plantar erythodysesthesia	283 (58.0)	80 (16.4)	6 (1.2)	0 (0.0)
Vomiting	143 (29.3)	22 (4.5)	93 (19.0)	4 (0.8)
Neutropenia	42 (8.6)	21 (4.3)	29 (5.9)	10 (2.0)
Hypokalemia	42 (8.6)	20 (4.1)	42 (8.6)	11 (2.2)
Fatigue	136 (27.9)	17 (3.5)	172 (35.1)	12 (2.4)
Nausea	218 (44.7)	12 (2.5)	192 (39.2)	4 (0.8)
Mucosal inflammation	93 (19.1)	11 (2.3)	33 (6.7)	1 (0.2)
Anemia	39 (8.0)	8 (1.6)	51 (10.4)	13 (2.7)
Increased ALT	43 (8.8)	7 (1.4)	83 (16.9)	14 (2.9)
Increased AST	46 (9.4)	4 (0.8)	110 (22.4)	21 (4.3)
Thrombocytopenia	12 (2.5)	1 (0.2)	137 (28.0)	63 (12.9)

*The safety population includes all patients who received at least one dose of the treatment, based on actual treatment received.
ALT = alanine aminotransferase, AST = aspartate aminotransferase, T-DM1 = trastuzumab emtansine

Table 11.12 Toxicities reported in the EMILIA trial, comparing lapatinib/capecitabine to T-DM1

	Lapatinib Plus Capecitabine (N=389)	**T-DM1 (N=397)**
Objective response, n (%)	120 (30.8)	173 (43.6)
95% CI	26.3–35.7	38.6–48.6
Difference in rates, % (95% CI)	12.7 (6.0–19.4)	
P value	0.0002	
Complete response, n (%)	2 (0.5)	4 (1.0)
Partial response, n (%)	118 (30.3)	169 (42.6)
Median duration of objective response, months (95% CI)	6.5 (5.5–7.2)	12.6 (8.4–20.8)

*The total number of patients in each group reflects those with measurable disease at baseline, as determined by independent review.
CI = confidence interval, T-DM1 = trastuzumab emtansine

2013. Marianne is a three-arm randomized open-label registrational trial examining the combination of T-DM1 plus the HER2-directed monoclonal antibody pertuzumab compared to T-DM1 plus placebo or combined trastuzumab plus a taxane as first-line treatment of recurrent or progressive locally advanced breast cancer or previously untreated MBC. The addition of pertuzumab, which like trastuzumab binds to HER2 but inhibits HER2 signaling by mechanisms distinct from trastuzumab, is

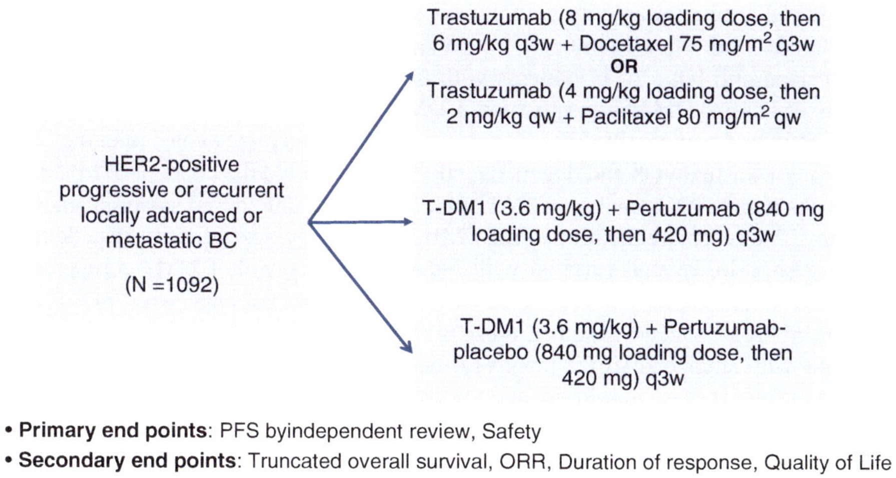

Fig. 11.7 Schema for the ongoing MARIANNE study, a randomized open-label multi-institutional phase III study of T-DM1 plus pertuzumab and T-DM1 plus pertuzumab–placebo versus the combination of trastuzumab plus a taxane for the treatment of patients with HER2-positive progressive or recurrent locally advanced breast cancer or newly diagnosed metastatic breast cancer

hypothesized to provide additional antitumor efficacy compared to T-DM1 alone. This is based in part on preclinical breast cancer models that showed synergistic antitumor effects when T-DM1 is combined with pertuzumab and clinical results from studies of pertuzumab combined with trastuzumab that demonstrated objective responses in patients who had prior disease progression on trastuzumab alone [36]. A phase Ib/II study of T-DM1 combined with pertuzumab (TDM4373g) as second-line and first-line treatment of HER2-positive MBC has been conducted and demonstrated the feasibility of combining the two agents at full single-agent doses from a safety and efficacy standpoint [23].

The primary endpoints of the MARIANNE study are PFS by independent review and safety. An important secondary endpoint of the MARIANNE study is the assessment of patients' quality of life through the use of patient-reported outcomes. Together with conventional measures of safety, these questionnaires will provide an opportunity to more fully describe the impact of treatment toxicities on the individual patient and determine the overall clinical benefit of T-DM1 with respect to disease-related toxicities [37].

Future Directions

Results of clinical studies conducted to date strongly support T-DM1 as an effective and tolerable therapeutic option against HER2-positive cancer. It is noteworthy that single-agent T-DM1, in the absence of additional systemic chemotherapy, has meaningful antitumor activity not only in patients with advanced disease who have been treated with a large number of anticancer therapies including prior trastuzumab and/or lapatinib but also in patients with *de novo* metastatic disease. Preliminary results of study TDM4450g, in which T-DM1 administered without systemic chemotherapy had comparable efficacy and fewer severe adverse events than the combination of trastuzumab and docetaxel, strongly supported the concept of treatment regimens using ADCs such as T-DM1 that are free of untethered systemic chemotherapy. The recent publication of the EMILIA trial provides definitive data demonstrating superior overall survival with reduced toxicity with T-DM1 compared to standard chemotherapy combined with lapatinib in patients with pre-treated advanced breast cancer. Together, these results demonstrate the utility of T-DM1 in patients with advanced HER2-positive breast cancer who, because of the advanced nature of their disease and frequent comorbidities, often require tolerable yet effective therapy. Regardless of the setting in which T-DM1 is administered, the potential minimal impact of T-DM1 treatment on patients' quality of life cannot be underestimated. Based on these data, several planned studies will also explore the use of T-DM1 in the adjuvant or neoadjuvant settings.

While evidence to date indicates that T-DM1 has an important role in the treatment of HER2-positive cancers, there remain a number of important questions as to how T-DM1 can be best used. First, additional work remains to assess combination therapies of T-DM1 with other anticancer agents. Ongoing studies are exploring the utility and feasibility of combining T-DM1 with chemotherapeutic agents such as paclitaxel and docetaxel, as well as other monoclonal antibodies such as pertuzumab (e.g., the phase III MARIANNE study). Additional combinations with other agents that specifically target molecular pathways critical to the survival and proliferation of breast cancers would also be of considerable scientific and clinical interest. Such novel combinations would constitute major steps in fulfilling the vision of effective therapy against HER2-positive breast cancer free of systemic chemotherapy.

Beyond the conceptual considerations, it should be noted that the optimal dose schedule as defined for single-agent studies of T-DM1 in advanced HER2-positive breast cancer could differ when combined with other agents. Further dose adjustments among the individual agents may be necessary to achieve the optimal balance of efficacy and safety and tolerability. Moreover, these considerations are particularly important as T-DM1 begins to be explored in earlier-line indications including the neoadjuvant and adjuvant settings. The potential for combined targeted approaches to treat HER2-positive breast cancer was recently exemplified by recent findings from neoadjuvant studies demonstrating the benefit of dual-HER2 inhibition. In one study, the addition of the HER2-directed monoclonal pertuzumab to trastuzumab and chemotherapy and, in a separate study, the addition of the oral receptor EGFR/HER2 tyrosine kinase inhibitor lapatinib to trastuzumab and chemotherapy resulted in improved pathologic complete response rates compared to trastuzumab plus chemotherapy alone [38, 39]. Even interactions of T-DM1 with commonly used conventional chemotherapy agents remain to be studied. Whether the sequential use of T-DM1 following anthracycline chemotherapy, for example, has any deleterious effects on cardiac function as was observed in patients treated with trastuzumab is an important question that requires further investigation.

While the clinical investigations of T-DM1 to date have been in HER2-positive breast cancer, the potential use of T-DM1 in other HER2-positive tumors remains unexplored. The recent demonstration that trastuzumab in combination with chemotherapy for the first-line treatment of HER2-positive gastric cancer [40] is demonstration of the value of HER2 suppression for cancers beyond breast cancer and suggests that the ability of T-DM1 to both inhibit HER2 and specifically deliver a potent cytotoxic agent makes it worthy of evaluation in gastric cancer [41]. On the other hand, optimization of T-DM1 dose schedules will be necessary. Not only, as previously mentioned, is the feasibility of combining T-DM1 with other anticancer agents not fully elucidated but the pharmacokinetics and pharmacodynamics of T-DM1, which to date have been assessed solely in HER2-positive breast cancer, are completely unknown in HER2-positive gastric cancer. Dose-finding studies, characterization of T-DM1 pharmacokinetics and pharmacodynamics, and clinical correlations to efficacy and tolerability in HER2-positive gastric cancer will be required.

In an era of personalized health care, identifying patients that could benefit from T-DM1 is critically important. Completed and ongoing studies of T-DM1 utilize HER2 expression as the single determinant of identifying patients eligible for T-DM1 treatment and preliminary data from study TDM4258g indicate that HER2 gene expression is a major determinant in T-DM1 efficacy. However, it remains to be seen if T-DM1 treatment would result in varying degrees of clinical benefit within the HER2-positive breast cancer population. For example, cancers that harbor potential resistance mechanisms to trastuzumab therapy such as activating mutations in the PI3K pathway [42] and/or expression of the truncated form of HER2 receptor (p95HER2) [43] could also be resistant to treatment with T-DM1. To answer specific hypotheses around these biologically important questions will require clinical trials designed to access or obtain tumor tissue at various time points throughout a patient's treatment course.

While the concept of ADCs is not new, only recently have developments in target selection, linker design, and payload optimization resulted in fulfilling their clinical potential. T-DM1 is a molecule unique even among ADCs because of the documented clinical benefit of the parent antibody trastuzumab on top of the benefits of targeted delivery of chemotherapy. The promising results of T-DM1 in clinical trials to date, and in particular the recent remarkable results of the EMILIA trial, are clear evidence of the potential of ADCs to be important players in the treatment of patients with cancer.

References

1. Hynes NE, Stern DF (1994) The biology of erbB-2/neu/HER-2 and its role in cancer. Biochim Biophys Acta 1198:165–184
2. Dawood S, Broglio K, Buzdar AU et al (2010) Prognosis of women with metastatic breast cancer by HER2 status and trastuzumab treatment: an institutional-based review. J Clin Oncol 28:92–98

3. Galsky MD, Von Hoff DD, Neubauer M et al (2012) Target-specific, histology-independent, randomized discontinuation study of lapatinib in patients with HER2-amplified solid tumors. Invest New Drugs 30(2):695–701. doi:10.1007/s10637-010-9541-0
4. Slamon DJ, Leyland-Jones B, Shak S et al (2001) Use of chemotherapy plus a monoclonal antibody against HER2 for metastatic breast cancer that overexpresses HER2. N Engl J Med 344:783–792
5. Romond EH, Perez EA, Bryant J et al (2005) Trastuzumab plus adjuvant chemotherapy for operable HER2-positive breast cancer. N Engl J Med 353:1673–1684
6. Marty M, Cognetti F, Maraninchi D et al (2005) Randomized phase II trial of the efficacy and safety of trastuzumab combined with docetaxel in patients with human epidermal growth factor receptor 2-positive metastatic breast cancer administered as first-line treatment: the M77001 study group. J Clin Oncol 23:4247–4250
7. Trastuzumab (Herceptin®) Investigator Brochure, Genentech, Inc., South San Francisco, CA, July 2007
8. Lapatinib (Tykerb®) Product Insert, GlaxoSmithKline, 2008
9. Johnston S, Pippen J, Pvot X et al (2009) Lapatinib combined with Letrozole versus letrozole and placebo as first-line therapy for postmenopausal hormone receptor-positive metastatic breast cancer. J Clin Oncol 27:5538–5546
10. Clinicaltrials.gov identifier numbers NCT00526669 and NCT00486954
11. Spector NL, Xia W, Burris H 3rd et al (2005) Study of the biologic effects of lapatinib, a reversible inhibitor of ErbB1 and ErbB2 tyrosine kinases, on tumor growth and survival pathways in patients with advanced malignancies. J Clin Oncol 23:2502–2512
12. Krop I, Beeram M, Modi S et al (2010) A phase I study of trastuzumab-DM1, a HER2 antibody-drug conjugate, given every 3 weeks to patients with HER2+ metastatic breast cancer. J Clin Oncol 28:2698–2704
13. Remillard S, Rebhun LI, Howie GS, Kupchan SM (1975) Antimitotic activity of the potent tumor inhibitor maytansine. Science 189:1002–1005
14. Cassady JM, Chan KK, Floss HG, Leistner E (2004) Recent developments in the maytansinoid antitumor agents. Chem Pharm Bull 52:1–26
15. Widdison WC et al (2006) Semisynthetic maytansine analogues for the targeted treatment of cancer. J Med Chem 49:4392–4408
16. Data-on-file, Genentech, Inc., South San Francisco, CA, July 2007
17. Lewis-Phillips GD, Li G, Dugger DL (2008) Targeting HER2-positive breast cancer with trastuzumab-DM1, an antibody-cytotoxic drug conjugate. Cancer Res 6:9280–9290
18. Junttila T, Fields C, G. Li, et al (2008) Trastuzumab-mertansine (T-DM1) retains all the mechanisms of action (MOA) of trastuzumab and is effective in combination with docetaxel. European Organization for Research and Treatment of Cancer Annual Meeting. Abstract #515, 2008
19. Younes A, Bartlett NL, Leonard JP et al (2010) Brentuximab Vedotin (SGN-35) for relapsed CD30-positive lymphomas. NEJM 363:1812–1821
20. Austin CD, De Maziere AM, Pisacane PI et al (2004) Endocytosis and sorting of ErbB2 and the site of action of cancer therapeutics trastuzumab and geldanamycin. Mol Biol Cell 15:5268–5282
21. Austin CD, Wen X, Gazzard L et al (2005) Oxidizing potential of endosomes and lysosomes limits intracellular cleavage of disulfide-based antibody-drug conjugates. PNAS 102: 17987–17992
22. Shen B-Q, Bumbaca D, Saad O et al (2011) Metabolic fate and pharmacokinetic characterization of trastuzumab emtansine (T-DM1): an emphasis on preclinical and clinical catabolism [Poster PIII-72]. Clin Pharmacol Ther 89(Suppl 1):S90
23. Dieras V, Harbeck N, Albain K et al (2010) A phase Ib/II trial of trastuzumab-DM1 with pertuzumab for patients with HER2-positive, locally advanced or metastatic breast cancer: interim efficacy and safety results [abstract P3-14-01]. Cancer Res 70(Suppl 2):291s
24. Krop IE, Modi S, Elias A et al (2010) A dose-escalation study of trastuzumab-DM1 (T-DM1), paclitaxel (T), and pertuzumab (P) in patients with HER2-positive, locally advanced or metastatic

breast cancer (MBC) previously treated with a trastuzumab-containing regimen. Abstract P3-14-10. Cancer Res 70(Suppl 2):295s
25. Holden SN, Beeram M, Krop IE, et al (2008) A phase I study of weekly dosing of trastuzumab-DM1 in patients with advanced HER2+ breast cancer. J Clin Oncol 26(Suppl): abstract 1029
26. Burris HA, Rugo HS, Vukelja SA et al (2011) Phase II study of the antibody drug conjugate trastuzumab-DM1 for the treatment of human epidermal growth factor receptor 2 (HER2)-positive breast cancer after prior HER2-directed therapy. J Clin Oncol 29:398–405
27. Krop I, LoRusso P, Miller KD, et al (2010) A phase 2 study of the HER2 antibody-drug conjugate trastuzumab-DM1 (T-DM1) in patients (pts) with HER2-positive metastatic breast cancer (MBC) previously treated with trastuzumab, lapatinib, and chemotherapy [abstract 2770]. Presented at 35th ESMO Congress, 8–12 October 2010, Milan, Italy
28. Therasse P, Arbuck SG, Eisenhauer EA et al (2000) New guidelines to evaluate the response to treatment in solid tumors. J Natl Cancer Inst 92:205–216
29. Wolff AC, Hammond M, Schwartz J et al (2007) American Society of Clinical Oncology/College of American Pathologists guideline recommendations for human epidermal growth factor receptor 2 testing in breast cancer. Arch Pathol Lab Med 131:18–43
30. Press MF, Sauter G, Bernstein L et al (2005) Diagnostic evaluation of HER-2 as a molecular target: an assessment of accuracy and reproducibility of laboratory testing in large, prospective, randomized clinical trials. Clin Cancer Res 11:6598–6607
31. LoRusso P et al (2010) Quantitative assessment of diagnostic markers and correlations with efficacy in two phase II studies of trastuzumab-DM1 (T-DM1) for patients (pts) with metastatic breast cancer (MBC) who had progressed on prior HER2-directed therapy. Abstract 1016. J Clin Oncol 28 15s: 118s
32. Tolcher AW, Ochoa L, Hammond LA et al (2003) Cantuzumab mertansine, a maytansinoid immunoconjugate directed to the CanAg antigen: a phase I, pharmacokinetic, and biologic correlative study. J Clin Oncol 21:211–222
33. Ewer SM, Ewer MS (2008) Cardiotoxicity profile of trastuzumab. Drug Saf 31:459–467
34. Lu D, Gupta M, Wang B, et al (2011) An integrated population pharmacokinetic model for a first-in-class HER2 targeted antibody-drug conjugate trastuzumab emtansine (T-Dm1): simultaneous modeling of T-DM1 and total trastuzumab pharmacokinetics in heavily pretreated HER2-positive metastatic breast cancer patients. Presented at The American Society of Clinical Pharmacology and Therapeutics 2011 Annual Meeting
35. Gupta M, LoRusso PM, Wang B et al (2012) Clinical implications of pathophysiological and demographic covariates on the population pharmacokinetics of trastuzumab-DM1, a HER2-targeted antibody-drug conjugate, in patients with HER2-positive metastatic breast cancer. J Clin Pharm 52(5):691–703
36. Hurvitz SA, Dirix L, Kocsis J et al (2011) Trastuzumab emtansine (T-DM1) versus trastuzumab + docetaxel in previously untreated HER2-positive metastatic breast cancer (MBC): primary results of a randomized, multicenter, open-label phase II study (TDM4450g/BO21976). ESMO Annual Meeting. Abstract 5001
37. Kirkova J, Davis MP, Walsh D et al (2006) Cancer symptom assessment instruments: a systematic review. J Clin Oncol 24:1459–1473
38. Baselga J et al (2010) First results of the NeoALTTO trial (BIG 01–06/EGF 106903): a phase III, randomized, open label, neoadjuvant study of lapatinib, trastuzumab, and their combination plus paclitaxel in women with HER2-positive primary breast cancer. SABCS 2010. Abstract 291
39. Gianni L, et al (2010) Neoadjuvant pertuzumab (P) and trastuzumab (H): antitumor and safety analysis of a randomized phase II study (NeoSphere). SABCS 2010. Abstract S3-2.
40. Bang Y-J, Cutsem EV, Feyereislova A et al (2010) Trastuzumab in combination with chemotherapy versus chemotherapy alone for treatment of HER2-positive advanced gastric or gastro-oesophageal junction cancer (ToGA): a phase 3, open-label, randomized controlled trial. Lancet 376:687–697
41. Nishiyama M, Eguchi H (2009) Pharmacokinetics and pharmacogenomics in gastric cancer chemotherapy. Adv Drug Deliv Rev 61:402–407

42. Berns K, Horlings HM, Hennessy BT et al (2007) A functional genetic approach identifies the PI3K pathway as a major determinant of trastuzumab resistance in breast cancer. Cancer Cell 12:395–402
43. Scaltriti M, Rojo F, Ocana A et al (2007) Expression of p95HER2, a truncated form of the HER2 receptor, and response to anti-HER2 therapies in breast cancer. JNCI 99:628–638
44. Verma S et al (2012) Trastuzumab Emtansine for HER2-Positive Advanced Breast Cancer. N Engl J Med
45. Bender BC et al (2012) A population pharmacokinetic/pharmacodynamic model of thrombocytopenia characterizing the effect of trastuzumab emtansine (T-DM1) on platelet counts in patients with HER2-positive metastatic breast cancer. Cancer Chemother Pharmacol
46. Baselga J et al (2012) Pertuzumab plus trastuzumab plus docetaxel for metastatic breast cancer. N Engl J Med 366(2):109–119

Chapter 12
CDX-011 (Glembatumumab Vedotin, CR011-vcMMAE)

Christos Vaklavas, Albert F. LoBuglio, Mansoor Saleh, Michael Yelin, and Andres Forero

Introduction

The development of monoclonal antibodies as cancer therapeutic agents has improved the outlook for many patients as evidenced by the number of such drugs that have been approved for oncologic indications [1]. Monoclonal antibodies allow selective killing of malignant cells (targeted therapy) with relative sparing of the normal tissues resulting in higher therapeutic efficacy and lower toxicity. The advances in the monoclonal antibody field have been expedited by the discovery of targets or pathways that are uniquely present or upregulated in cancer cells along with the advances in the technology used for the production of human or "humanized" reagents [2]. An additional strategy to enhance monoclonal antibody therapy is to utilize these reagents to selectively deliver radioisotopes (radioimmunotherapy) or cytotoxic agents (antibody–drug conjugates) to tumor cells [3, 4]. CDX-011 is a recently described antibody–drug conjugate in early clinical trials.

CDX-011

CDX-011 (glembatumumab vedotin, CR011-vcMMAE) is an antibody–drug conjugate comprised of a fully human IgG_2 monoclonal antibody (CR011) directed against the extracellular domain of glycoprotein nonmetastatic B (GPNMB) and conjugated to the tubulin-binding cytotoxic compound monomethylauristatin E (MMAE) via a protease-sensitive valine–citrulline (vc) linker. The average MMAE:CR011 molar ratio is approximately 4.5:1; thus, there is an average of 4 or 5 MMAE molecules delivered to tumor cells per antibody interaction [5].

C. Vaklavas (✉) • A.F. LoBuglio • M. Saleh • M. Yelin • A. Forero
Comprehensive Cancer Center, University of Alabama at Birmingham, Birmingham, AL, USA
e-mail: cvaklavas@uabmc.edu

G.L. Phillips (ed.), *Antibody-Drug Conjugates and Immunotoxins: From Pre-Clinical Development to Therapeutic Applications*, Cancer Drug Discovery and Development, DOI 10.1007/978-1-4614-5456-4_12,

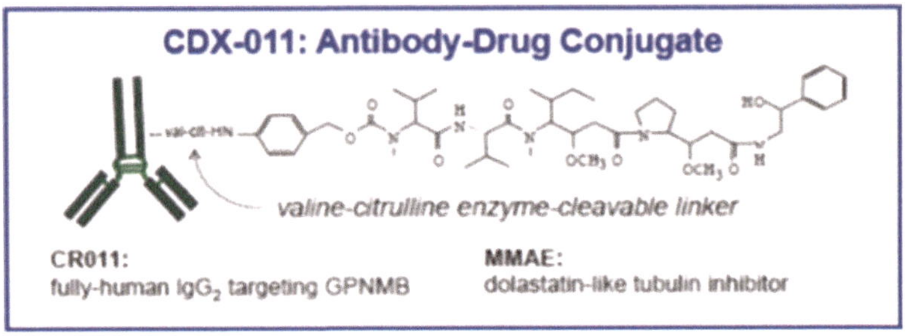

Fig. 12.1 CDX-011 structure. CDX-011consists of the fully human mAb CR011, a linker (consists of a thiol-reactive maleimide, a caproyl spacer, the dipeptide valine–citrulline, and *p*-aminobenzyloxycarbonyl), and the small molecule anti-tubulin agent monomethylauristatin E. Source: Image Provided by Celldex Therapeutics

The Antibody, CR011

CR011 is a fully human IgG2 monoclonal antibody generated in the human IgG2-bearing XenoMouse strains developed by Abgenix (Fremont, CA) via immunization with recombinant extracellular domain of the human GPNMB [5]. These genetically engineered XenoMouse strains possess an immune system in which the mouse antibody-producing genes have been inactivated and functionally replaced by most of the human antibody-producing genes; thus, the strains still recognize human antigens as foreign, but instead of producing mouse antibodies they produce high-affinity fully human antibodies (different strains produce different classes of IgG antibodies) [6, 7]. In the case of CR011, the generated hybridoma cell lines were subsequently screened for antibody reactivity and specificity to the extracellular domain of human and cloned GPNMB. The antibody selected for further characterization and expansion had a dissociation constant of 52 nmol/L for the purified extracellular domain of GPNMB and was designated CR011 [5].

The Conjugate, CDX-011 (CR011-vcMMAE or Glembatumumab Vedotin)

Although CR011 was able to bind GPNMB on melanoma cell lines, the antibody did not inhibit cell growth or induce apoptosis [5]. Thus, it was decided to generate an antibody–drug conjugate to combine the tumor targeting specificity of CR011 with the cytotoxic activity of the MMAE compound [5]. CDX-011 was generated by covalently coupling CR011 to MMAE (monomethyl auristatin E) via a cathepsin B-cleavable valine–citrulline (vc) peptide linker (Fig. 12.1). Monomethyl auristatin E (MMAE) is a synthetic derivative of dolastatin 10, a natural cytostatic pseudopeptide originally isolated from the marine shell-less mollusk *Dorabella auricularia* [8].

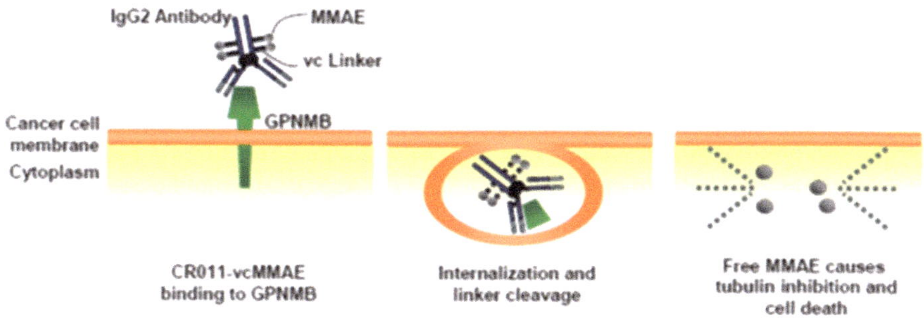

Fig. 12.2 CDX-011 mechanism of action. The cytotoxin MMAE is released from the antibody–drug conjugate intracellularly via lysosomal protease cleavage at the valine–citrulline dipeptide. Source: Image Provided by Celldex Therapeutics

MMAE exerts its potent cytostatic effect by inhibiting microtubule assembly, tubulin-dependent GTP hydrolysis, and polymerization. MMAE–antibody–drug conjugates have demonstrated potent in vitro (very low IC_{50}) and in vivo antitumor activity in multiple malignancies [9, 10]. Importantly, the conjugation of MMAE to CR011 potently and specifically inhibited the growth of GPNMB-positive melanoma cell lines in vitro (SK-Mel-2 and SK-Mel-5) but not GPNMB-negative cell lines [5]. In addition, in a melanoma xenograft model, CR011-vcMMAE induced significant dose-proportional antitumor effects, including complete regressions, at doses as low as 1.25 mg/kg [5]. Similar preclinical observations have been seen in GPNMB-positive breast cancer cell lines [11]. Once CDX-011 binds to the surface antigen, the antibody–drug conjugate migrates to the lysosomes where the active cytotoxic compound is released with the action of lysosomal enzymes (Fig. 12.2) [12]. Although the peptide-based linker provides a highly stable bond under physiologic conditions, it facilitates rapid and efficient drug cleavage upon internalization of the immunoconjugate by the target tumor cell [13]. In addition, this stable linker decreases levels of the circulating unbound cytotoxic agent resulting in decreased nonselective toxicity [13].

The Target, Glycoprotein Nonmetastatic B

CDX-011 is directed against glycoprotein nonmetastatic B (GPNMB), also known as osteoactivin; dendritic cell–heparin integrin ligand (DC-HIL); or hematopoietic growth factor inducible neurokinin-1 type (HGFIN). GPNMB is encoded by the GPNMB gene on chromosome 7p15, a locus involved in the human inherited disease cystoid macular edema also known as dominant cystoid macular dystrophy [14]. GPNMB was initially identified as a gene that was differentially expressed among melanoma cell lines with high and low metastatic potential [15]. The encoded protein is a type I transmembrane protein, which shows closest homology (by 26% amino acid sequence) to the melanocyte/melanoma specific protein pMEL17 [15].

In sequencing and cloning the extracellular domain of GPNMB, two alternative splice variants of the protein were identified [5], 560 or 572 amino acids each one. The extracellular domain of the GPNMB contains a putative heparin binding site, many N-glycosylation sites (play a role in modulating protein stability, conformation, and protein:protein interactions), a SIG domain (determines the entry of GPNMB into the secretory pathway), an Arg-Gly-Asp (RGD) motif (responsible for integrin-mediated cell adhesion), a GAP1 and GAP2 domain separated by a KRG (kringle-like) domain (involved in protein–protein interactions), and a polycystic kidney disease domain (mediates the interaction between the GPNMB expressed on antigen-presenting cells and syndecan-4 expressed on activated T cells) [16–19].

GPNMB is normally expressed in various tissues including the bone (osteoclasts and osteoblasts), hematopoietic system (dendritic cells and macrophages), breast epithelia, and the skin (epidermal Langerhans cells and melanocytes) [20–27]. GPNMB was shown to be upregulated or aberrantly expressed in several malignant tumors including hepatocellular carcinoma [28], gliomas [29–31], breast carcinoma [32, 33], and melanoma (cutaneous and uveal) [34–36]. In preclinical studies of breast cancer, GPNMB expression was shown to play a significant role in skeletal metastases, and invasion; in addition, GPNMB in breast cancer can promote tumor angiogenesis by two interrelated mechanisms: upregulation of stromal VEGF expression and chemoattraction of endothelial cells by GPNMB ectodomain shedding [37, 38]. Studies in breast cancer have identified a correlation between high GPNMB expression and features of aggressive phenotype including ER-negative status, increasing grade, and p53 mutational status [32, 39]. GPNMB is highly expressed in triple negative breast cancer and is associated with increased risk of recurrence [39]. In melanoma, GPNMB expression has been seen preferentially in low-metastatic cell lines; transfection of partial GPNMB cDNA into highly metastatic melanoma cell line resulted in slower subcutaneous tumor growth in nude mice [15]. In addition, overexpression of GPNMB promoted growth of melanoma cells by inhibiting the activation of tumor-reactive T cells via an interaction with syndecan-4 [40]. Finally, GPNMB was shown to interact with the surface of endothelial cells [22], a finding that may have implications for GPNMB-expressing melanoma cell transendothelial migration and metastasis [36]. In hepatocellular carcinoma GPNMB levels of expression were higher in well-differentiated tumors, and in glioblastomas GPNMB expression is associated with poor clinical outcomes. A recent report suggests that GPNMB may be upregulated by pharmacologic interventions (such as ERK or p38 MAPK pathway inhibitors); this phenomenon may enhance sensitivity of tumor cells to CDX-011 [41].

Clinical Trials with CDX-011

CDX-011 has been evaluated in two phase I/II clinical trials: one in advanced melanoma and one in advanced/metastatic breast cancer [42–47]. Enrollment has been completed in both trials.

Table 12.1 Antitumor activity of CDX-011 in metastatic melanoma

	Dose and schedule of CDX-011			Strong (3+, 90%) GPNMB expression ($n=7$)
	1.88 mg/kg q3w ($n=34$)	1.5 mg/kg weekly x2 q3w ($n=6$)	1.0 mg/kg weekly ($n=15$)	
ORR	5 (15%)	2 (33%)	3 (20%)	2 (29%)
PR or SD ≥ 12 weeks	20 (59%)	3 (50%)	5 (33%)	6 (86%)
Median PFS (months)	3.9	3.0	1.4	4.9

ORR objective response rate (all partial responses), *PR* partial response; *SD* stable disease, *PFS* progression-free survival

CDX-011 in Melanoma

CDX-011 has been evaluated for the treatment of unresectable stage III or IV melanoma [45]. The phase I portion of the study was designed to evaluate safety of CDX-011 and to establish the MTD using a standard 3 × 3 dose escalation design at several dose schedules; in addition, pharmacokinetic parameters were evaluated. The primary objective of the expansion phase II portion of the study was to estimate objective response rate; in addition, the phase II portion had secondary objectives including toxicity, progression-free survival, stable disease, and immunogenicity.

The study enrolled a total of 117 patients, 79 of whom were treated with the every 3-week intravenous schedule. Sixty four percent of the patients were male, the median age was 62 years, 89% had stage IV disease, and 50% had M1c. The median number of prior cancer therapies for metastatic disease was 1 with a range of 0–8. Dose-limiting toxicities on the every 3-week schedule included hand-foot syndrome, skin rash, erythema multiforme, and neutropenic fever. MTD was established at 1.88 mg/kg [45]. The more frequent dose schedules had more severe dose-limiting toxicities (epidermal necrolysis, hyperglycemia, acute renal failure, and rash) with MTD of 1 mg/kg weekly and 1.5 mg/kg weekly for 2 of 3 weeks, respectively. Treatment-related adverse events of grade 3 severity or greater included rash (20%), neutropenia (15%), fatigue (8%), neuropathy (7%), pruritus (3%), diarrhea (3%), myalgias, and arthralgias (3% each). Forty two tumor specimens were available for GPNMB expression analysis; 5/7 patients with M1c disease stained strongly positive. The patients with strong GPNMB expression may have enhanced efficacy, but patient numbers were small.

As seen in Table 12.1, the objective response rate in the expansion phase of the study using the every 3-week dose schedule was 15% (5/34), while 59% of the patients achieved clinical benefit (partial response or stable disease for at least 12 weeks) [45]. The more frequent dosing schedules had similar response rate but shorter progression-free survival [45]. Interestingly, patients who developed rash while on treatment did better than those with no rash. For the every 3-week schedule, the half-life of the antibody drug conjugate increased with dose (range, 16–38 h; dosing, 0.03–1.88 mg/kg). The emergence of anti-CDX-011 antibodies was seen in approximately 7% of treated patients.

CDX-011 in Breast Cancer

CDX-011 has also been evaluated in a phase I/II study that enrolled patients with advanced/metastatic breast cancer [46]. The study consisted of a standard 3 + 3 dose escalation portion to evaluate the safety of the antibody–drug conjugate and to establish the MTD, followed by a phase II expansion portion at the MTD to further assess safety and efficacy (12-week progression-free rate). Dose escalation proceeded through the predefined maximum dose of 1.88 mg/kg (the "phase II dose"). However, patients with preexisting grade II or greater neuropathy were excluded from the trial because of initial experience with worsening of their neuropathy [47].

A total of 42 patients were enrolled in the study, including 14 patients enrolled in the phase I portion. Patients enrolled in the trial had a median of 7 prior anticancer regimens, 83% had liver and/or lung metastasis, 27% were HER2 positive, and 32% had triple negative breast cancer. The toxicity profile of the CDX-011 showed significant overlap between the two clinical trials (melanoma and breast cancer) [46]. CDX-011 was well tolerated; treatment-related adverse events ≥ grade 3 severity included neutropenia (21%), neuropathy (7%), nausea (5%), vomiting (5%), asthenia (5%), fatigue (2%), and rash (5%). Four patients discontinued therapy due to adverse events (neuropathy, rash, dermatologic bullae, and acute renal failure). Of the 14 patients in whom GPNMB expression was evaluated, 10 (71%) were positive.

The primary efficacy endpoint of the study was disease progression-free rate at 12 weeks with 35% of the phase II population achieving the primary efficacy endpoint (Table 12.2) [46]. The objective response rate for patients treated at the phase II dose (including those treated at 1.88 mg/kg in the dose escalation portion) was 12%. The response rate among a small number of GPNMB-expressing patients in either the stroma or the tumor cells was higher (Table 12.2). The progression-free survival among the GPNMB-expressing patients was 3.8 months (significant GPNMB stromal expression) and 4.0 months (significant GPNMB tumor cell expression). As listed in Table 12.2, 7/10 (70%) triple negative breast cancer patients had progression-free survival greater than 12 weeks. These triple negative breast cancer patients had mean progression-free survival of 4.1 months compared to 2.1 months for the group as a whole.

The activity of CDX-011 in patients with significant stromal expression of GPNMB may be due to both a "bystander effect", in which MMAE is released from the GPNMB-expressing stromal cells, killing neighboring tumor cell populations, as well as direct depletion of supporting stromal cells. Both patients with tumor tissue assessed by IHC who achieved confirmed objective partial responses showed significant tumor cell and/or stromal expression of GPNMB, and continued on treatment from 27 to 54+ weeks.

Table 12.2 Antitumor activity of CDX-011 in metastatic breast cancer

	All patients ($n=34$)	TNBC ($n=10$)	Stromal expression[a] GPNMB[a] ($n=6$)	Tumor cell expression[b] GPNMB[b] ($n=5$)	Stromal or tumor cell expression GPNMB ($n=9$)
ORR	4 (12%)	2 (20%)	2 (33%)	1 (20%)	2 (22%)
PFS > 12 weeks	13 (38%)	7 (70%)	4 (67%)	3 (60%)	6 (67%)
Median PFS (months)	2.1	4.1	3.8	4.0	4.0

ORR objective response rate; *PFS* progression-free survival; *TNBC* triple negative breast cancer

[a]Stromal expression (≥2+)

[b]Tumor cell expression (≥60%, ≥1–2+)

Future Directions

The preliminary efficacy data of CDX-011 seen in the phase I/II clinical trials conducted in metastatic melanoma and breast cancer and the safety profile of the antibody–drug conjugate warrant further development of CDX-011 in both tumors as a single agent and in combination with other therapeutic modalities. Although the data are limited, both trials suggest that expression of GPNMB may be an important biomarker for selection of patients for therapy.

In breast cancer, a phase II trial of CDX-011 in heavily pretreated, metastatic breast cancer patients who are refractory/resistant to chemotherapy has been initiated; the endpoints of the study are overall response rate, duration of response, progression-free survival, and overall survival. One hundred and twenty patients will be enrolled and their tumors are required to have significant GPNMB expression. In addition, preclinical observations provide rationale for combining CDX-011 with targeted antiangiogenic therapies such as bevacizumab as well as therapies targeting the RANK–RANKL pathway such as denosumab (GPNMB was shown to promote angiogenesis via upregulation of VEGF expression in the stroma [37, 38] as well as promote the formation of osteolytic metastases in association with RANKL [20]).

Further evaluations in melanoma are being considered, possibly focusing on patients with strong tumoral GPNMB expression and/or combination therapy protocols, such as with ipilimumab. In addition, GPNMB many be an appealing target in other malignancies including hepatocellular carcinomas and glioblastomas.

References

1. Reichert JM, Valge-Archer VE (2007) Development trends for monoclonal antibody cancer therapeutics. Nat Rev Drug Discov 6:349–356
2. Oldham RK, Dillman RO (2008) Monoclonal antibodies in cancer therapy: 25 years of progress. J Clin Oncol 26(11):1774–1777
3. Goldenberg DM, Sharkey RM, Paganelli G, Barbet J, Chatal JF (2006) Antibody pretargeting advances cancer radioimmunodetection and radioimmunotherapy. J Clin Oncol 24(5):823–834
4. Cartwer PJ, Senter PD (2008) Antibody-drug conjugates for cancer therapy. Cancer J 14(3): 154–169
5. Tse KF, Jeffers M, Pollack VA et al (2006) CR011, a fully human monoclonal antibody-auristatin E conjugate, for the treatment of melanoma. Clin Cancer Res 12:1373–1382
6. Mendez MJ, Green LL, Corvalan JR et al (1997) Functional transplant of megabase human immunoglobulin loci recapitulates human antibody response in mice. Nat Genet 15:146–156
7. Yang XD, Jia XC, Corvalan JR et al (1999) Eradication of established tumors by a fully human monoclonal antibody to the epidermal growth factor receptor without concomitant chemotherapy. Cancer Res 59:1236–1243
8. Pettit GR, Kamano Y, Herald CL et al (1987) The isolation and structure of a remarkable marine animal antineoplastic constituent: dolastatin 10. J Am Chem Soc 109:6883–6885
9. Francisco JA, Cerveny CG, Meyer DL et al (2003) cAC10-vcMMAE, an anti-CD30-monomethyl auristatin E conjugate with potent and selective antitumor activity. Blood 102:1458–1465

10. Gerber HP, Kung-Sutherland M, Stone I et al (2009) Potent antitumor activity of the anti-CD19 auristatin antibody drug conjugate hBU12-vcMMAE against rituximab-sensitive and -resistant lymphomas. Blood 113:4352–4361
11. Rose AAN, Dong Z, MacDonald PA, Russo C, Bertos NR, Simantov R, Park M, Siegel PM. (2009) GPNMB is novel pro-angiogenic factor and therapeutic target in breast cancer. Montreal international symposium in angiogenesis and metastasis (Abstract #P21)
12. Sutherland MS, Sanderson RJ, Gordon KA et al (2006) Lysosomal trafficking and cysteine protease metabolism confer target-specific cytotoxicity by peptide-linked anti-CD30-auristatin conjugates. J Biol Chem 281:10540–10547
13. Doronina SO, Toki BE, Torgov MY et al (2003) Development of potent monoclonal antibody auristatin conjugates for cancer therapy. Nat Biotechnol 21:778–784
14. Kremer H, Pinckers A, van den Helm B, Deutman AF, Ropers HH, Mariman ECM (1994) Localizaion of the gene for dominant cystoid macular dystrophy on chromosome 7p. Hum Mol Genet 3(2):299–302
15. Weterman MA, Ajubi N, van Dinter IM et al (1995) nmb, a novel gene, is expressed in low-metastatic human melanoma cell lines and xenografts. Int J Cancer 60:73–81
16. Hoashi T, Sato S, Yamaguchi Y et al (2010) Glycoprotein nonmetastatic melanoma protein b, a melanocytic cell marker, is a melanosome-specific and proteolytically released protein. FASEB J 24:1616–1629
17. Tomihari M, Hwang SH, Chung JS et al (2009) Gpnmb is a melanosome-associated glycoprotein that contributes to melanocyte/keratinocyte adhesion in a RGD-dependent fashion. Exp Dermatol 18:586–595
18. Shikano S, Bonkobara M, Zukas PK et al (2001) Molecular cloning of a dendritic cell-associated transmembrane protein, DC-HIL, that promotes RGD-dependent adhesion of endothelial cells through recognition of heparan sulfate proteoglycans. J Biol Chem 276:8125–8134
19. Chung JS, Dougherty I, Cruz PD Jr et al (2007) Syndecan-4 mediates the coinhibitory function of DC-HIL on T cell activation. J Immunol 179:5778–5784
20. Sheng MH, Wergedal JE, Mohan S et al (2008) Osteoactivin is a novel osteoclastic protein and plays a key role in osteoclast differentiation and activity. FEBS Lett 582:1451–1458
21. Abdelmagid SM, Barbe MF, Arango-Hisijara I et al (2007) Osteoactivin acts as downstream mediator of BMP-2 effects on osteoblast function. J Cell Physiol 210:26–37
22. Shikano S, Bonkobara M, Zukas PK, Ariizumi K (2001) Molecular cloning of a dendritic cell-associated transmembrane protein, DC-HIL, that promotes RGDdependent adhesion of endothelial cells through recognition of heparan sulfate proteoglycans. J Biol Chem 276:8125–8134
23. Abdelmagid SM, Barbe MF, Rico MC et al (2008) Osteoactivin, an anabolic factor that regulates osteoblast differentiation and function. Exp Cell Res 314:2334–2351
24. Selim AA, Abdelmagid SM, Kanaan RA et al (2003) Anti-osteoactivin antibody inhibits osteoblast differentiation and function in vitro. Crit Rev Eukaryot Gene Expr 13:265–275
25. Ripoll VM, Meadows NA, Raggatt LJ et al (2008) Microphthalmia transcription factor regulates the expression of the novel osteoclast factor GPNMB. Gene 413:32–41
26. Ripoll VM, Irvine KM, Ravasi T et al (2007) Gpnmb is induced in macrophages by IFN-gamma and lipopolysaccharide and acts as a feedback regulator of proinflammatory responses. J Immunol 178:6557–6566
27. Chung JS, Bonkobara M, Tomihari M et al (2009) The DC-HIL/syndecan-4 pathway inhibits human allogeneic T-cell responses. Eur J Immunol 39:965–974
28. Onaga M, Ido A, Hasuike S et al (2003) Osteoactivin expressed during cirrhosis development in rats fed a choline-deficient, L-amino acid-defined diet, accelerates motility of hepatoma cells. J Hepatol 39:779–785
29. Loging WT, Lal A, Siu IM et al (2000) Identifying potential tumor markers and antigens by database mining and rapid expression screening. Genome Res 10:1393–1402
30. Kuan CT, Wakiya K, Dowell JM et al (2006) Glycoprotein nonmetastatic melanoma protein B, a potential molecular therapeutic target in patients with glioblastoma multiforme. Clin Cancer Res 12:1970–1982

31. Rich JN, Shi Q, Hjelmeland M et al (2003) Bone-related genes expressed in advanced malignancies induce invasion and metastasis in a genetically defined human cancer model. J Biol Chem 278:15951–15957
32. Rose AA, Grosset AA, Dong Z et al (2010) Glycoprotein nonmetastatic B is an independent prognostic indicator of recurrence and a novel therapeutic target in breast cancer. Clin Cancer Res 16:2147–2156
33. Rose AA, Pepin F, Russo C et al (2007) Osteoactivin promotes breast cancer metastasis to bone. Mol Cancer Res 5:1001–1014
34. Okamoto I, Pirker C, Bilban M et al (2005) Seven novel and stable translocations associated with oncogenic gene expression in malignant melanoma. Neoplasia 7:303–311
35. Williams MD, Esmaeli B, Soheili A et al (2010) GPNMB expression in uveal melanoma: a potential for targeted therapy. Melanoma Res 20:184–190
36. Tomihari M, Chung JS, Akiyoshi H et al (2010) DC-HIL/glycoprotein Nmb promotes growth of melanoma in mice by inhibiting the activation of tumor-reactive T cells. Cancer Res 70:5778–5787
37. Rose AA, Annis MG, Dong Z et al (2010) ADAM10 releases a soluble form of the GPNMB/Osteoactivin extracellular domain with angiogenic properties. PLoS One 5:e12093
38. Ghilardi C, Chiorino G, Dossi R et al (2008) Identification of novel vascular markers through gene expression profiling of tumor-derived endothelium. BMC Genomics 9:201
39. Rose AN, Grosset AA, Dong Z, Russo C, MacDonald PA, Bertos NR, St-Pierre Y, Simantov R, Hallett M, Park M, Gaboury L, Siegel PM (2010) Glycoprotein nonmetastatic B Is an independent prognostic indicator of recurrence and a novel therapeutic target in breast cancer. Clin Cancer Res 16:2147–2156
40. Tomihari M, Chung JS, Akiyoshi H, Cruz PD, Ariizumi K (2010) DC-HIL/glycoprotein Nmb promotes growth of melanoma in mice by inhibiting the activation of tumor-reactive T cells. Cancer Res 70(14):5778–5787
41. Qian X, Mills E, Torgov M, LaRochelle WJ, Jeffers M (2008) Pharmacologically enhanced expression of GPNMB increases the sensitivity of melanoma cells to the CR011-vcMMAE antibody-drug conjugate. Mol Oncol 2:81–93
42. A Phase I/II Study of CR011-vcMMAE in subjects with unresectable Stage III or Stage IV melanoma (NCT00412828), 2010
43. A Phase I/II Study of CR011-vcMMAE in patients with locally advanced or metastatic breast cancer (NCT00704158), 2010
44. A Phase II, randomized, multicenter study of CDX-011 (CR011-vcMMAE) in patients with advanced GPNMB-expressing breast cancer (NCT01156753), 2010
45. Hamid O, Sznol M, Pavlick AC et al (2010) Frequent dosing and GPNMB expression with CDX-011 (CR011-vcMMAE), an antibody-drug conjugate (ADC), in patients with advanced melanoma. 2010 ASCO annual meeting, Chicago, IL. J Clin Oncol 28:15s (Suppl; Abstr 8525)
46. Saleh MN, Bendell JC, Rose A et al (2010) Correlation of GPNMB expression with outcome in breast cancer (BC) patients treated with the antibody-drug conjugate (ADC), CDX-011 (CR011-vcMMAE). 2010 ASCO annual meeting, Chicago, IL. J Clin Oncol 28:15s (Suppl; Abstr 1095)
47. Burris H, Saleh M, Bendell J, Hart L, Rose AAN, Dong Z, Siegel PM, Crane MF, Donovan D, Crowley E, Simantov R, Vahdat L (2010) A Phase I/II Study of CR011-vcMMAE (CDX-011), an antibody-drug conjugate, in patients with locally advanced or metastatic breast cancer. SABCS 2009 (Abstract # 6096)

Chapter 13
Case Study: An Antibody–Drug Conjugate Targeting MUC16 for Ovarian Cancer

Douglas Leipold and William G. Mallet

Tumors can arise from healthy tissues due to dysregulation of key cellular pathways and abnormal responses to extracellular cues. The cells that comprise a malignant tumor bear molecular signatures that can either betray their tissue of origin or result from their abnormal physiology. Specifically, tumor cells express surface antigens that may be virtually absent from, or have a restricted distribution in, normal tissues. Expression of some of these surface antigens, notably growth factor receptors such as Met, IGF-1R, VEGF-R, and the ErbB/HER family, may provide a growth or survival advantage to the tumor cells [1]. For other antigens, the reason for their selective expression by tumors is much less clear. In either case, the surface antigen may represent a molecular address for targeting tumor cells with antibodies (a "tumor antigen"). A therapeutic strategy based on this concept uses antibodies conjugated to cytotoxic agents to deliver the agents selectively to the tumor cells and spare the normal tissues [2, 3]. This chapter will describe the preclinical development strategies, including target validation, in vitro characterization, and linker-drug impact on in vivo pharmacology and safety considerations of antibody–drug conjugates (ADC) targeting the ovarian cancer surface antigen, MUC16.

The selection criteria for an ADC target antigen are discussed elsewhere in this volume. Briefly, the optimal properties include:

1. Selective overexpression of the target antigen in tumors versus normal tissues
2. Absence from critical normal tissues
3. Normal physiological function that is not vital or disrupted by antibody binding

D. Leipold (✉)
Department of Pharmacokinetics and Pharmacodynamics, Genentech, Inc.,, South San Francisco, CA 94080, USA
e-mail: leipold.doug@gene.com

W.G. Mallet
Department of Oncology Biologics, Novartis Institutes of BioMedical Research, Emeryville, CA 94608, USA

G.L. Phillips (ed.), *Antibody-Drug Conjugates and Immunotoxins: From Pre-Clinical Development to Therapeutic Applications*, Cancer Drug Discovery and Development, DOI 10.1007/978-1-4614-5456-4_13, © Springer Science+Business Media New York 2013

4. Absolute expression levels allowing delivery of cytotoxic doses of ADC-bound drugs
5. Plasma membrane expression providing access to the ADC
6. Endocytosis at a rate such that sufficient amounts of cytotoxic agent are delivered into the cell

MUC16 satisfies many of these criteria. Beyond these considerations, the target antigen should be sufficiently immunogenic that one can obtain a panel of specific antibodies for lead ADC selection. Historically, ADC targets have been single-pass or GPI-anchored targets [4], having a relatively large extracellular domain (ECD) that can be used as an antigen for antibody production, and MUC16 falls into this group. Recent advances in antibody discovery (including phage and yeast display libraries and DNA immunization) may facilitate the development of ADCs against polytopic membrane proteins (such as G-protein coupled receptors and most transporters).

Approximately 10 years ago, we undertook an effort to identify novel tumor antigens using transcript profiling. The correlation of transcript and protein levels is far from perfect, but overall those genes that are highly transcribed are also translated to protein [5]. Transcript profiling can be performed at a large scale, analyzing thousands of transcripts across a broad sampling of normal tissues and tumors. Another major advantage of transcript profiling is that the target genes need not be well characterized, and indeed promising antigens can be identified in the absence of any antibodies or any proteomic analyses. Our profiling of the known transcriptome across a wide range of human malignancies and normal tissues revealed a number of antigens with selective overexpression in cancers. Among these, the overexpression of MUC16 (probe 220196_at) in ovarian cancers was notable (Fig. 13.1) and consistent with an extensive literature.

The gene product now known as MUC16 was initially discovered as the target antigen of an antibody, OC125, generated by immunization of mice with a human ovarian cancer cell line, OVCA 433 [6]. The antigen recognized by OC125 was determined to be a glycoprotein (named "CA125") that was preferentially detected in epithelial ovarian cancers (EOC) and cell lines derived from EOC [7–9]. CA125 was detected both at the surface of cells and in the conditioned medium. In part due to the very large size of this antigen, proposed full-length sequences were not reported until many years later, when the gene encoding the CA125 antigen was described as a mucin, MUC16, characterized by extensive N- and O-linked glycosylation but little sequence identity with other mucins [10]. The consensus MUC16 gene (RefSeq NM_024690.2/NP_078966.2) encodes a predicted 14,507 amino acid polypeptide [11–13]; several full-length sequences have been proposed, but the basic organization and properties of these variants are very similar. CA125 now commonly refers to the ECD of MUC16 that is shed into systemic circulation of patients with EOC and various other pathologies; this shed ECD is a frequently used marker of EOC progression and response to therapy [6, 7, 14]. Within the ECD is a stretch of at least eleven tandem repeating SEA (sea urchin sperm protein, enterokinase, agrin) domains of 154–156 amino acids each; the polypeptide sequence of a given SEA repeat domain is approximately 70–90% identical with the sequence of

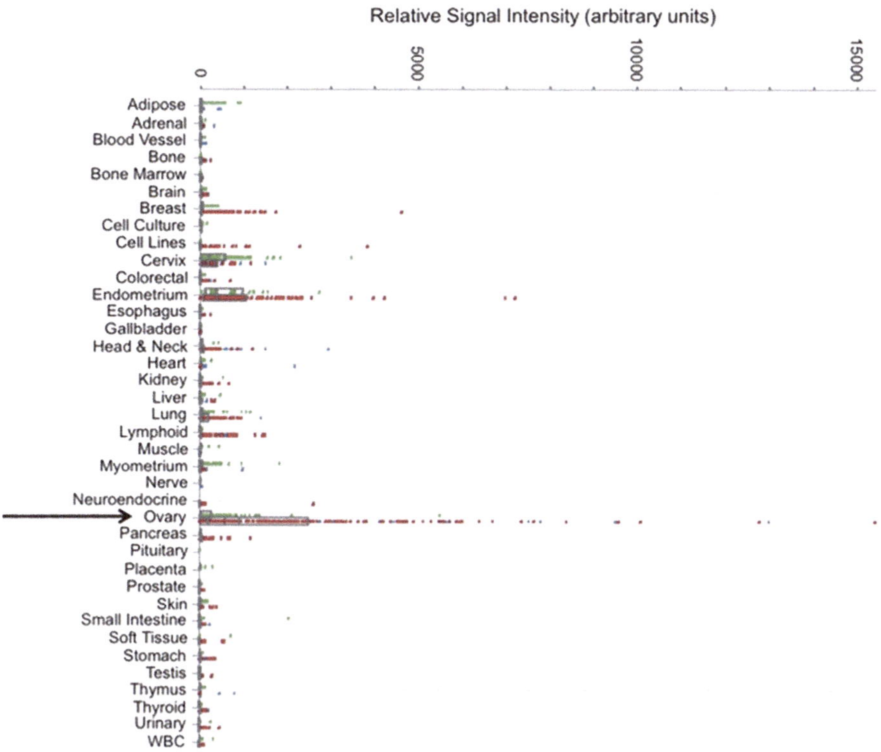

Fig. 13.1 Micro-array profile of MUC16 transcript across gynecologic malignancies and normal tissues. *Green dots* represent MUC16 gene expression in normal tissue; *red dots* represent MUC16 gene expression in malignant tissue. *Arrow* denotes ovarian tissue

any other SEA repeat domain [11, 13]. By immunohistochemistry (IHC) analysis using commercial reagents, we confirmed the selective overexpression of MUC16 in EOC (for example, >90% of serous EOC, the most common histological subtype) as reported in the literature [7–9]. We also detected MUC16 expression in a significant fraction of pancreas adenocarcinomas, again consistent with published reports [15]. Surface expression was confirmed by flow cytometry using commercially available antibodies.

This focus on expression level may yield target antigens that are not "drivers" of the cancer, i.e., do not have an indispensible function in carcinogenesis. There exists no selective pressure to maintain expression of an antigen that is truly a "passenger" on the tumor cell without a vital function. Although CA125 was first identified as a serum marker for ovarian cancer about 30 years ago, the function of MUC16 in the disease is poorly understood. MUC16 expression does not appear to be critical for tumor cell growth or survival (in contrast with Her2), but recent reports have implicated MUC16 and/or CA125 in promoting tumor invasion and suppressing NK-mediated tumor killing [16–21]. Specifically, Manish Patankar and colleagues have reported that MUC16 or CA125 binds to Siglec-9 expressed on $CD16^{+}/CD56^{dim}$ NK cells, inducing their conversion by an unknown mechanism into the less cytolytic $CD16^{-}/CD56^{bright}$ NK cells [16, 17, 20]. Alternatively, the same research lab has suggested that the engagement of NK cells by MUC16 directly inhibits NK-tumor cell "synapse" formation and subsequent NK-mediated cytolysis [19]. Intriguingly, MUC16 has been shown to interact in vitro with mesothelin [18, 21], a cell surface protein that is also overexpressed in epithelial cancers of the ovary and pancreas [56]. This interaction may promote tumor cell invasion or otherwise influence tumor–stromal interactions. Hence, MUC16 may not be readily disposed of by the tumor. Ideally, preclinical efficacy models will provide an indication of whether or not the tumors lose expression of the target antigen as a mechanism of resistance to the ADC.

While MUC16 function in tumor progression remains incompletely understood, the prevalence of this antigen has been exploited through multiple strategies. Oregovomab is a mouse monoclonal antibody that binds to circulating CA125 [22–25]. The CA125–oregovomab immune complex is proposed to elicit an immune response against the tumor. A similar antibody strategy is represented by abagovomab, an anti-idiotypic antibody that is also designed to induce antitumor host immunity [26, 27]. Both of these agents are in advanced clinical studies [28, 57]. The cell surface expression of MUC16, its high prevalence in EOC, and its limited expression in normal tissues suggest a great opportunity to develop an ADC targeting MUC16-positive cancers. An ADC therapeutic is not designed to disrupt target function, but even so, the biology of the antigen must still be considered at some level. We and others have found MUC16 expressed in the fallopian tube and ovarian surface epithelium and in the epithelia of bronchioles and the cornea [8, 29–32], albeit at lower levels than as detected in EOC. It must be assumed that MUC16 has a function in normal tissues, and an antibody may adversely influence that function; this would have to be determined in the course of safety studies with the appropriate models.

Two separate panels of antibodies against MUC16 were developed: one directed against a portion of the ECD C-terminal to the SEA repeats and the second directed against the shed CA125 (presumably comprising most of the ECD, including the SEA repeats) [33]. No antibody on its own exhibited any antitumor activity in vitro or in xenograft tumor studies. This result is expected when the target antigen is not a driver of cell growth. Alternative mechanisms of antitumor activity, such as antibody-dependent cellular cytotoxicity (ADCC), do not apply to cells growing on plastic or in soft agar, although ADCC can inhibit tumor growth in immune-compromised mice. The antibodies appear to be internalized quite slowly, presumably reflecting the intrinsic rate of MUC16 endocytosis. When OVCAR-3 cells were incubated continuously with the antibodies in immuno-fluorescent microscopy studies, cell surface staining predominated after two hours, and internal vacuolar labeling (evidence of antibody internalization and delivery to endosomes) was marked only after an overnight incubation. In principle, different antibodies against the same target antigen can exhibit different rates of internalization. Given that an ADC is designed to deliver a cytotoxic agent inside the cell, an antibody that exhibits rapid internalization might be favored, and there are data to support this preference [34]. However, rapid endocytosis is not a prerequisite for an antibody in the context of an ADC; endocytic rate is only one component of cytotoxic drug delivery via ADCs. Indeed, rapid internalization may be a consequence of an activity such as receptor activation or cross-linking, and such an activity may not be desirable. If comparing two antibodies, both specific for the target antigen and having similar affinities and species cross-reactivities, and not differing in properties such as receptor agonism, it is reasonable to select the more rapidly internalizing antibody. With sufficient cell surface antigen expression levels, a slowly internalizing antibody may still be able to deliver sufficient drug to produce a therapeutic effect. Inefficient delivery requires a very potent drug, as discussed elsewhere in this volume.

Although the anti-MUC16 antibodies shared certain properties, we expected that using different antigens in the two antibody campaigns would yield antibodies recognizing different sequences. Each of the MUC16-specific antibodies detected the antigen when used to probe Western blots following reducing SDS-PAGE. We took advantage of this property to determine the sequences recognized by each antibody through expression of different MUC16 fragments. Antibodies from the first panel recognized non-repeating epitopes. Among the first panel, antibody 11D10 recognized MUC16 with highest affinity and was selected for further evaluation. Epitope mapping demonstrated that this antibody bound within an 82 amino acid sequence C-terminal to the last conserved SEA domain (Fig. 13.2a); this epitope was shared by several other antibodies among the first panel. Antibody 3A5 from the second panel recognized a repeating motif within the SEA domains. Using constructs with specific deletions and substitutions with alanine ("alanine scanning"), we further defined the residues that are critical for 3A5 binding. Specifically, we found that a conserved MxxP motif (where at least one "x" is His or Arg) was particularly important for 3A5 binding (Fig. 13.2b, c). Based on the structure of a mouse MUC16 SEA domain [35], this sequence forms a "tight turn" between two alpha helices. The epitopes of other antibodies from the second panel could not be defined, presenting a significant challenge for ADC development. The major issue is that antigen specificity is difficult to demonstrate if the epitope is unknown. A heavily glycosylated protein such as MUC16 may share so-called "glycotopes" with other cell surface proteins that we do not wish to target with an ADC. Both 11D10 and 3A5 were easily validated as specific antibodies against MUC16. Additionally, epitope information is valuable for assessing the species cross-reactivity of an antibody in preparation for preclinical testing, particularly in the case of a very large protein such as MUC16. Full-length clones of MUC16 do not exist, so the ability to focus on a defined sequence greatly facilitated the cloning and expression of orthologous rat and cynomolgus monkey sequences. The use of this information in preclinical studies is illustrated later in this chapter.

In flow cytometry studies, both 11D10 and 3A5 bound to the surface of cells that express MUC16, as is required for an ADC strategy; MUC16-negative cells were not recognized by these antibodies [33]. These antibodies could then be used to identify cell lines that can serve as models for preclinical studies. The model cell lines should have antigen expression levels that are comparable to the levels detected

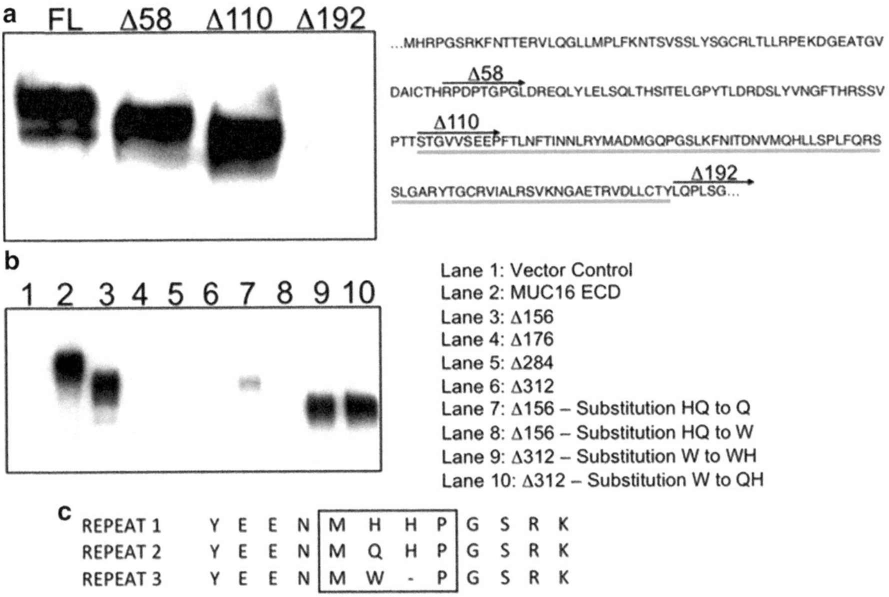

Fig. 13.2 (**a**) 11D10 binds to a unique epitope of MUC16 and 3A5 binds to a repeating epitope. Lysates from 293S cells expressing a partial MUC16 sequence lacking SEA domains ("FL") and successive deletions from the N-terminus of that MUC16 sequence ("Δ58" etc.) were blotted and probed with murine 11D10. Loss of 11D10 binding from Δ110 to Δ192 defines the 11D10 epitope. (**b**) Deletion and mutation constructs were expressed transiently in 293S cells. Conditioned media were collected, blotted, and probed with 3A5. *Lane 1*: vector control, *lane 2*: MUC16 ECD; *lanes 3–6*: successive deletions. Substitution of "QH" in Δ156 (*lane 3*) with "Q" or "W" (*lanes 7 and 8*) greatly reduces 3A5 binding. Substitution of "W" in Δ312 (*lane 6*) with "WH" or "QH" (*lanes 9 and 10*) restores 3A5 binding. No effect on 11D10 binding following aforementioned deletions or substitutions (data not shown). (**c**) Alignment of repeats around the critical residues in the "MxxP" motif (in *boxed* area) for 3A5 binding

in the target tumors. A risk to using cell lines with atypically high antigen expression is that the activity of an ADC against such a line may not be relevant to the activity against tumors having substantially lower antigen expression. Ovarian cancer cells such as OVCAR-3 [36] and PE01 [37] express surface MUC16 [33, 38]. We were fortunate that both 3A5 and 11D10 proved to be sensitive reagents for IHC in paraffin-embedded sections, exhibiting staining patterns and distributions that were very similar to those obtained using commercially available anti-MUC16 antibodies (Fig. 13.3) [7–9]. We could then show that paraffin-embedded pellets of OVCAR-3 and PE01 cells stained with intensities similar to ovarian cancer sections; that is, these cell lines can serve as relevant preclinical models. Xenograft tumors derived from these cell lines likewise expressed relevant levels of MUC16.

The flow cytometry and IHC studies also revealed that 3A5 detected full-length, endogenous MUC16 with a stronger signal than 11D10 by either method (Fig. 13.4) [33]. Although the apparent monomeric binding affinity of 3A5 is somewhat weaker

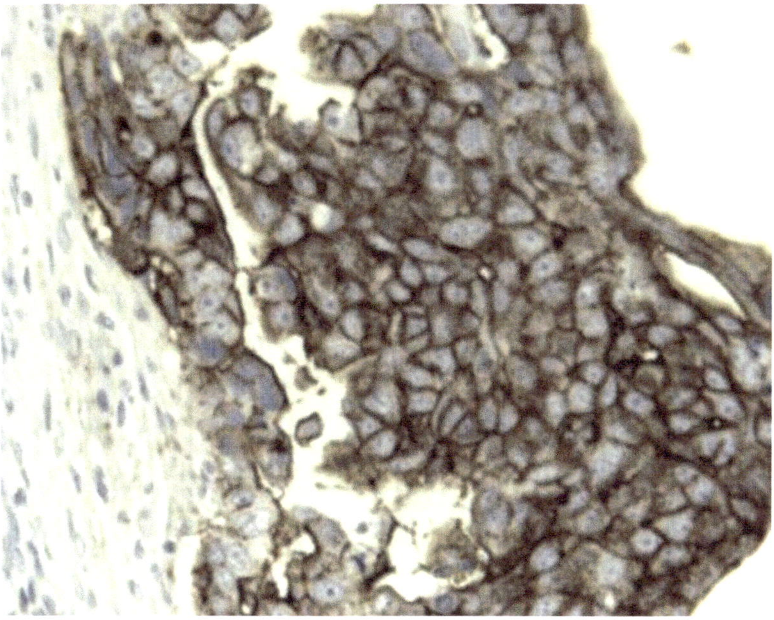

Fig. 13.3 Immunohistochemistical (*IHC*) staining with 3A5 antibody of ovarian adenocarcinoma tissue demonstrates specificity with staining of epithelial cells (*Brown* (*DAB*: 3,3′-diaminobenzidine) stain) and a lack of staining of stromal cells

than 11D10, 3A5 can bind multiple times to each MUC16 surface protein; therefore more 3A5 than 11D10 binds to a MUC16-expressing ovarian cancer. We demonstrated this by flow cytometry using cells expressing recombinant MUC16 constructs lacking the 3A5 epitope SEA domain or having a single SEA domain, and cells expressing endogenous (presumably full-length) MUC16. 3A5 failed to bind to the most truncated form of MUC16 (which was recognized by 11D10); 3A5 and 11D10 gave comparable binding to the single-repeat construct; and 3A5 bound much more extensively than 11D10 to OVCAR-3 cells. This finding was confirmed by ELISA using CA125, where the data indicated that 11D10 binds to a single epitope on CA125 whereas 3A5 can bind approximately eight times per CA125 molecule. Finally, Scatchard binding analyses on OVCAR-3 cells gave similar results [33].

Since more 3A5 antibodies bind to ovarian cancer cells than 11D10, we expected that ADCs using 3A5 would have superior activity. The behavior of antibodies in vivo can be influenced by factors that are not assessable in vitro, notably pharmacokinetics; a rapidly clearing antibody (for example due to binding shed antigen) may not achieve the duration of exposure sufficient to inhibit tumor growth. To minimize differences in pharmacokinetics, two antibodies must be compared under the same format. Both 11D10 and 3A5 were cloned, and human Fc chimeric forms of each were expressed and conjugated to auristatins. The auristatins, structurally related to dolastatin-10, inhibit cell division by disrupting tubulin polymerization. Our colleagues at Seattle Genetics have characterized two auristatins, monomethyl

a

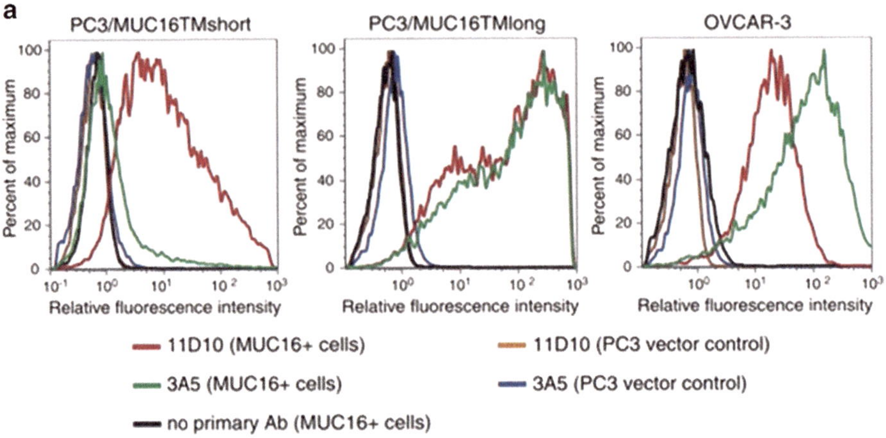

b

	11D10	3A5
Serous cystadenocarcinoma	17/26	24/25
Endometrioid adenocarcinoma	13/22	16/20
Clear cell carcinoma	3/8	5/10
Mucinous adenocarcinoma	1/9	0/8
Normal Tissue	None	None

Fig. 13.4 Relative binding of anti-MUC16 3A5 and 11D10 to MUC16 expressed at the surface of cells or recombinant MUC16 ECD proteins and differential IHC staining incidence with 11D10 and 3A5 antibodies. (**a**) Cells expressing MUC16 endogenously (OVCAR-3) or by stable transfection (PC3/MUC16TMshort and PC3/MUC16TMlong) were incubated with human Fc chimeric forms of antibodies (4 Ag/mL). Relative binding was determined using a fluorescent anti-human Fc secondary antibody. *Red line*, cells labeled with 11D10; green line, cells labeled with 3A5; *black line*, cells stained only with the fluorescent secondary antibody (*Ab*); *brown line*, PC3 vector control cells stained with 11D10 (same plot used in all histograms); *blue line*, PC3 vector control cells stained with 3A5 (same plot used in all histograms) (taken from Chen et al. [33]); (**b**) 3A5 antibody labels a higher proportion of ovarian cancer tissue samples compared to 11D10 antibody

auristatins E and F (MMAE and MMAF), which differ in their membrane permeabilities but both can be incorporated into highly active ADCs [33, 39]. We found that ovarian cancer cell lines are generally sensitive to MMAE, as expected given the sensitivity of ovarian cancer cell lines to antimitotic drugs in vitro and the high initial response rates of ovarian cancers to first-line chemotherapy with paclitaxel and carboplatin (Fig. 13.5) [40, 41]. Both 3A5 and 11D10 were conjugated using two formats: A protease-labile dipeptide linker attached to MMAE ("MC-VC-PABC-MMAE") and a relatively stable alkyl ketone linker attached to MMAF ("MC-MMAF"). In both formats, the release of an active agent within the target cell is thought to require delivery of the ADC to lysosomes [39, 42, 43]. Both 3A5 and 11D10 are transported to lysosomes after internalization (Fig. 13.6), with no apparent difference in rate.

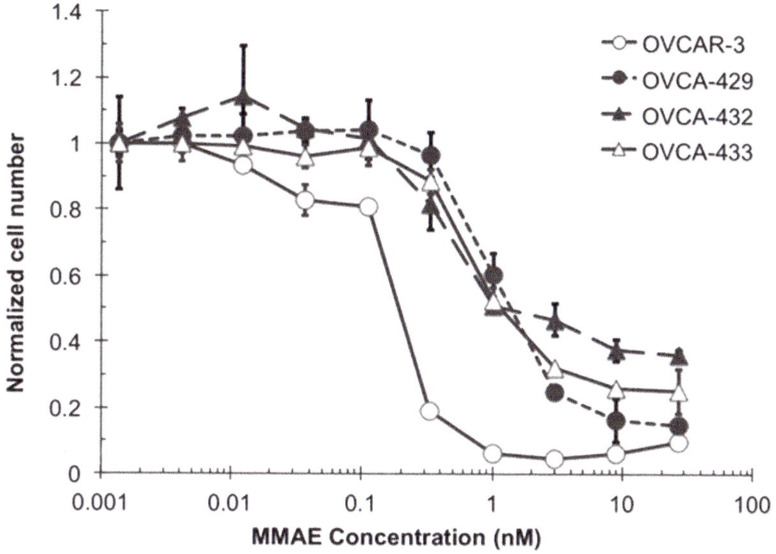

Fig. 13.5 Ovarian cancer cell lines are sensitive to free MMAE. Normalized cell proliferation in several OVCAR-3 cell lines: OVCAR-3 (*open circles*), OVCAR-429 (*closed circles*), OVCAR-432 (*closed triangles*), OVCAR-433 (*open triangles*) in the presence of increasing MMAE concentrations (0.001–27 nM)

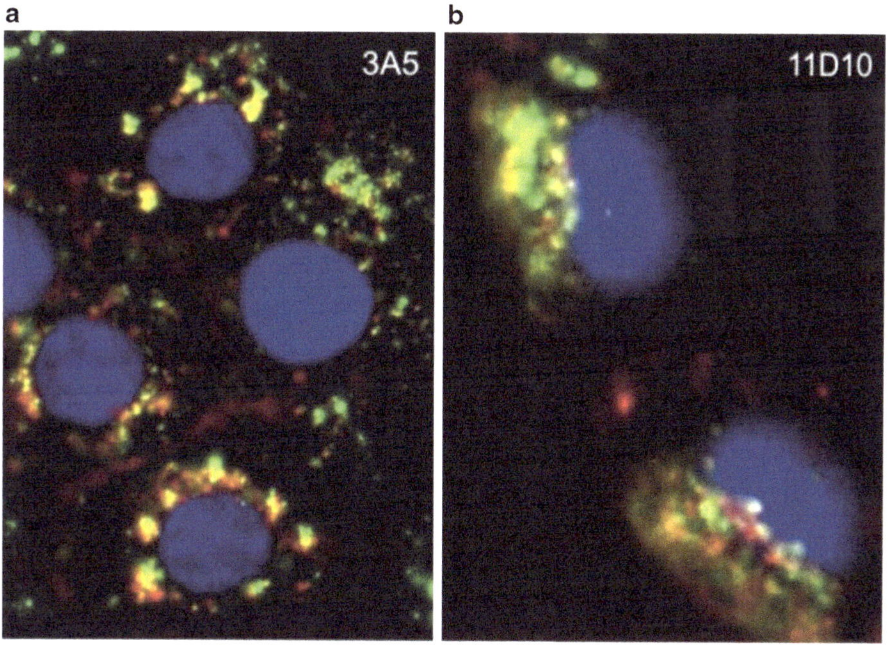

Fig. 13.6 (**a**, **b**) 11D10 and 3A5 antibodies delivery to the lysosomes after a 20-h incubation was determined using a fluorescent antibody against human Fc. Localization of lysosomes was determined using a labeled Dextran (*green*) and a fluorescent antibody against chimeric IgG. In the pseudo-colored images 11D10 and 3A5 are *red*, Dextran (lysosome) is *green*, and DAPI (nuclei) is *blue*. Delivery of internalized anti-muc16 to lysosomes of OVCAR-3 cells is indicated by the *yellow color*

The 3A5 and 11D10 ADCs were compared in vitro and in vivo using OVCAR-3 cells. To evaluate the ADCs in a relevant tumor model, OVCAR-3 cells were transduced with firefly luciferase. These cells were then injected into the peritoneal cavity, where they formed tumors that are reminiscent of human ovarian cancer with respect to disease progression, ascites formation, and sites of metastases [44]. Tumor growth and response to ADC dosing were determined by measuring bioluminescence after injection of luciferin. When administered to OVCAR-3 cells in culture and to OVCAR-3/luciferase intraperitoneal tumors, the 3A5 ADCs (MC-VC-PABC-MMAE and MC-MMAF) were more efficacious in vitro and in vivo than the corresponding 11D10 ADCs [33]. The ability to bind to a repeating epitope presumably explains the far greater activity of the 3A5-derived ADCs. Indeed, PC3 cells engineered to express a truncated MUC16 having equivalent binding to 11D10 and 3A5 were slightly more sensitive in vitro to the 11D10 ADCs, likely reflecting their higher affinity relative to the 3A5 ADCs [33].

Although less efficacious, an ADC using 11D10 could still be preferred over a 3A5 ADC if the 11D10 ADC were much better tolerated. However, pilot safety studies in Sprague-Dawley rats showed no advantage of the 11D10 conjugates; indeed, the 3A5 conjugates were slightly better tolerated. The toxicities (mainly liver function and myelosuppression) were the same for the two antibodies. Given its superior efficacy, 3A5 was selected for anti-MUC16 ADC development. Subsequent studies with conjugates of humanized 3A5 have confirmed and extended these findings.

As previously mentioned, along with the greater cell surface binding, 3A5 also interacts with CA125 to a greater degree than does 11D10. The potential complication of shed ECD binding is not peculiar to MUC16; ECD shedding is a common property of membrane proteins, including ADC targets such as Her2/ErbB2 and mesothelin [45, 46]. The additional fact that 3A5 can bind multiple times to a single CA125 molecule prompted us to examine this interaction in greater detail. Levels of CA125 are measured using immuno-assays and are expressed in terms of U/mL; it is almost certain that CA125 cannot be defined as a single molecular entity. In advanced EOC, serum CA125 can range from below detection to 10,000 U/mL or higher and correlate roughly with MUC16 expression [9, 47]. Peritoneal CA125 levels can exceed serum levels [14]. It is clear that CA125 potentially could limit the therapeutic effects of an anti-MUC16 ADC, through binding the ADC in circulation both to prevent tumor targeting and to form an immune complex that may increase ADC toxicities. To assess the risk to the 3A5 ADC imposed by CA125, we first determined how a given U/mL level translated to 3A5 binding and immune complex formation. In vitro, co-incubation of a 3A5 ADC with CA125 shifts the IC_{50} for cell proliferation (Fig. 13.7). Even so, maximal inhibition is observed at 1 μg/mL ADC in the presence of 1,000 or 4,000 U/mL CA125. Direct chromatographic measurement of immune complex formation demonstrated that approximately 80% of the antibody remained free when 1 μg/mL of 3A5 was mixed with 1,000 U/mL CA125, and approximately 50% of the antibody remained free when 0.1 μg/mL of 3A5 was mixed with 1,000 U/mL CA125, consistent with the in vitro proliferation findings [44]. Since circulating ADC levels can remain above 1 μg/mL for several days following administration of a therapeutic

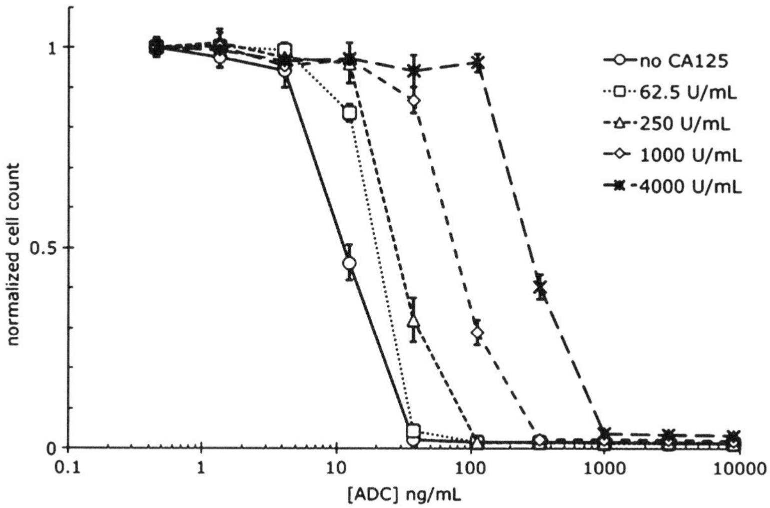

Fig. 13.7 Anti-muc16 ADC demonstrates in vitro potency at effective concentrations in the presence of increasing CA125 concentrations. Normalized cell proliferation of OVCAR-3 cells in the presence of increasing Anti-muc16 ADC concentrations (0.5–9,000 ng/mL) incubated with 0 U/mL (*circle*), 62.5 U/mL (*square*), 250 U/mL (*triangle*), 1,000 U/mL (*diamond*), 4,000 U/mL (*asterisk*)

dose [38], we predict that clinically relevant levels of CA125 would not be sufficient to compete for 3A5 ADC delivery to tumors.

We have further evaluated 3A5 and the ADC in preclinical models where circulating CA125 is generated by peritoneal OVCAR-3 tumors and have observed that the antibody can indeed form a complex with CA125 in the blood [44]. Our data are consistent with the immune complex clearing relatively rapidly through the liver. Notably, the immune complex was only detected with sub-efficacious 3A5 doses (75 μg/kg) or when the complex was formed ex vivo prior to dosing. At efficacious dose levels (1–10 mg/kg for an ADC), the immune complex was not detected. Again, this result indicates that immune complex formation will probably not limit the ability of therapeutic doses of 3A5 ADC to reach the tumor of a patient with CA125 levels in the typical range for ovarian cancers. Likely, a small fraction of total 3A5 formed immune complexes that were rapidly cleared, making detection unfeasible. The bulk of administered 3A5 was well in excess of CA125 binding sites and accumulated over time in the tumor compartments. Under these conditions, the pharmacokinetics of total 3A5 were typical of an antibody in mice. We assessed the safety liabilities of immune complex formation using a nude rat OVCAR-3 xenograft tumor model with circulating CA125 [33]. The 3A5 ADC safety findings were consistent with an irrelevant ADC at the same dose (likely related to the cytotoxic component of the ADC) and there were no findings indicative of organ-specific immune complex deposition at either the low or high dose of the 3A5 ADC. Finally, the 3A5 ADCs were potently active in peritoneal OVCAR-3 xenograft models, albeit with lower levels of circulating CA125.

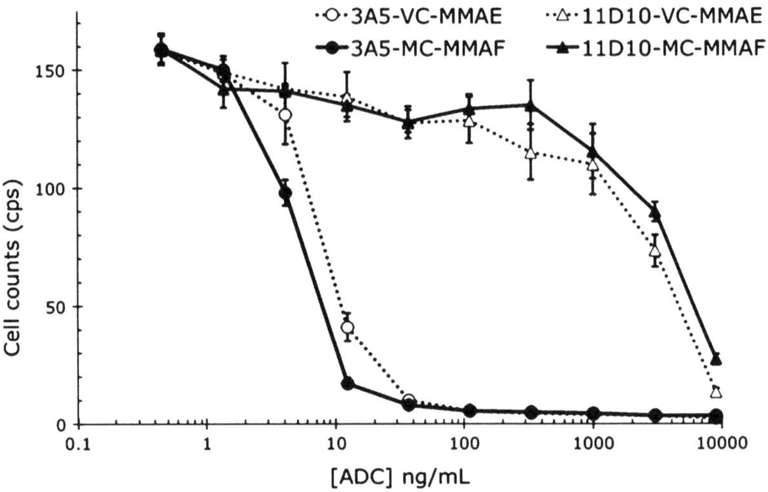

Fig. 13.8 In vitro potencies of MUC16 VC-MMAE and MC-MMAF are comparable. Cell proliferation in OVCAR-3 cells in the presence of increasing concentrations (0.5–9,000 ng/mL) of 3A5-VC-MMAE (*open circles*), -MC-MMAF (*closed circles*) and 11D10-VC-MMAE (*open triangles*), -MC-MMAF (*closed triangles*)

All of these studies suggest that circulating CA125 is not likely to compromise the therapeutic value of the 3A5 ADC. However, the course of a xenograft tumor in an immune-compromised rodent is very different from the human disease, particularly with respect to antigen shedding and clearance. Since the risk created by immune complex formation depends on many variables, including levels of circulating antigen, antibody affinity, and ADC dose, the potential impact of ECD shedding on efficacy and safety should be evaluated for each target antigen.

Following the selection of 3A5 for anti-MUC16 ADC development, the next steps would be to understand the therapeutic index for each of the two 3A5 ADC candidates (MC-VC-PAB-MMAE and MC-MMAF), by further characterizing the efficacy, safety, as well as pharmacokinetics of the ADCs. Following the path of antibody selection, the two 3A5 ADC candidates were initially tested for in vitro activity against OVCAR-3 cells. As demonstrated in Fig. 13.8, there is no apparent difference between the two linker-drugs ADC candidates when comparing the two ADCs in an in vitro potency assay. However, the similarity in potency between the MC-VC-PAB-MMAE and MC-MMAF conjugates in the in vitro activity assay did not translate into similar efficacies in vivo. Using an OVCAR-3 mammary fat pad transplant model (previously described in [33]), a single dose of 3A5-VC-MMAE demonstrates tumoristasis at a significantly lower dose compared to the more stable linker drug, MC-MMAF (Fig. 13.9). In Chen et al., this improved potency of 3A5-VC-MMAE compared with 3A5-MC-MMAF was also observed following multiple doses. Although we do not know precisely why 3A5-VC-MMAE exhibits superior efficacy in vivo, the two ADC formats differ in some important respects. Specifically, the primary metabolite of 3A5-VC-MMAE after lysosomal digestion is believed to be MMAE, a membrane-permeable molecule that could act on

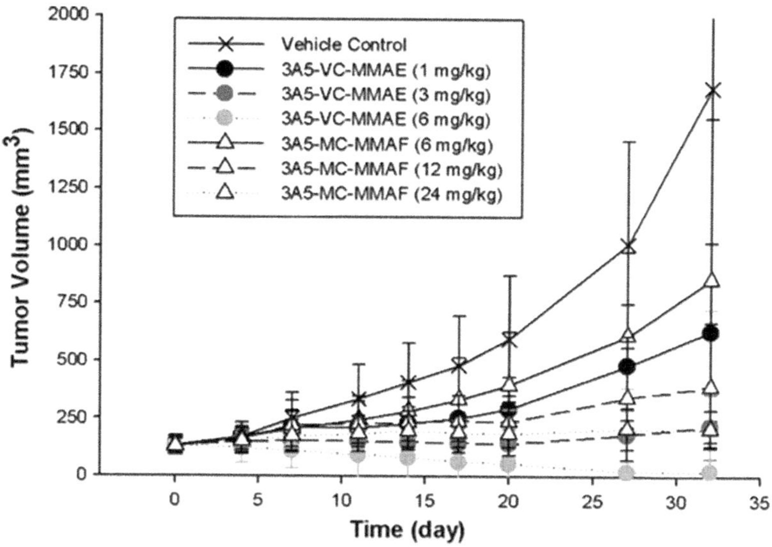

Fig. 13.9 In vivo dose ranging study in tumor-bearing mice: 3A5-VC-MMAE was approximately 8-fold more potent than 3A5-MC-MMAF on dose comparison basis

neighboring cells (the so-called "bystander" effect), whereas 3A5-MC-MMAF is metabolized into cysteine-MC-MMAF, a much less membrane-permeable molecule [48]. These findings highlight some of the limitations of using in vitro potency assays to screen or evaluate different linker-drugs.

As with any monoclonal antibody therapy, including ADCs, selecting a pharmacologically relevant animal species for testing the safety and pharmacokinetics to support preclinical testing is vital and can be challenging. For toxicology studies of antibodies, the relevant species is/are selected based on anticipated ability to predict toxicities in humans, assuming that the toxicological liabilities of the antibody are related to its pharmacological activity. In the case of an ADC, the pharmacological and toxicological activity of the antibody and cytotoxic agent (in this case, MMAE) should be considered. The unconjugated (naked) antibody of an ADC may have little or no pharmacological and thus toxicological activity, as is the case with the 3A5 antibody. Therefore, the most relevant species are simply those that express the desired epitope and demonstrate a similar tissue cross-reactivity profile to human tissues. For determination of the most relevant species, binding of 3A5 was assessed against recombinant MUC16 ECD proteins of rat, cynomolgus monkey, and humans. Using surface plasmon resonance-based technology, 3A5 bound to MUC16 ECD proteins of all species tested (rat, cynomolgus monkey, and human), suggesting that both rat and monkey are relevant binding species. Comparisons of the binding affinities were also similar between the ADCs and 3A5, suggesting that the conjugation of MMAE did not affect the antibody's binding affinity to MUC16.

As previously mentioned, the publication of full-length clones of MUC16 greatly facilitated the cloning and expression of orthologous rat and cynomolgus monkey

HUMAN 1	P	F	T	L	N	F	T	I	T	N	L	Q	Y	E	E	D	M	R	R	P	G	S	R	K	F	N	T	T	E	R	V
HUMAN 2	L	F	T	I	N	F	T	I	T	N	L	R	Y	E	E	N	M	H	H	P	G	S	R	K	F	N	T	T	E	R	V
HUMAN 3	L	F	T	L	N	F	T	I	T	N	L	R	Y	E	E	N	M	Q	H	P	G	S	R	K	F	N	T	T	E	R	V
MONKEY 1	P	F	T	L	N	F	T	I	N	N	L	R	Y	E	E	D	M	G	R	P	G	S	R	K	F	S	T	T	E	R	V
MONKEY 2	L	F	T	L	N	F	T	I	T	N	L	W	Y	E	E	S	M	H	H	P	G	S	G	K	F	N	T	T	E	R	V
MONKEY 3	P	F	T	L	N	F	T	I	T	N	L	R	Y	E	E	N	M	Q	H	P	G	S	R	K	F	N	T	T	E	R	V
RAT 1	H	F	T	I	N	F	T	I	I	N	L	K	F	E	E	D	M	R	N	P	G	S	R	K	F	N	I	T	Q	R	T
RAT 2	P	F	T	I	N	F	T	V	T	N	L	E	Y	V	E	D	M	G	H	P	G	S	R	K	F	N	A	T	E	R	V
RAT 3	P	F	T	I	N	F	T	V	T	N	L	E	F	E	K	D	M	R	Y	P	G	S	R	K	F	N	I	T	E	R	I

Fig. 13.10 Critical 3A5 binding residues are conserved in MUC16 mucin repeats. Comparison of rat, cynomolgus monkey, and human 3A5 binding residues. *Boxed* amino acids denote locations in which 3A5 binding is reduced when changed to an alanine

sequences using conventional methods. Comparison of the amino acid residues in the cynomolgus monkey and human MUC16 mucin repeats demonstrated that the critical 3A5 binding residues were highly conserved across the two species. In comparison, the rat ortholog demonstrated lower sequence homology to human across these conserved muc16-binding regions (Fig. 13.10). Therefore, on the basis of these data, the cynomolgus was considered the more pharmacologically relevant species, despite both rat and cynomolgus monkey demonstrating binding to 3A5.

Finally, understanding the expression of the antigen distribution in different tissues is also of importance in providing an integrated evaluation of safety findings. Comparison of MUC16 tissue expression between cynomolgus monkey and human tissues was conducted by immunohistochemical staining using 3A5; the expression of MUC16 in cynomolgus monkey tissues was similar to expression in human tissues, with no notable differences in MUC16 expression [33].

Using the cynomolgus monkey as a model, the next step was to determine which linker-drug would be better tolerated. However, prior to initiating any tolerability and safety studies, it is also important to consider the implications of the linker stability and pharmacokinetics between these two linker-drugs: 3A5-VC-MMAE AND 3A5-MC-MMAF. The impact of in vivo linker stability on efficacy and tolerability of ADCs has been well established [49, 50]. Early versions of reducible disulfide and acid-labile hydrazone linkers had significant liabilities with unintended cleavage of the linkers at nontarget sites [51]. As a result, linker-drugs have been developed to balance stability in circulation and enzymatic lability at the site of action, of which the "VC-MMAE" and "MC-MMAF" are two linker-drug counterweights in this delicate balance. The "VC-MMAE" linker-drug, as noted previously, is considered an enzymatically "cleavable" linker and free MMAE is released by intracellular proteases such as cathepsin B [42, 52]. Conversely, the "MC-MMAF" linker is chemically stable, and does not release free MMAF, but rather releases "cys-MC-MMAF" through degradation of the monoclonal antibody [39]. However, despite these differences, the pharmacokinetics of both the "VC-MMAE" and "MC-MMAF" ADCs were bi-exponential and demonstrated expected monoclonal antibody pharmacokinetic behavior as characterized by limited distribution and relatively slow clearance [48, 53].

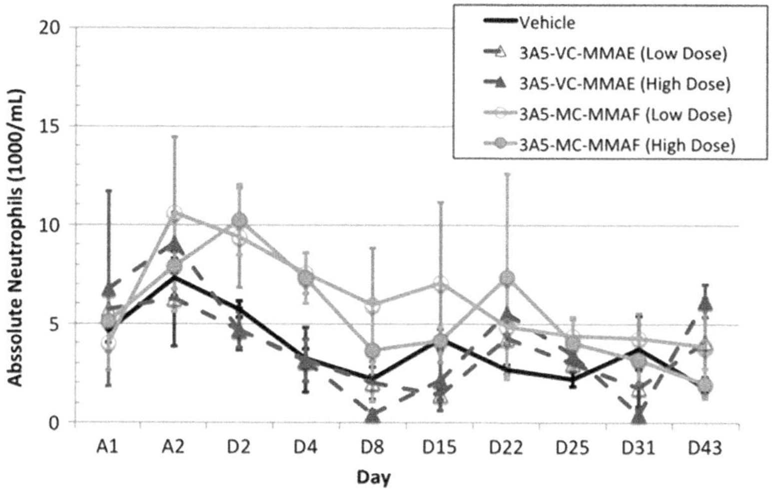

Fig. 13.11 Changes in neutropenia over time following two doses of 3A5 ADCs every 3 weeks in cynomolgus monkeys. *Arrows* denote approximate dosing days. *A*, acclimation period (i.e. prior to first dose of ADC). *D*, day based on initial administration of ADC on Day 1

ADC linker-drug selection will have specific importance in the tolerability of the different ADCs. The more enzymatically labile linker-drugs may have the tendency to release the potent free drug at nontarget sites, and thus may be more toxic, on a dose-based comparison with the enzymatically stable linker-drugs. In one report, the enzymatically labile linker-drug conjugated with MMAF attained an MTD of 50 and 15 mg/kg in mice and rats, respectively, while MMAF conjugated with the stable "MC" linker attained a three- and fivefold higher MTD in mice and rats, respectively [39]. Similarly, at equivalent doses of approximately 20 mg/kg of an anti-CD22 "VC-MMAE" and "MC-MMAF", the "VC-MMAE" linker-drug had identifiable hepatic and hematologic toxicities in rats administered a single IV dose, while the more stable linker appeared to be better tolerated [34]. With the cynomolgus monkey identified as the most pharmacologically relevant species, a multiple-dose safety/tolerability study was conducted with 3A5-VC-MMAE and 3A5-MC-MMAF. In the study, cynomolgus monkeys were administered intravenously two doses every 3 weeks of 3A5-VC-MMAE or 3A5-MC-MMAF. Given the observed lower potency, the doses of 3A5-MC-MMAF were markedly higher at approximately 20 and 40 mg/kg, while 3A5-VC-MMAE was administered at approximately sixfold lower doses, 3 and 6 mg/kg. As expected, for the auristatin conjugates (both MMAE and MMAF), there was reversible myelotoxicity to varying degrees at the different doses. At the high dose of 3A5-VC-MMAE, an apparent transient decrease in the neutrophils was observed, while at the lower dose, the decrease was less demonstrative (Fig. 13.11). A similar trend was noted with the doses of 3A5-MC-MMAF; however, the magnitude was not as significant compared to the 3A5-VC-MMAE conjugates (Fig. 13.11). The more pronounced myelotoxicity in the 3A5-VC-MMAE is consistent with the

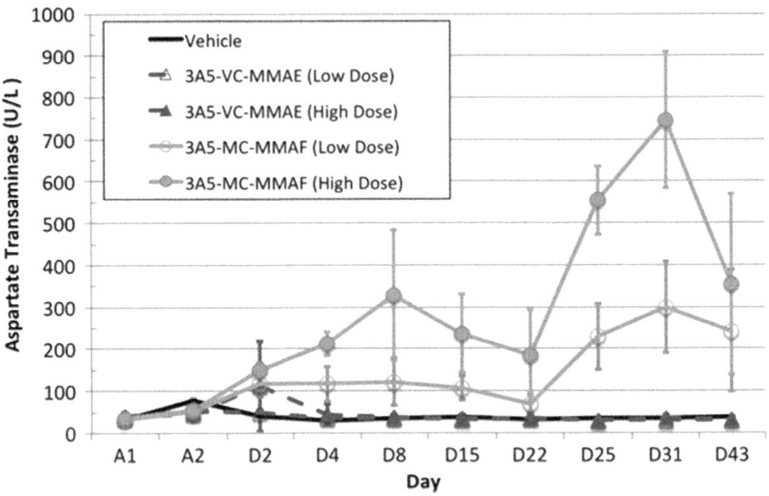

Fig. 13.12 Changes in aspartate transaminase (*AST*) over time following two doses of 3A5 ADCs every 3 weeks in cynomolgus monkeys. *Arrows* denote approximate dosing days. *A*, acclimation period (i.e., prior to first dose of ADC). *D*, day based on initial administration of ADC on Day 1

known toxicities of MMAE and the enzymatic lability of the linker [54, 55]. The myelotoxicity is most likely an antigen-independent toxicity, as MUC16 is not expressed on granulocytes [33]. No other notable drug-related toxicity findings were observed with the 3A5-VC-MMAE conjugates.

Beyond the myelotoxicity, the primary toxicity observed with the 3A5-MC-MMAF conjugate was liver toxicity as evidenced by a sustained and cumulative elevation of serum aspartate transaminase levels at both doses (Fig. 13.12). Increases in serum gamma-glutamyltransferase, serum chemistry marker of hepatic impairment, were also noted at both doses of 3A5-MC-MMAF (data not shown). These serum chemistry alterations correlated to histologic findings in the liver. By comparison, 3A5-VC-MMAE did not demonstrate any apparent liver toxicity at either dose (Fig. 13.12). These safety findings in the monkey were not confounded by any detectable host immune response to the 3A5 drug conjugates.

Thus following final selection of the antibody, 3A5, determination of the linker-drug was based upon the same criteria used in the development of any new molecular entity, that is, a balance of the efficacy and toxicity of each linker-drug. For VC-MMAE, although the linker-drug appeared to have more notable, although transient, neutropenia, the VC-MMAE linker-drug was also significantly more potent in efficacy models, with tumoristasis observed at a single dose of 3 mg/kg. Conversely, the MC-MMAF linker-drug safety profile included both neutropenia (up to approximately 40 mg/kg) and hepatotoxicity, and was significantly less potent in efficacy models (tumoristasis was apparent 24 mg/kg at a both single dose) than VC-MMAE. Lastly it should be noted that understanding and comparing the potencies of different linker-drugs likely entail comparisons based on their exposures rather than strictly a dose-based comparison. However, for the MUC16 conjugates exposure-based comparisons did not facilitate any greater delineation between linker-drugs as other aforementioned factors had greater influence.

The MUC16 example illustrates the potential of the ADC strategy to target a well-validated antigen. The overexpression of MUC16 in ovarian cancer has long been appreciated and was readily confirmed using straightforward mRNA expression profiling. However, a more careful consideration of the MUC16 protein structure was required for the identification of an antibody that could mediate cell killing in relevant models. In vitro data were decisive for selection of the antibody, but we evaluated the specific ADC formats based on both efficacy and safety in vivo. Furthermore, we developed in vitro and in vivo models to investigate the potential impact of ECD shedding, an issue that is perhaps apparent for, but not exclusive to, MUC16. In summary, each step along the preclinical path for MUC16 ADC development has required us to identify the right tools to answer the right questions.

References

1. Hanahan D, Weinberg RA (2000) The hallmarks of cancer. Cell 100(1):57–70
2. Carter PJ, Senter PD (2008) Antibody-drug conjugates for cancer therapy. Cancer J 14(3): 154–169
3. Senter PD (2009) Potent antibody drug conjugates for cancer therapy. Curr Opin Chem Biol 13(3):235–244
4. Teicher BA (2009) Antibody-drug conjugate targets. Curr Cancer Drug Targets 9(8):982–1004
5. Greenbaum D, Colangelo C, Williams K et al (2003) Comparing protein abundance and mRNA expression levels on a genomic scale. Genome Biol 4(9):117
6. Bast RC Jr, Feeney M, Lazarua H et al (1981) Reactivity of a monoclonal antibody with human ovarian carcinoma. J Clin Invest 68:1331–1337
7. Høgdall EVS, Christensen L, Kjaer SK et al (2007) CA125 expression pattern, prognosis and correlation with serum CA125 in ovarian tumor patients. Gynecol Oncol 104(3):508–515
8. Kabawat SE, Bast RC, Welch WR et al (1983) Immunopathologic characterization of a monoclo- nal antibody that recognizes common surface antigens of human ovarian tumors of serous, endometrioid, and clear cell types. Am J Clin Pathol 79:98–104
9. Rosen DG, Wang L, Atkinson JN et al (2005) Potential markers that complement expression of CA125 in epithelial ovarian cancer. Gynecol Oncol 99(2):267–277
10. Dekker J, Rossen JWA, Buller HA et al (2002) The MUC family: an obituary. Trends Biochem Sci 27(3):126–131
11. O'Brien TJ, Beard JB, Underwood LJ et al (2002) The CA 125 gene: a newly discovered extension of the glycosylated N-terminal domain doubles the size of this extracellular superstructure. Tumor Biol 23:154–169
12. Yin BWT, Lloyd KO (2001) Molecular cloning of the CA125 ovarian cancer antigen: identification as a new mucin, MUC16. J Biol Chem 276:27371–27375
13. Yin BWT, Dnistrian A, Lloyd KO (2002) Ovarian cancer antigen CA125 is encoded by the MUC16 mucin gene. Int J Cancer 98:737–740
14. Hunter VJ, Weinberg JB, Haney AF et al (1990) CA 125 in peritoneal fluid and serum from patients with benign gynecologic conditions and ovarian cancer. Gynecol Oncol 36(2):161–165
15. Macdonald F, Downing R, Allum WH (1988) Expression of CA125 in pancreatic carcinoma and chronic pancreatitis. Br J Cancer 58(4):505–506

16. Belisle JA, Gubbels JAA, Raphael CA et al (2007) Peritoneal natural killer cells from epithelial ovarian cancer patients show an altered phenotype and bind to the tumour marker MUC16 (CA125). Immunology 122(3):418–429
17. Belisle JA, Horibata S, Gubbels JAA et al (2010) Identification of Siglec-9 as the receptor for MUC16 on human NK cells, B cells, and monocytes. Mol Cancer 9(1):118
18. Gubbels JAA, Belisle J, Onda M et al (2006) Mesothelin-MUC16 binding is a high affinity, N-glycan dependent interaction that facilitates peritoneal metastasis of ovarian tumors. Mol Cancer 5(1):50
19. Gubbels JA, Felder M, Horibata S et al (2010) MUC16 provides immune protection by inhibiting synapse formation between NK and ovarian tumor cells. Mol Cancer 9(1):11
20. Patankar M, Jing Y, Morrison J et al (2005) Potent suppression of natural killer cell response mediated by the ovarian tumor marker CA125. Gynecol Oncol 99(3):704–713
21. Rump A, Morikawa Y, Tanaka M et al (2004) Binding of ovarian cancer antigen CA125/MUC16 to mesothelin mediates cell adhesion. J Biol Chem 279(10):9190–9198
22. Berek JS, Taylor PT, Gordon A et al (2004) Randomized, placebo-controlled study of oregovomab for consolidation of clinical remission in patients with advanced ovarian cancer. J Clin Oncol 22:3507–3516
23. Berek J, Taylor P, McGuire W, Smith L, Schultes B, Nicodemus C (2009) Oregovomab maintenance monoimmunotherapy does not improve outcomes in advanced ovarian cancer. J Clin Oncol 27:418–425
24. Ehlen TG, Hoskins PJ, Miller D et al (2005) A pilot phase 2 study of oregovomab murine monoclonal antibody to CA125 as an immunotherapeutic agent for recurrent ovarian cancer. Int J Gynecol Cancer 15(6):1023–1034
25. Schultes BC, Baum RP, Niesen A et al (1998) Anti-idiotype induction therapy: anti-CA125 antibodies (Ab3) mediated tumor killing in patients treated with Ovarex mAb B43.13 (Ab1). Cancer Immunol Immunother 46(4):201–212
26. Reinartz S, Kohler S, Schlebusch H et al (2004) Vaccina- tion of patients with advanced ovarian carcinoma with the anti-idiotype ACA125: immunological response and survival (phase Ib/II). Clin Cancer Res 10:1580–1587
27. Sabbatini P, Dupont J, Aghajanian C et al (2006) Phase I study of abagovomab in patients with epithelial ovarian, fallopian tube, or primary peritoneal cancer. Clin Cancer Res 12(18): 5503–5510
28. Oei AL, Sweep FC, Thomas CMG et al (2008) The use of monoclonal antibodies for the treatment of epithelial ovarian cancer. Int J Oncol 32:1145–1157
29. Argüeso P, Spurr-Michaud S, Russo CL, Tisdale A, Gipson IK (2003) MUC16 mucin is expressed by the human ocular surface epithelia and carries the H185 carbohydrate epitope. Invest Ophthalmol Vis Sci 44:2487–2495
30. Nouwen EJ, Pollet DE, Eerdekens MW et al (1986) Immunohistochemical localization of placental alkaline phosphatase, carcinoembryonic antigen, and cancer antigen 125 in normal and neoplastic human lung. Cancer Res 46(2):866–876
31. Nouwen EJ, Hendrix PG, Dauwe S, Eerdekens MW, De Broe ME (1987) Tumor markers in the human ovary and its neoplasms. A comparative immunohistochemical study. Am J Pathol 126:230–242
32. Nouwen EJ, Dauwe S, De Broe ME (1990) Occurrence of the mucinous differentiation antigen CA125 in genital tract and conductive airway epithelia of diverse mammalian species (rabbit, dog, monkey). Differentiation 45:192–198
33. Chen Y, Clark S, Wong T et al (2007) Armed antibodies targeting the mucin repeats of the ovarian cancer antigen, MUC16, are highly efficacious in animal tumor models. Cancer Res 67(10):4924–4932
34. Polson AG, Calemine-Fenaux J, Chan P et al (2009) Antibody-drug conjugates for the treatment of non-hodgkin's lymphoma: target and linker-drug selection. Cancer Res 69(6):2358–2364
35. Maeda T, Inoue M, Koshiba S et al (2004) Solution structure of the SEA domain from the murine homologue of ovarian cancer antigen CA125 (MUC16). J Biol Chem 279: 13174–13182

36. Hamilton TC, Young RC, McKoy WM et al (1983) Characterization of a human ovarian carcinoma cell line (NIH:OVCAR-3) with androgen and estrogen receptors. Cancer Res 43(11):5379–5389
37. Langdon SP, Lawrie SS, Hay FG, Hawkes MM, Mcdonald A, Hayward IP, Schol DJ, Leonard RCF, Smyth JF (1988) Characterization and properties of nine human ovarian adenocarcinoma cell lines. Cancer Res 48:6166–6172
38. Junutula JR, Raab H, Clark S et al (2008) Site-specific conjugation of a cytotoxic drug to an antibody improves the therapeutic index. Nat Biotechnol 26(8):925–932
39. Doronina SO, Mendelsohn BA, Bovee TD et al (2006) Enhanced activity of monomethylauristatin F through monoclonal antibody delivery: effects of linker technology on efficacy and toxicity. Bioconjug Chem 17(1):114–124
40. McGuire WP, Markman M (2003) Primary ovarian cancer chemotherapy: current standards of care. Br J Cancer 89:S3–S8
41. Smith JA, Ngo H, Martin MC, Wolf JK (2005) An evaluation of cytotoxicity of the taxane and platinum agents combination treatment in a panel of human ovarian carcinoma cell lines. Gynecol Oncol 98(1):141–145
42. Doronina SO, Toki BE, Torgov MY et al (2003) Development of potent monoclonal antibody auristatin conjugates for cancer therapy. Nat Biotechnol 21(7):778–784
43. Okeley NM, Miyamoto JB, Zhang X et al (2010) Intracellular activation of SGN-35, a potent anti-CD30 antibody-drug conjugate. Clin Cancer Res 16(3):888–897
44. Pastuskovas CV, Mallet W, Clark S et al (2010) Effect of immune complex formation on the distribution of a novel antibody to the ovarian tumor antigen CA125. Drug Metab Dispos 38(12):2309–2319
45. Hassan R, Remaley AT, Sampson ML et al (2006) Detection and quantitation of serum mesothelin, a tumor marker for patients with mesothelioma and ovarian cancer. Clin Cancer Res 12(2):447–453
46. Mehta RR, McDermott JH, Heiken TJ, Marler KC, Patel MK, Wild LD et al (1998) Plasma c-erbB-2 levels in breast cancer patients: prognostic significance in predicting response to chemotherapy. J Clin Oncol 16:2409–2416
47. Bast RC Jr, Klug TL, StJohn E, Jenison E, Niloff JM, Lazarus H, Berkowitz RS, Leavitt T, Griffiths CT, Parker L, Zurawski VR Jr, Knapp RC (1983) A radioimmunoassay using a monoclonal antibody to monitor the course of epithelial ovarian cancer. N Engl J Med 309:883–887
48. Alley SC, Zhang X, Okeley NM et al (2009) The pharmacologic basis for antibody-auristatin conjugate activity. J Pharmacol Exp Ther 330(3):932–938
49. Alley SC, Benjamin DR, Jeffrey SC et al (2008) Contribution of linker stability to the activities of anticancer immunoconjugates. Bioconjug Chem 19(3):759–765
50. Dosio F, Brusa P, Cattel L (2011) immunotoxins and anticancer drug conjugate assemblies: the role of the linkage between components. Toxins 3(7):848–883
51. Thorpe PE, Wallace PM, Knowles PP et al (1987) New coupling agents for the synthesis of immunotoxins containing a hindered disulfide bond with improved stability in vivo. Cancer Res 47(22):5924–5931
52. Francisco JA (2003) cAC10-vcMMAE, an anti-CD30-monomethyl auristatin E conjugate with potent and selective antitumor activity. Blood 102(4):1458–1465
53. Sanderson RJ, Hering MA, James SF et al (2005) In vivo drug-linker stability of an anti-CD30 dipeptide-linked auristatin immunoconjugate. Clin Cancer Res 11(2 Pt 1):843–852
54. Mirsalis JC, Schindler-Horvat J, Hill JR et al (1999) Toxicity of dolastatin 10 in mice, rats and dogs and its clinical relevance. Cancer Chemother Pharmacol 44(5):395–402
55. Younes A, Bartlett NL, Leonard JP et al (2010) Brentuximab vedotin (SGN-35) for relapsed CD30-positive lymphomas. N Engl J Med 363(19):1812–1821
56. Frierson HF, Jr et al (2003) Large-scale molecular and tissue microarray analysis of mesothelin expression in common human carcinomas. Human Pathology 34:605–609
57. Frederick PJ, Straughn JM, Jr, Alvarez RD et al (2009) Preclinical studies and clinical utilization of monoclonal antibodies in epithelial ovarian cancer. Gynecologic Oncology 113:384–390

Chapter 14
EphA2 Immunoconjugate

Zhan Xiao, Dowdy Jackson, and David A. Tice

Introduction to the Eph Family of Receptors

Eph (erythropoietin-producing hepatocellular) family receptors represent the largest family of the receptor tyrosine kinases (RTKs). In humans, it consists of 16 members which, based on sequence homologies of the extracellular domains (ECD) and ligand-binding preferences, are divided into two subfamilies: EphA subclass (EphA1-10) and EphB subclass (EphB1-6) [1, 2].

As shown in Fig. 14.1 all Eph receptors share the same overall structural organization: Ligand-binding domain is located on the N-terminus of the ECD, which is followed by a cysteine-rich domain and two fibronectin-type III repeats. On the cytoplasmic side, Eph receptors consist of a tyrosine kinase domain immediately following the juxtamembrane region. A sterile-alpha-motif (SAM) domain and a PDZ-binding motif are located to the C-terminus of the kinase domain.

The ligands of the Eph receptors are called Ephrins and consist of eight members in humans. They are also classified into two subfamilies, EphrinA (1–5) and EphrinB (1–3). Both subfamilies are anchored to the plasma membranes, but EphrinAs are attached through a GPI linker whereas EphrinBs are anchored through a transmembrane domain [3, 4]. One unique feature of the Ephrin ligands is that besides stimulating receptors leading to downstream pathway activation in Eph-expressing cells (forward-signaling pathway), Eph binding can also trigger a reverse-signaling pathway into Ephrin-expressing cells. EphrinB ligands contain cytoplasmic tails with conserved motifs implicated in several intracellular signaling pathways. It is not clear whether or not EphrinA ligands can sustain reverse signaling as they lack

Z. Xiao • D.A. Tice (✉)
MedImmune, 1 MedImmune Way, Gaithersburg, MD 20878, USA
e-mail: ticed@medimmune.com

D. Jackson
Agensys, Inc., 2105 Colorado Ave, Santa Monica, CA 90404, USA

G.L. Phillips (ed.), *Antibody-Drug Conjugates and Immunotoxins: From Pre-Clinical Development to Therapeutic Applications*, Cancer Drug Discovery and Development,
DOI 10.1007/978-1-4614-5456-4_14, © Springer Science+Business Media New York 2013

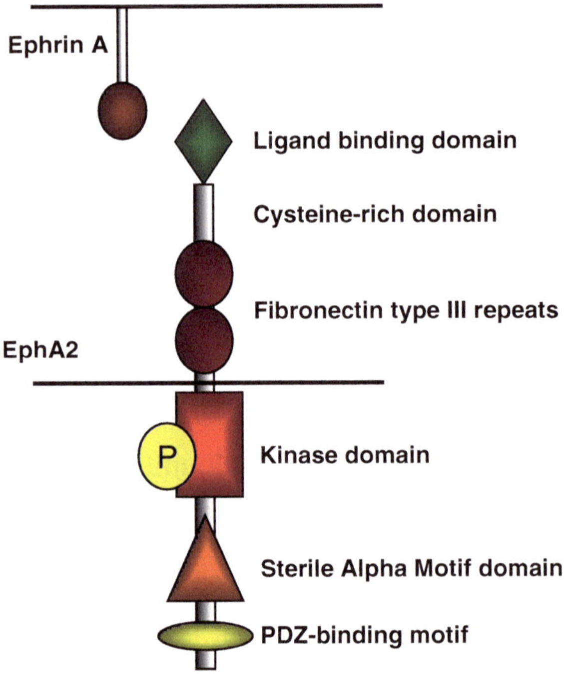

Fig. 14.1 Structural features of EphA2 receptor tyrosine kinase

cytoplasmic domains. Another salient feature of Ephrins is that some level of clustering of soluble ligands, such as dimerization through Fc-fusion, or membrane anchoring is required to achieve optimal stimulation effects [4–6].

EphrinAs usually interact with EphAs whereas EphrinBs normally bind to EphBs, but this rule is not absolute. Some promiscuity has been observed in terms of certain EphrinA ligands binding to EphBs: EphrinA5 binds to EphB2 in addition to EphAs [7]. Also, within each ligand–receptor class, the pairings could be highly promiscuous [8].

Expressions of Ephs and ephrins are developmentally regulated: highly expressed during embryonic stages and development but generally at lower levels in normal adult tissues [9, 10]. The most established functions of Eph/Ephrins in normal physiology involve pathway selection by axons, the guidance of cell migration, the establishment of regional pattern in the nervous system, formation and remodeling of synaptic connections, and nervous system repair [9, 11]. Consistent with these roles, the Ephrin/Eph interaction is known to mediate cell–cell repulsion, regulate and restrict cell migration, and define clear boundaries between different anatomical compartments in developing organs such as brains or cardiovascular systems [11, 12].

Even though Ephs belong to the RTK superfamily, they have a unique bifunctionality that is not often seen with other RTKs. RTKs usually act as oncogenes to promote the tumorigenic processes through induction of Ras/MEK/ERK or PI3K/AKT pathways. In contrast, many Eph receptors have been shown to play dichotomous roles to both promote and suppress oncogenesis in different cellular contexts.

EphB2 was found to act as a tumor suppressor in prostate [13, 14] and colorectal cancers [15–17], potentially as a result of its ability to inhibit the Ras/MEK pathway [18]. In contrast, EphB2 is overexpressed in several solid tumors and promote the invasion and growth of glioblastoma cells through activation of the R-Ras pathway [19, 20]. EphB4, a close homolog of EphB2, can be overexpressed and contribute to tumorigenesis in colorectal and ovarian cancers [21, 22], but suppresses mammary carcinogenesis through Abl/Crk pathway [23]. Additionally, our unpublished data indicate that EphB4 activation may show antiangiogenic effect by suppressing the growth of endothelial cells (Xiao unpublished data).

EphA2

EphA2 was initially cloned in 1990 by the screening of a human epithelial cancer cell line (Hela cells) cDNA library using degenerate probes to highly conserved regions of protein tyrosine kinases and represents the second Eph family member to be cloned after EphA1. In the human genome, the EphA2 gene is located on chromosome 1 and encodes a RTK of 976 amino acids with an apparent molecular weight of 130–150 kDa and 90% sequence identity to the mouse EphA2. The overall sequence homology with other Ephs is 25–35%, but the tyrosine kinase domain shows the highest local sequence homology [24, 25].

Genetic deletion of EphA2 in mouse does not cause any overt abnormalities. The mice are fertile, develop, and grow normally [16, 17, 26]. This was attributed to potential functional overlap or redundancy among the Eph family members. But EphA2 deletion led to markedly enhanced susceptibility to chemical-induced skin carcinogenesis. EphA2-null mice developed skin tumors with an increased frequency and shortened latency. Moreover, these tumors grew faster and were twice as likely to show invasive malignant progression [16, 17].

EphA2 shows a highly controlled expression pattern in embryogenesis and early stages of development. Its transcripts are first detected in gastrulation stage embryos (6.5–7.5 days post coitum) in ectodermal cells adjacent to the distal region of the primitive streak. Later on EphA2 exhibits a dynamic and spatially restricted expression pattern in the prospective hindbrain region. By the 10-somite stage, EphA2 mRNA in these cells is downregulated [25]. A later study confirmed these findings by showing that EphA2 was expressed in blastocyst and later restricted to the primitive streak, node, and to regions of the hindbrain in 6.5- to 10.5-day embryos [26]. These observations suggest that EphA2 may be involved in cell–cell interactions guiding early hindbrain development.

EphA2 mRNA levels have been analyzed in adult human tissues using Northern blot. High expression was confined to several epithelial tissues with relatively high proliferation rate such as skin, colon, lung, ovary, and bladder. EphA2 mRNA was detectable in kidney, brain, spleen, and submaxillary gland, but was present at very low levels in heart, skeletal muscle, liver, testes, and thymus [24]. An independent study using qRT-PCR revealed similar findings [10]. However, the EphA2 protein expression, as assessed by IHC, may be disconnected from the RNA profile: Although kidney only has modest RNA expression, it showed the strongest staining in EphA2 IHC. Tissues with the highest RNA levels, such as lung or colon, only showed relatively light staining [24]. Therefore there exists a nonlinear relationship between mRNA and protein levels for EphA2.

In contrast to its limited expression patterns in normal tissues, EphA2 has been found to be overexpressed in a vast majority of solid tumor types, in both cell lines and primary tumor samples, at both the mRNA and protein levels: breast, prostate, ovarian, glioblastoma, pancreas, renal, lung, melanoma, gastric, bladder, colorectal, and esophageal cancers. (For general review, see [27, 28].) The extents of EphA2 overexpression are especially impressive in prostate cancers (85% [29]), ovarian cancers (76% [30]), pancreatic cancers (95% [31]), and glioblastoma mutiformae (61% [32]).

In addition to the wide tumor overexpression pattern, EphA2 has been established as a prognostic marker for increased invasion and metastasis, and decreased survival in a majority of these tumor types: in prostate cancer, EphA2 is overexpressed more in metastatic than noninvasive cells [29, 33]; in breast cancer, EphA2 is highly upregulated in more invasive and tumorigenic breast cancer cells [34]; in lung cancer, high levels of EphA2 predict shorter survival and brain metastases [35]; in esophageal cancer, EphA2 expression is correlated with lymph node metastasis and poor survival rates [36]; in ovarian cancer, EphA2 overexpression is significantly associated with higher grade, advanced disease stage, and shorter survival [30, 37]; in melanoma, EphA2 is expressed and phosphorylated specifically in aggressive metastatic melanoma cells and functions in vasculogenic mimicry [38]; and in GBM, increased EphA2 expression is significantly associated with poor survival and adverse patient outcome [39]. All these results strongly indicate that EphA2 plays functional roles in these tumors.

Furthermore, ectopic expression of EphA2 in MCF10A normal mammary epithelial cells induced malignant transformation [40]. Conversely, overexpression of a kinase-deficient and hence dominant-negative EphA2 with cytoplasmic domain deletion suppressed the growth of 4 T1 breast cancer cells [41]. Combined, these lines of evidence suggest that EphA2 may qualify as an attractive cancer target whose inhibition may confer anti-solid-tumor effects.

Therapeutic Targeting of EphA2

Small Molecule Tyrosine Kinase Inhibitors

Tyrosine kinase activity is essential to the oncogenic capacity of RTKs; therefore, tyrosine kinase inhibitors (TKIs) could be an efficient way to suppress EphA2 activity and achieve antitumor activity. Dasatinib, an orally active TKI developed to target multiple kinases including the Bcr-abl and Src family kinases, also inhibits EphA2 tyrosine kinase activity. Consequently, treating breast cancer cells in vitro with dasatinib reduced EphA2 expression, phosphorylation, and associated kinase activity [42]. However, due to its rather promiscuous nature and inhibition of a wide range of kinase targets, extreme caution should be taken when assigning the potent in vitro/in vivo antitumor efficacy of dasatinib to its inhibition of EphA2. Other TKIs have been developed to target EphA2, but like dasatinib they are not highly selective inhibitors.

EphA2-Targeted Peptides

Two related peptides, YSA and SWL, have been identified that selectively bind the ligand-binding domain of EphA2, but not other Eph receptors. Consequently, both peptides behave as ligand mimetic in activating EphA2 and inhibiting downstream oncogenic signaling pathways in PC3 cancer cells. The two peptides are quite stable in conditioned cell culture medium and show promise for delivering drugs and imaging agents to EphA2-expressing tumors [43].

Monoclonal Antibodies

Monoclonal antibodies (mAb) can be generated against the ECD of EphA2 by either immunizing mice with recombinant ECD protein or phage-panning against ECD protein [44]. The mAb leads were selected based on the ability to inhibit metastatic properties of the cancer cells while minimizing damage to nontransformed cells. The mAbs were found to inhibit the soft agar colonization by the highly metastatic MDA-MB-231 breast cancer cells, but did not affect monolayer growth by nontransformed MCF-10A breast epithelial cells. They also prevented tumor cells from forming tubular networks on reconstituted basement membranes, a key indicator of metastatic character. The proposed mechanism of action involves mAb induction of EphA2 phosphorylation and followed by internalization and subsequent degradation, similar to antitumor effect achieved by antisense RNA of EphA2 [44].

Another commercially developed EphA2 mAb, 1C1, failed to confer substantial antitumor effect in monotherapy setting. However, 1C1 showed synergistic interaction with the HER2 mAb trastuzumab in abrogating resistance of HER2-amplified breast cancers to this drug [45]. This finding is consistent with the preferential overexpression of EphA2 in trastuzumab-resistant cancers. However, other studies have suggested that stimulation of EphA2 results in activation of FAK and has no effect on in vivo tumor growth [46]. These discrepancies make the functional significance of EphA2 in tumor progression unclear, such that the development path for traditional therapeutic antibody approaches may be challenging.

Alternatively, selective targeting and potent suppression of tumor growth was achieved using an EphA2/CD3 bi-specific single-chain antibody construct [47]. An EphA2-specific single-chain antibody (scFv) was selected for the recognition of an epitope of EphA2 that is preferentially exposed on malignant cells; this was fused to a CD3-specific single-chain antibody targeting CD3 on T cells to generate bscEphA2xCD3. The resultant bi-specific mAb redirected unstimulated human T cells to lyse EphA2-expressing tumor cells both in vitro and in vivo with high potency.

MEDI-547

EphA2 as an Immunoconjugate Target

Antibodies coupled to cytotoxics provide a mechanism to circumvent the uncertainty around EphA2 biology. Antibody–drug conjugates (ADC) represents a marriage between the highly tumor-selective but less potent mAb and the highly potent but non-tumor-selective small molecule cytotoxic payloads. Linking the toxic payload to a tumor-specific mAb essentially ensures that only tumor tissues will be targeted sparing normal, non-target-expressing tissues of any toxicity. More importantly, the ADC platform greatly expands the potential target list from obligatory cancer “drivers” exposed on the cell surface (a very limited number) to a much larger collection of cell surface molecules that are differentially expressed in tumor versus normal tissues.

Based on the basic rationale of the ADC platform, the most critical requirement of an ADC target is high tumor-selective expression and low/preferentially null normal tissue expression. EphA2 is overexpressed in a vast majority of solid tumor types, in both cell lines and primary tumor samples, satisfying this key requirement. However, it is unknown whether the low levels of EphA2 protein found on some normal tissues will present any problems with toxicity when using an ADC approach.

Another key determinant of ADC sensitivity is target internalization which is a prerequisite for most ADCs to efficiently cleave the linker to release the drug inside the cells. Internalization can be achieved through either spontaneous target recycling via the endo-lysosomal pathways or mAb-induced internalization. Theoretically the former case is more desirable as it places less stringent requirements on the selection of the mAb. It is not clear if EphA2 undergoes robust endocytosis on its own. However, both EphrinA ligand and EphA2 mAbs have demonstrated superb abilities to induce rapid internalization and degradation of EphA2, indicating that this target could be highly amenable to the ADC approach [48–52].

Lead Identification

Several approaches were taken to derive antibodies against EphA2. Antibodies were obtained from mouse immunizations with EphA2 ECD [53] and then later humanized [54]. In addition human antibody fragments were derived from phage libraries and later converted to human IgG1 [49]. In both approaches, mAbs were identified that activated and degraded the receptor. Activation was assessed by measuring the amount of tyrosine phosphorylation that occurred on the C-terminal tail of the receptor acutely after addition of the antibody on cells. Degradation was measured in a variety of assays by determining the absolute levels of EphA2 remaining in the whole cell lysate or on the cell surface. These two parameters served as a surrogate for antibody-induced internalization and lysosomal targeting of the receptor on tumor cells.

Several considerations contributed to the selection of a suitable payload. As EphA2 is expressed on many epithelial-derived solid tumor types, the mechanism of action of the payload must be compatible with standard of care for these patients. Taxanes are commonly used alone or in combination with other cytotoxic agents for many of the lead indications, including ovarian and prostate cancer, making the choice of microtubule disrupting agents a logical decision. Another consideration in the choice of payload is whether bystander activity is desired. Given that EphA2 expression is fairly homogeneous in most tumor types, this was not a major factor in choosing the payload.

In collaboration with Seattle Genetics, Inc., five antibodies were directly conjugated to a variety of payloads available at the time. The payloads were all based on potent dolastatin 10 analogs, a microtubule disrupting agent that failed in clinical development as a single agent [55]. The antibodies were conjugated to three payloads. These were based on the pairwise combination of two linkers, valine–citrulline (vc) and maleimidocaproyl (mc), and two drugs, monomethyl auristatin F (MMAF) and monomethyl auristatin E (MMAE). One combination, maleimidocaproyl monomethyl auristatin E, was previously shown to be ineffective as a conjugate and thus not pursued. The drug to antibody ratio was held constant at 4.

The criteria for selection of the lead antibody drug conjugate targeting EphA2 were based on therapeutic index. Therapeutic index provides a measure of several attributes of each ADC including serum stability, biodistribution, tumor penetration, as well as other pharmacokinetic properties in addition to potency and toxicity. Thus, the use of therapeutic index eliminates the need to do these tests independently or identify in vitro surrogate assays to simulate these properties. However, it is important to establish that the animal model is suitable by establishing comparable expression profiles of the antigen as well as sensitivity to the drug payload. In development of MEDI-547, murine models were used due to ease of use and comparable EphA2 expression profiles. However, the therapeutic index was exaggerated in this species due to the lower sensitivity of mice to this class of compound [56].

EphA2 antibodies conjugated to vcMMAF had a much smaller therapeutic index compared to either mcMMAF or vcMMAE (Table 14.1). This emphasized the utility of comparing both activity and toxicity since comparisons based on activity alone would not have allowed the distinction between vcMMAF and mcMMAF.

Table 14.1 Therapeutic index calculated for different payloads conjugated to an EphA2 antibody 1C1

	Dose needed to induce complete response of PC3 tumors (mg/kg)	Dose causing >15% body weight loss in mice (mg/kg)	Therapeutic index
1C1-vcMMAE	3	60	20
1C1-vcMMAF	6	30	5
1C1-mcMMAF	6	>180	>30

Therapeutic index: Tox dose/efficacious dose

Development of MEDI-547

A human IgG_1 mAb, 1C1, selectively bound to EphA2 amongst a panel of EphA and EphB receptors and has an acceptable binding affinity for human, mouse, rat, and Cynomolgus monkey EphA2 ($K_d = 1$ nM). 1C1 is rapidly internalized by EphA2-expressing cells and induces receptor phosphorylation and degradation. When attached to mcMMAF payload, 1C1 provided the best overall drug-like properties and therapeutic index. Thus MEDI-547 is comprised of the antibody 1C1 with an average of four MMAF molecules covalently attached to cysteine residues via the mc linker (Fig. 14. 2, [49]).

The addition of the payload mcMMAF to the cysteines of 1C1 did not impair antibody binding to EphA2. Surface plasmon resonance studies were used to compare the binding affinities of 1C1 and MEDI-547 for human, mouse, rat, or Cynomolgus monkey recombinant EphA2. In addition, MEDI-547 and 1C1 were labeled with europium and the binding affinities to cell surface human, rat, and Cynomolgus monkey EphA2 were measured. MEDI-547 binds to both recombinant and cell surface EphA2 from each species with binding affinities comparable to 1C1. These studies confirmed that the conjugation reaction did not reduce the binding affinity of 1C1 to EphA2.

If an ADC is to be effective in killing the antigen-expressing cells, it must be internalized and reach the proper intracellular compartment to release its drug payload. 1C1 and MEDI-547 are rapidly internalized 10–15 min after they bind to EphA2 on the surface of human tumor cells. Furthermore, MEDI-547 and 1C1 colocalize to lysosomes approximately 2 h after internalization by PC3 cells (Fig. 14.3). Almost complete degradation of EphA2 protein can be observed following in vitro treatment of tumor cells with MEDI-547 or 1C1, further supporting the evidence for lysosomal trafficking of the receptor. This is also true in vivo where a single dose of 5 mg/kg in tumor bearing animals results in degradation of EphA2 as soon as one hour and as long as 6 days post dosing. As shown previously, the localization of ADCs to the lysosome is critical to the release of the active drug payload, cys-mcMMAF [57].

MEDI-547 inhibited the growth of EphA2-expressing cells, in a dose-dependent manner, while non-EphA2-expressing cells were unaffected. EphA2 receptor density did not correlate with MEDI-547 IC_{50} values. In subsequent studies, RNA

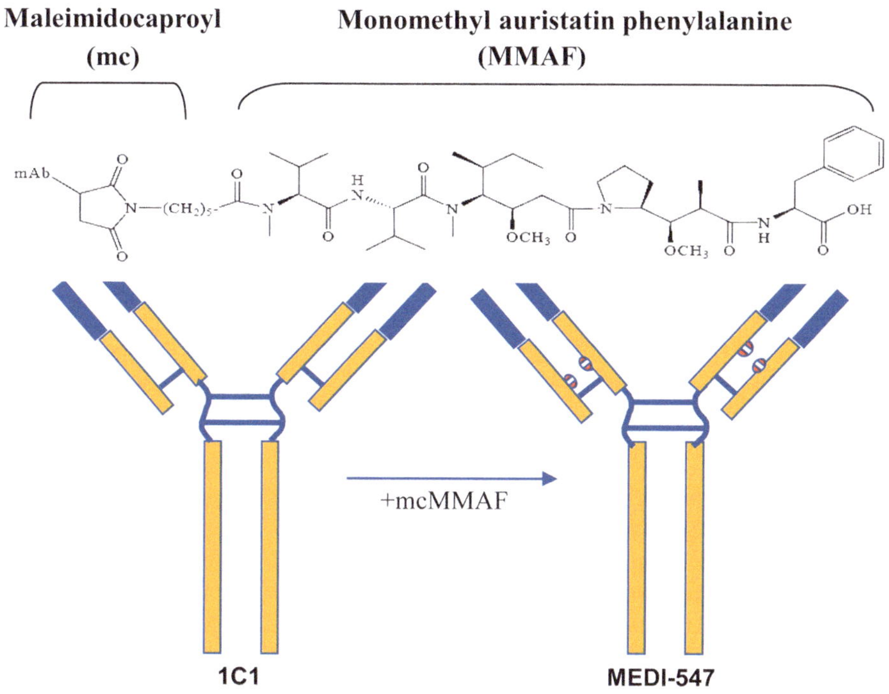

Fig. 14.2 MEDI-547 anti-EphA2 antibody drug conjugate

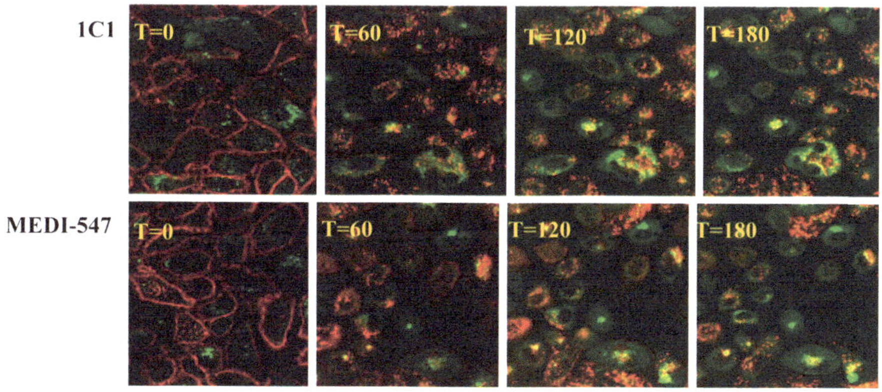

Fig. 14.3 Anti-EphA2 antibody internalization in tumor cells. PC3 cells were stained for EphA2 (*red*) and a lysosome marker (*green*) and then incubated at 37°C for the time indicated (minutes)

interference was used to reduce EphA2 receptor levels in PC3 cells. In these studies MEDI-547 did not inhibit the growth of PC3 cells with low levels of EphA2 expression. These data show that EphA2 expression is critical for MEDI-547 activity and a minimum receptor density is also required. Furthermore MEDI-547 kills

Table 14.2 Effect of drug efflux pump modulation on cell viability following drug treatment

Treatment	MDA-MB231 IC_{50} (nM)	MDA-MB231 -MDR1 IC_{50} (nM)	MDA-MB231-MDR1 + verapamil (10 mM) IC_{50} (nM)	Resistance (fold)
MEDI-547	0.22	1.45	0.19	7
mcMMAF	>10,000	>10,000	>10,000	N/A
1C1-vcMMAE	0.37	>100	21.29	N/A
MMAE	0.48	24.30	0.98	51
Paclitaxel	1.55	96.10	1.61	62
Vinblastine	0.11	5.22	0.25	47
Doxorubicin	6.92	35.65	4.47	5
Cisplatin	574.70	605.40	486.90	N/A

Resistance (fold): IC_{50} for MDA-MB231 + MDR1/IC_{50} for MDA-MB231

EphA2-expressing cells by inducing apoptotic cell death as evidenced by the activation of caspase 3/7 [49].

Tumors can develop resistance mechanisms against a variety of chemotherapeutic drugs. One mechanism of drug resistance is the upregulation of drug efflux pumps, which prevents the intracellular accumulation of the cytotoxic drug [58, 59]. P-glycoprotein (PGP), which is produced by the multidrug resistance-1 gene (MDR-1), is one of the most commonly studied drug efflux pumps. PGP expression has been shown to lead to tumor resistance of some well-known chemotherapeutic drugs, including paclitaxel. We used MDA-MB231 cells that overexpressed MDR-1 to explore the effect MDR expression may have on MEDI-547 activity (Table 14.2). MEDI-547 can kill the parental MDA-MB231 cells, but is less potent against the MDA-MB231-MDR1 cells. The IC_{50} value, in the presence of verapamil, which blocks PGP activity, is comparable to the parental MDA-MB231 cell line, suggesting that mcMMAF may be a weak PGP substrate. In contrast when 1C1 was conjugated to the valine–citrulline monomethyl auristatin E (vcMMAE) payload, the MDA-MB231-MDR1 cells were resistant to 1C1-vcMMAE. The addition of verapamil enhances the killing but not to the same level as the parental cell line. These data suggest that mcMMAF may be preferable to vcMMAE when targeting tumor cells expressing MDR1.

MEDI-547 can also selectively inhibit the growth of EphA2-expressing human tumor cells in vivo. In tumor bearing nude mice, complete growth suppression was observed at doses as low as 1 mg/kg delivered weekly for 4 weeks. Tumor regression was observed at only 3 mg/kg with the same weekly regimen. Dose-dependent inhibition of tumor growth was observed only in the MEDI-547-treatment group and not in any of the control arms. In addition, when tenfold excess 1C1 was dosed in combination with MEDI-547, MEDI-547 was unable to inhibit tumor growth, demonstrating that MEDI-547 is inhibiting tumor growth via the EphA2 receptor. No weight loss or other adverse effects were observed in the study [49].

Since dolastatin-10, the parent compound of mcMMAF, was reported to be less toxic in mice as compared to other species [56], MEDI-547 was used to treat established

EphA2-expressing (F98) and non-EphA2-expressing (RG2) syngeneic rat tumors in Fischer 344 rats. MEDI-547 inhibited the growth of F98 tumors but did not inhibit the growth of the non-EphA2-expressing RG2 tumors. Interestingly, EphA2 was expressed in the RG2 tumor vasculature, although this does not appear to be sufficient to confer inhibition of RG2 tumor growth [49]. Even in the more sensitive species a therapeutic index could still be established. These studies supported the IND-enabling safety evaluation of MEDI-547 in rodents and non-human primates leading to a phase I clinical trial in humans.

References

1. Kullander K, Klein R (2002) Mechanisms and functions of Eph and ephrin signalling. Nat Rev Mol Cell Biol 3:475–486
2. Murai KK, Pasquale EB (2003) 'Eph'ective signaling: forward, reverse and crosstalk. J Cell Sci 116:2823–2832
3. Beckmann MP, Cerretti DP, Baum P et al (1994) Molecular characterization of a family of ligands for eph-related tyrosine kinase receptors. EMBO J 13:3757–3762
4. Davis S, Gale NW, Aldrich TH et al (1994) Ligands for EPH-related receptor tyrosine kinases that require membrane attachment or clustering for activity. Science 266:816–819
5. Egea J, Nissen UV, Dufour A et al (2005) Regulation of EphA4 kinase activity is required for a subset of axon guidance decisions suggesting a key role for receptor clustering in Eph function. Neuron 47:515–528
6. Vearing CJ, Lackmann M (2005) Eph receptor signalling: dimerisation just isn't enough. Growth Factors 23:67–76
7. Himanen JP, Chumley MJ, Lackmann M et al (2004) Repelling class discrimination: ephrin-A5 binds to and activates EphB2 receptor signaling. Nat Neurosci 7:501–509
8. Gale NW, Yancopoulos GD (1997) Ephrins and their receptors: a repulsive topic? Cell Tissue Res 290:227–241
9. Flanagan JG, Vanderhaeghen P (1998) The ephrins and Eph receptors in neural development. Annu Rev Neurosci 21:309–345
10. Hafner C, Schmitz G, Meyer S et al (2004) Differential gene expression of Eph receptors and ephrins in benign human tissues and cancers. Clin Chem 50:490–499
11. Pasquale EB (2008) Eph-ephrin bidirectional signaling in physiology and disease. Cell 133:38–52
12. Zisch AH, Pasquale EB (1997) The Eph family: a multitude of receptors that mediate cell recognition signals. Cell Tissue Res 290:217–226
13. Huusko P, Ponciano-Jackson D, Wolf M et al (2004) Nonsense-mediated decay microarray analysis identifies mutations of EPHB2 in human prostate cancer. Nat Genet 36:979–983
14. Kittles RA, Baffoe-Bonnie AB, Moses TY et al (2006) A common nonsense mutation in EphB2 is associated with prostate cancer risk in African American men with a positive family history. J Med Genet 43:507–511
15. Alazzouzi H, Davalos V, Kokko A et al (2005) Mechanisms of inactivation of the receptor tyrosine kinase EPHB2 in colorectal tumors. Cancer Res 65:10170–10173
16. Guo DL, Zhang J, Yuen ST et al (2006) Reduced expression of EphB2 that parallels invasion and metastasis in colorectal tumours. Carcinogenesis 27:454–464
17. Guo H, Miao H, Gerber L, Singh J, Denning MF, Gilliam AC, Wang B (2006) Disruption of EphA2 receptor tyrosine kinase leads to increased susceptibility to carcinogenesis in mouse skin. Cancer Res 66(14):7050–7058

18. Elowe S, Holland SJ, Kulkarni S, Pawson T (2001) Downregulation of the Ras-mitogen-activated protein kinase pathway by the EphB2 receptor tyrosine kinase is required for ephrin-induced neurite retraction. Mol Cell Biol 21(21):7429–7441
19. Zou JX, Wang B, Kalo MS, Zisch AH, Pasquale EB, Ruoslahti E (1999) An Eph receptor regulates integrin activity through R-Ras. Proc Natl Acad Sci USA 96:13813–13818
20. Nakada M, Niska JA, Tran NL, McDonough WS, Berens ME (2005) EphB2/R-Ras signaling regulates glioma cell adhesion, growth, and invasion. Am J Pathol 167:565–576
21. Kumar SR, Masood R, Spannuth WA et al (2007) The receptor tyrosine kinase EphB4 is over-expressed in ovarian cancer, provides survival signals and predicts poor outcome. Br J Cancer 96:1083–1091
22. Kumar SR, Scehnet JS, Ley EJ, Singh J et al (2009) Preferential induction of EphB4 over EphB2 and its implication in colorectal cancer progression. Cancer Res 69(9):3736–3745
23. Noren NK, Foos G, Hauser CA, Pasquale EB (2006) The EphB4 receptor suppresses breast cancer cell tumorigenicity through an Abl-Crk pathway. Nat Cell Biol 8:815–825
24. Lindberg RA, Hunter T (1990) cDNA cloning and characterization of eck, an epithelial cell receptor protein-tyrosine kinase in the eph/elk family of protein kinases. Mol Cell Biol 10:6316–6324
25. Ruiz JC, Robertson EJ (1994) The expression of the receptor-protein tyrosine kinase gene, eck, is highly restricted during early mouse development. Mech Dev 46:87–100
26. Chen J, Nachabah A, Scherer C et al (1996) Germ-line inactivation of the murine Eck receptor tyrosine kinase by gene trap retroviral insertion. Oncogene 12:979–988
27. Ireton RC, Chen J (2005) EphA2 receptor tyrosine kinase as a promising target for cancer therapeutics. Curr Cancer Drug Targets 5(3):149–157
28. Wykosky J, Debinski W (2008) The EphA2 receptor and ephrinA1 ligand in solid tumors: function and therapeutic targeting. Mol Cancer Res 6(12):1795–1806
29. Zeng G, Hu Z, Kinch MS et al (2003) High-level expression of EphA2 receptor tyrosine kinase in prostatic intraepithelial neoplasia. Am J Pathol 163:2271–2276
30. Thaker PH, Deavers M, Celestino J et al (2004) EphA2 expression is associated with aggressive features in ovarian carcinoma. Clin Cancer Res 10:5145–5150
31. Mudali SV, Fu B, Lakkur SS, Luo M, Embuscado EE, Iacobuzio-Donahue CA (2006) Patterns of EphA2 protein expression in primary and metastatic pancreatic carcinoma and correlation with genetic status. Clin Exp Metastasis 23:357–365
32. Wykosky J, Gibo DM, Stanton C, Debinski W (2005) EphA2 as a novel molecular marker and target in glioblastoma multiforme. Mol Cancer Res 3:541–551
33. Walker-Daniels J, Coffman K, Azimi M et al (1999) Overexpression of the EphA2 tyrosine kinase in prostate cancer. Prostate 41:275–280
34. Fox BP, Kandpal RP (2004) Invasiveness of breast carcinoma cells and transcript profile: Eph receptors and ephrin ligands as molecular markers of potential diagnostic and prognostic application. Biochem Biophys Res Commun 318:882–892
35. Kinch MS, Moore MB, Harpole DH (2003) Predictive value of the EphA2 receptor tyrosine kinase in lung cancer recurrence and survival. Clin Cancer Res 9:613–618
36. Miyazaki T, Kato H, Fukuchi M, Nakajima M, Kuwano H (2003) EphA2 overexpression correlates with poor prognosis in esophageal squamous cell carcinoma. Int J Cancer 103: 657–663
37. Han L, Dong Z, Qiao Y (2005) The clinical significance of EphA2 and Ephrin A-1 in epithelial ovarian carcinomas. Gynecol Oncol 99:278–286
38. Hess AR, Seftor EA, Gardner LM et al (2001) Molecular regulation of tumor cell vasculogenic mimicry by tyrosine phosphorylation: role of epithelial cell kinase (Eck/EphA2). Cancer Res 61:3250–3255
39. Wang LF, Fokas E, Bieker M et al (2008) Increased expression of EphA2 correlates with adverse outcome in primary and recurrent glioblastoma multiforme patients. Oncol Rep 19:151–156
40. Zelinski DP, Zantek ND, Stewart JC, Irizarry AR, Kinch MS (2001) EphA2 overexpression causes tumorigenesis of mammary epithelial cells. Cancer Res 61:2301–2316

41. Fang WB, Brantley-Sieders DM, Parker MA, Reith AD, Chen J (2005) A kinase-dependent role for EphA2 receptor in promoting tumor growth and metastasis. Oncogene 24:7859
42. Huang F, Reeves K, Han X (2007) Identification of candidate molecular markers predicting sensitivity in solid tumors to dasatinib: rationale for patient selection. Cancer Res 67: 2226–2238
43. Mitra S, Duggineni S, Koolpe M, Zhu X, Huang Z, Pasquale EB (2010) Structure-activity relationship analysis of peptides targeting the EphA2 receptor. Biochemistry 49(31):6687–6695
44. Carles-Kinch K, Kilpatrick KE, Stewart JC, Kinch MS (2002) Antibody targeting of the EphA2 tyrosine kinase inhibits malignant cell behavior. Cancer Res 62(10):2840–2847
45. Zhuang G, Brantley-Sieders DM, Vaught D, Yu J, Xie L, Wells S et al (2010) Elevation of receptor tyrosine kinase EphA2 mediates resistance to trastuzumab therapy. Cancer Res 70(1):299–308
46. Kiewlich D, Zhang J, Gross C et al (2006) Anti-EphA2 antibodies decrease EphA2 protein levels in murine CT26 colorectal and human MDA-231 breast tumors but do not inhibit tumor growth. Neoplasia 8:18–30
47. Hammond SA, Lutterbuese R, Roff S et al (2007) Selective targeting and potent control of tumor growth using an EphA2/CD3-Bispecific single-chain antibody construct. Cancer Res 67(8):3927–35
48. Zhuang G, Hunter S, Hwang Y, Chen J (2007) Regulation of EphA2 receptor endocytosis by SHIP2 lipid phosphatase via phosphatidylinositol 3-Kinase-dependent Rac1 activation. J Biol Chem 282(4):2683–2694
49. Jackson D, Gooya J, Mao S, Kinneer K, Xu L, Camara M et al (2008) A human antibody-drug conjugate targeting EphA2 inhibits tumor growth in vivo. Cancer Res 68(22):9367–9374
50. Wykosky J, Palma E, Gibo DM, Ringler S, Turner CP, Debinski W (2008) Soluble monomeric EphrinA1 is released from tumor cells and is a functional ligand for the EphA2 receptor. Oncogene 27(58):7260–75273
51. Lee JW, Han HD, Shahzad MM, Kim SW, Mangala LS, Nick AM et al (2009) EphA2 immunoconjugate as molecularly targeted chemotherapy for ovarian carcinoma. J Natl Cancer Inst 101(17):1193–1205
52. Lee JW, Stone RL, Lee SJ, Nam EJ, Roh JW, Nick AM et al (2010) EphA2 targeted chemotherapy using an antibody drug conjugate in endometrial carcinoma. Clin Cancer Res 16(9):2562–2570
53. Coffman KT, Hu M, Carles-Kinch K et al (2003) Differential EphA2 epitope display on normal versus malignant cells. Cancer Res 63:7907–7912
54. Dall'Acqua WF, Damschroder MM, Zhang J et al (2005) Antibody humanization by framework shuffling. Methods 36(1):43–60
55. Doronina SO, Toki BE, Torgov MY, Mendelsohn BA, Cerveny CG, Chace DF et al (2003) Development of potent monoclonal antibody auristatin conjugates for cancer therapy. Nat Biotechnol 21(7):778–84
56. Mirsalis JC, Schindler-Horvat J, Hill JR, Tomaszewski JE, Donohue SJ, Tyson CA (1999) Toxicity of dolastatin 10 in mice, rats and dogs and its clinical relevance. Cancer Chemother Pharmacol 44(5):395–402
57. Doronina SO, Mendelsohn BA, Bovee TD, Cerveny CG, Alley SC, Meyer DL et al (2006) Enhanced activity of monomethylauristatin F through monoclonal antibody delivery: effects of linker technology on efficacy and toxicity. Bioconjug Chem 17(1):114–124
58. Mansouri A, Henle KJ, Nagle WA (1992) Multidrug resistance: prospects for clinical management. SAAS Bull Biochem Biotechnol 5:48–52
59. Patwardhan G, Gupta V, Huang J, Gu X, Liu YY et al (2010) Direct assessment of P-glycoprotein efflux to determine tumor response to chemotherapy. Biochem Pharmacol 80(1):72–79

Chapter 15
Anti-PSMA Antibody-Drug Conjugates and Immunotoxins

Philipp Wolf

Introduction

Prostate cancer is the most commonly diagnosed cancer with about 25% of all incident cases in men of the Western world and represents the second leading cause of cancer deaths [1]. Patients with localized tumors can be curatively treated by radical prostatectomy or radiation therapy. However, there is still a significant proportion of patients who present or progress to advanced metastatic disease, for which no curative treatment exists. First-line therapy for advanced prostate cancer is androgen deprivation, but almost all carcinomas progress to an androgen-independent stage. From then on, chemotherapy is the only available effective therapy, which leads to an improvement of the quality of life and to a modest overall survival benefit [2]. Due to the significant morbidity and mortality rate, many approaches are focused on new therapeutic strategies for the management of prostate cancer, including the development of ADCs.

Prostate cancer represents a qualified antibody target for several reasons. First, metastases are typically of small volume allowing sufficient antigen access and antibody penetration. Second, metastases are predominantly localized in the bone marrow or in lymph nodes, sites that generally receive high levels of circulating antibodies. Third, serum prostate-specific antigen (PSA) represents an early indicator for advanced or relapsed disease and allows the rapid monitoring of therapeutic efficacy. Finally, with the prostate-specific membrane antigen (PSMA), a protein exists on the surface of prostate cancer cells, which is especially well suited as a target antigen.

P. Wolf (✉)
Department of Urology, Experimental Urology, University Medical Center Freiburg, Breisacher Strasse 117, D-79106 Freiburg, Germany
e-mail: philipp.wolf@uniklinik-freiburg.de

G.L. Phillips (ed.), *Antibody-Drug Conjugates and Immunotoxins: From Pre-Clinical Development to Therapeutic Applications*, Cancer Drug Discovery and Development, DOI 10.1007/978-1-4614-5456-4_15,

The Prostate-Specific Membrane Antigen

Structure and Function

The gene encoding PSMA consists of 19 exons spanning about 60 kb of genomic DNA and was mapped to chromosome 11p11-p12 [3]. The cDNA sequence of PSMA codes for a type II membrane glycoprotein of 750 amino acids (aa), which is highly expressed on prostate epithelial cells. It consists of a small intracellular domain of 19 aa, which contains an internalization signal (MWNLL) [4], a transmembrane domain of 24 aa, and a large extracellular domain of 707 aa. The extracellular domain was crystallized and determined to fold into three distinct domains: the protease domain (aa 56–116 and 352–591), the apical domain (aa 117–351), and the C-terminal domain (aa 592–750). Based on the structural data, it was demonstrated that PSMA is expressed as a homodimer in a compact 3D structure. Furthermore, it was shown that PSMA is highly glycosylated with oligosaccharides accounting up to 25% of the molecular weight and that glycosylation is essential for proper folding [5, 6].

PSMA hydrolyzes carboxy-terminal glutamate residues and has also been designated human glutamate carboxypeptidase II (GCP II, EC 3.4.17.21). Carboxypeptidase activity was manifested in vitro as both folate hydrolase activity and *N*-acetylated alpha-linked acidic dipeptidase (NAALADase) activity [7, 8]. PSMA is thought to play a role in the folate metabolism of the prostate. However, its exact function in this organ remains unclear.

Unlike other prostate-related antigens, like PSA, prostatic acidic phosphatase, or prostate secretory protein, PSMA is not shed into circulation. Moreover, it undergoes constitutive internalization, which is enhanced after antibody binding [9]. It can therefore be speculated that PSMA has transport function for a yet unidentified ligand and that antibodies might act as surrogates to induce internalization. In a recent study with fluorescence-labeled copolymer–anti-PSMA antibody conjugates, the subcellular trafficking of PSMA in prostate cancer cells was analyzed. It could be demonstrated that after antibody binding, multiple receptor-mediated endocytic pathways, including clathrin-mediated endocytosis, macropinocytosis, and clathrin- and caveolae-independent endocytosis, were used [10].

Expression

Bostwick et al. performed an immunohistochemical study with the anti-PSMA mAb 7/E11 on specimen from 184 patients with prostate adenocarcinomas. He found that the average number of stained cells was lower in benign epithelium (69.5%, range 20–90%) and high-grade prostatic intraepithelial neoplasia (PIN; 77.9%, range 30–100%) than in adenocarcinomas (80.2%, range 30–100%). With rare exceptions, basal cells were negative, and no immunoreactivity of the prostate stroma, urothelium, or normal vasculature was monitored [11]. Other immunohistochemical studies with different mAbs against PSMA showed a heterogeneous, weak to moderate staining of the normal acinar prostate epithelial cells and an extensive staining in adenocarcinomas and metastases [12, 13]. An overview of studies that have assessed PSMA expression in benign and malignant prostate tissues [11–24] is given in Table 15.1.

PSMA expression in benign and malignant prostate-related tissues was also compared at the mRNA level by real-time PCR. In this study, a significant higher PSMA expression in carcinomas compared to benign prostate hyperplasia (BPH) could be measured. Additionally, a direct correlation between the highest number of PSMA transcripts and the Gleason score, which is used for the grading of prostate cancer, was determined for the adenocarcinomas [24]. Ross and colleagues demonstrated that PSMA expression correlates with adverse traditional prognostic factors, like tumor grade, pathological stage, aneuploidy, and biochemical recurrence, and therefore independently predicts disease outcome [19]. It was demonstrated that PSMA regulates the interleukin-6 (IL-6) and chemokine CCL5 expression by activating the MAPK pathways in prostate tumor cells, which may have influence on their proliferation and survival [25]. However, the specific biochemical function of PSMA in malignant transformation of prostate epithelial cells remains unclear to date.

There is also some extraprostatic PSMA expression in different human tissues. A cytoplasmatic staining of secretory cells of the salivary glands without participation of excretory duct cells was detected by immunohistochemical analyses [12]. This confirmed the detection of PSMA mRNA and protein in tissue extracts from this organ [26, 27]. Nevertheless, PSMA function in salivary glands is unknown to date.

In several studies, PSMA was also detected in duodenal brush border cells [12, 21], where it was found to act as a folate hydrolase [28]. The PSMA expression in this organ is of concern, but it is restricted to the villus and not to crypt cells. Thus, it would be unlikely that anti-PSMA ADCs that were effective would eliminate the intestinal crypt stem cell population.

PSMA expression was also described for s subset of proximal renal tubules [13, 20, 21]. Proximal tubule cells of the kidney have been shown to play a role in folate reabsorption at the apical membrane, which may explain the PSMA expression in this tissue.

It has to be considered that PSMA expression is not fully prostate specific as originally thought. This is also true for the expression in brain and colon, which is controversially discussed [12, 13, 21, 27, 29, 30]. Application of anti-PSMA ADCs could induce tissue damage in PSMA-expressing normal organs. However, potential side effects of anti-PSMA ADCs on these tissues in vivo are unknown.

Interestingly, PSMA was also found to be expressed in the neovascular endothelium of many solid tumors, including kidney, colon, lung, bladder, pancreas, breast, and melanoma, without expression in the corresponding tumor cells or normal vascular endothelium [13, 20, 21, 31, 32]. In this respect, it is presumed that PSMA participates in β1 integrin signaling and PAK activation in endothelial cells, leading to changes in cytoskeletal organization and finally cell invasion and angiogenesis [33].

Table 15.1 PSMA expression in benign and malignant prostate tissues as determined by immunohistochemical studies with different anti-PSMA mAbs

		PSMA-binding epitope		Prostate						
mAb	Immunization	Intra-/ extracellular	Residues	Normal	BPH	PIN	Cancer	Lymph node metastases	Bone metastases	Refs.
7/E11-C5	LNCaP cells	Intra	1–6	7/7	7/7	–	11/11	–	–	[14]
				2/2	–	–	10/10	–	–	[15]
				12/12	22/27	21/21	157/165	72/79	7/7	[16]
				–	–	–	25/25	–	–	[17]
				–	–	–	33/35	7/8	8/18	[13]
				232/232			232/232	98%		[18]
				184/184	–	129/129	184/184	–	–	[11]
				–	–	–	136/136	–	–	[19]
				–	–	–	21/21	–	–	[20]
				28/28	–	–	12/12	–	–	[21]
				–	–	–	–	6/6	7/7	[23]
				23/23	–	–	23/23	–	–	[22]
PM2J004.5	PCa plasma membranes	Intra	–	28/28	–	–	12/12	–	–	[21]
				–	–	–	–	6/6	7/7	[23]
PEQ226.5	PCa plasma membranes	Extra	134–437	28/28	–	–	12/12	–	–	[21]
E99	PCa epithelial cells	Extra	153–347	–	–	–	21/21	–	–	[20]
J451	PCa epithelial cells	Extra	C-terminus	–	–	–	21/21	–	–	[20]
				28/28	–	–	12/12	–	–	[21]
J533	PCa epithelial cells	Extra	153–347	–	–	–	21/21	–	–	[20]
J591	PCa epithelial cells	Extra	153–347	–	–	–	21/21	–	–	[20]
				28/28	–	–	12/12	–	–	[21]
				–	3/7	–	14/14	–	–	[24]
24.4E6	PSMA peptides	Extra	638–657	23/23	–	–	19/19	–	–	[22]
3/A12	Native LNCaP cell lysate	Extra	–	14/14	–	–	17/17	5/5	–	[12]
3/E7	Native LNCaP cell lysate	Extra	–	14/14	–	–	17/17	5/5	–	[12]
3/F11	Native LNCaP cell lysate	Extra	–	14/14	–	–	17/17	5/5	–	[12]

MAb monoclonal antibody; *PCa* prostate cancer; *BPH* benign prostate hyperplasia; *PIN* prostatic intraepithelial neoplasia

Because there is a clear difference in PSMA expression between tumor-associated and normal blood vessels, PSMA represents a potential unique antiangiogenic target. This is in contrast to current endothelial target antigens, such as vascular epidermal growth factor receptors, CD31, or alpha-v-beta-3 integrins, that are upregulated in malignancies but are also present in the normal endothelium.

Anti-PSMA Antibodies

The first mAb against PSMA, named 7E11, was published in 1987 [14]. This mAb was used for the initial validation of PSMA in vivo. However, molecular mapping revealed that 7E11 recognizes the N-terminus (MWNLLH) of the intracellular domain of PSMA (Table 15.1) [34] and is therefore not able to target viable cells for the delivery of cytotoxic agents.

In the following years, great efforts were undertaken to develop mAbs against the extracellular domain of PSMA. Whereas PSMA-binding mAbs could easily be generated, only few mAbs binding to cell-adherent PSMA were isolated [20, 35–41]. The reason for this is that the specific three-dimensional structure of the high-glycosylated PSMA homodimer on the cell surface, presenting unique binding epitopes, is lost after isolation with ionizing detergents [42]. Therefore, only mAbs elicited with native PSMA after host immunization with prostate cancer cells, cell membranes, or cell lysates may recognize and strongly bind to PSMA-expressing prostate cancer cells (Table 15.1). This squares with the fact that mAbs raised with PSMA peptides showed multiple cross-reactivities with extraprostatic tissues of many different organs [22].

Anti-PSMA Antibody–Drug Conjugates

PSMA was identified as a valuable target antigen for the generation of antibody–drug conjugates (ADCs) against prostate cancer, since it is highly organ specific, present at the cell surface at all tumor stages, overexpressed in advanced and metastatic disease, not shed into circulation, and internalized after antibody binding. Moreover, due to PSMA expression in the neovasculature of solid tumors, clinical applications using anti-PSMA ADCs are seen not to be limited to the treatment of prostate cancer but also to the angiogenesis targeting of solid tumors [43].

In the last years, various types of anti-PSMA ADCs (radioimmunoconjugates, immunotoxins, and targeted virotherapeutic agents) were generated by coupling radionuclides, chemotherapeutic agents, plant toxins, bacterial toxins, zootoxins, or viruses to anti-PSMA mAbs or antibody fragments and tested in preclinical or clinical trials. Figure 15.1 gives an overview of anti-PSMA ADCs published to date.

Anti-PSMA Radioimmunoconjugates

Radioimmunoconjugates consist of antibody-coupled radionuclides with the biologic effect of high linear energy transfer radiation as is seen with alpha and beta particles. The advantage of a targeted radiotherapy with such agents is that smaller amounts of drug can be given as compared to conventional radiation therapy. Furthermore, the effect of the radionuclide is not only restricted to cells presenting the target antigen but also for neighboring cells (bystander or crossfire effect).

Initial immunoscintigraphy trials of prostate cancer were performed with the ^{111}In-labeled form of 7E11 (ProstaScint®, 7E11/CYT-356, capromab pendetide) [44–47]. In these studies, it could be shown that ProstaScint® imaging was more sensitive compared to the computed tomography and magnetic resonance imaging for the detection of metastatic prostate cancer in soft tissues [48]. ProstaScint® has therefore received approval from the US Food and Drug Administration (FDA) for the detection and imaging of soft-tissue metastases [49]. However, since the binding epitope of 7E11 is on the intracellular domain of PSMA, it was suggested that 7E11 only binds to PSMA molecules in damaged, dead, or dying cells and is not capable to bind to viable cells. This provides a rationale to explain why ProstaScint® is more effective at identifying metastases in well-vascularized soft tissues than in bone, in which metastatic lesions tend to be relatively small and do not characteristically have a high percentage of necrotic or apoptotic cells. Indeed, early clinical trials using the ^{90}Y-labeled 7E11 for radioimmunotherapy resulted in no objective or biochemical (PSA) remissions [50, 51].

Therefore, radioimmunotherapeutic studies with mAbs binding to the extracellular domain of PSMA were performed. The ^{64}Cu-labeled mAbs 3/A12, 3/E7, and 3/F11 were used in positron emission tomography for the imaging of prostate cancer tumors in the SCID mouse xenograft model [52, 53]. Whereas excellent uptakes of the mAbs between 31.6% and 35.1% ID/g after 48 h were seen in PSMA-expressing tumors of the androgen-independent growing LNCaP subline C4-2, the activity in PSMA-negative DU145 xenografts remained at the background levels.

The mAb 3/F11 was chosen for radioimmunotherapy in first preclinical experiments [54]. For this, it was labeled with the beta-particle emitter ^{177}Lu using the highly stable chelator 1,4,7,10-tetraazacyclodecane-*N*,*N′*,*N″*,*N‴*-tetraacetic acid (DOTA). Flow cytometric analyses indicated that the DOTA labeling affected neither the PSMA specificity nor the binding capacity of 3/F11. Biodistribution data in mice showed that the tumor uptake of ^{177}Lu-DOTA-3/F11 gradually increased with time. A more than 70-fold activity compared to the muscle and a more than 4.5-fold activity compared to the blood were measured 72 h after injection. Remarkably, the treatment of mice bearing small C4-2 xenografts with a single dose of 1 MBq ^{177}Lu-DOTA-3/F11 resulted in a more than twofold enhanced mean survival and in a delay of tumor growth compared to the control group. However, mice treated with higher doses of ^{177}Lu-DOTA-3/F11 apparently died of myelotoxicity, which is the predominant limiting factor in radioimmunotherapeutic approaches with ^{177}Lu [55].

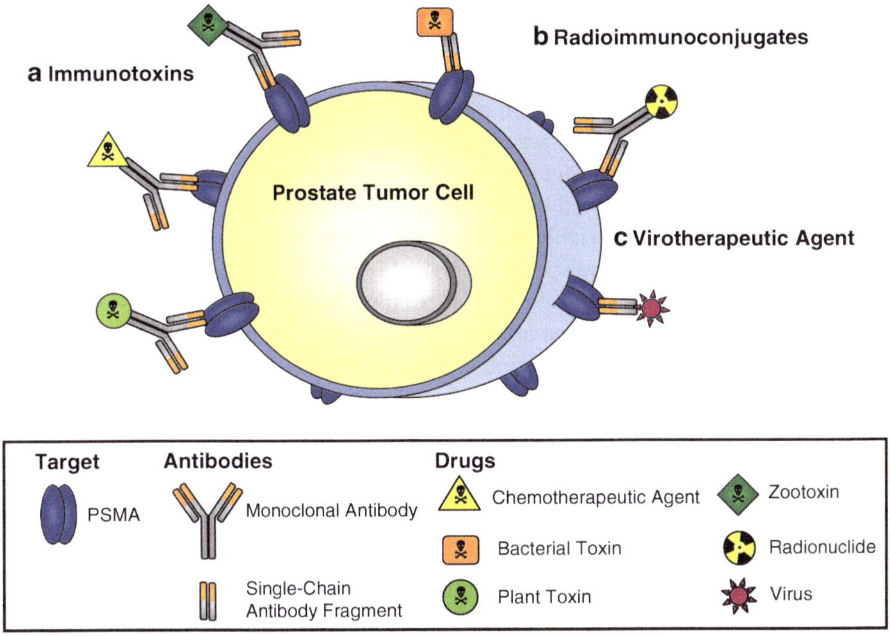

Fig. 15.1 Anti-PSMA ADCs for the targeting of prostate cancer cells. (**a**) Immunotoxins. Anti-PSMA immunotoxins were generated by linking toxins of different origin to monoclonal antibodies or single-chain antibody fragments. (**b**) Radioimmunoconjugates. PSMA-expressing prostate tumor cells were targeted by monoclonal antibodies covalently linked to cytotoxic radionuclides. (**c**) Virotherapeutic agent. A targeted virotherapeutic agent was created by linking the coat protein of measles virus to an anti-PSMA single-chain antibody fragment for the induction of cytopathic toxicity

The anti-PSMA mAb J591 was also used for the construction of radioimmunoconjugates, which were extensively studied in preclinical and clinical trials. An alpha-particle-emitting radioimmunoconjugate was prepared by linking the anti-PSMA mAb J591 to ^{213}Bi using *N*-[2-amino-3-(*p*-isothiocyanatophenyl)propyl]-*trans*-cyclohexane-1,2-diamine-*N*,*N*′,*N*′,*N*″,*N*″-pentaacetic acid (SCN-CHXA″-DTPA) as chelating agent. ^{213}Bi is a short-lived radionuclide that emits high-energy alpha particles with an effective range of 0.07–0.1 mm that are ideally suited for treating single-celled neoplasms and micrometastases. [^{213}Bi]J591 was specifically cytotoxic to PSMA-expressing LNCaP prostate cancer cells and led to a significant improvement of median tumor-free survival of nude mice with i.m. LNCaP xenografts. Furthermore, a significant reduction of PSA serum levels in treated animals was measured [56].

In a study of Smith-Jones and colleagues, the ^{131}I-labeled mAbs J415, J591, and 7E11 were tested in nude mice with LNCaP xenografts. Higher tumor-to-blood ratios with ^{131}I-J591 and ^{131}I-415 than with ^{131}I-7E11 were reached, and tumor uptake of ^{131}I-J591 was almost 20 times higher in LNCaP tumors than in PSMA-negative PC-3 and DU145 tumors. Autoradiographic studies confirmed that the intracellular binding mAb 7E11 distinctly favored localization to areas of necrosis whereas the extracellular binding mAbs J415 and J591 demonstrated a preferential accumulation in areas of viable tumor [56].

In another preclinical radioimmunotherapy study, the humanized or "deimmunized" form of J591 (huJ591) was used. Deimmunization was done by fusion of a human IgG1 backbone to further reduce the immunogenic potential of this antibody in humans. This was followed by site-directed mutagenesis of putative B and T cell reactive epitopes of the variable domains. HuJ591 was observed to retain the properties in terms of affinity and specificity to PSMA. ^{131}I-hu591 and ^{90}Y-DOTA-huJ591 were tested in nude mice bearing LNCaP xenografts and effected a 15–90% reduction in the mean tumor volume after single-dose application of 3.7–11.1 MBq and 3.7–7.4 MBq, respectively. Additionally, the median survival increased 2–3 times relative to untreated controls [57].

In a first phase I clinical trial, ^{90}Y-labeled huJ591 was tested in 29 prostate cancer patients [58]. Initially, patients received the mAb labeled with the gamma-emitting radionuclide ^{111}In to determine pharmacokinetics, biodistribution, and dosimetry. Total-body images with a gamma camera demonstrated significant metabolism of the radioimmunoconjugate in the liver and to a lesser extend in the kidneys and spleen. In addition, metastases in both bone and soft tissues were specifically targeted. ^{90}Y-labeled huJ591 was administered at different initial doses one week later. The maximal tolerated dose was determined to be 17.5 mCi/m^2. No antihuman antibody responses were observed. PSA stabilization was noted in six patients, and two patients showed an 85% and 70% decline in PSA serum levels lasting 8 and 8.6 months, respectively.

In another phase I study, 35 prostate cancer patients received ^{177}Lu-labeled hu591 at different doses between 10 and 75 mCi/m^2 to assess safety, dosimetry, and pharmacokinetics. All patients treated with a dose of 75 mCi/m^2 developed grade 3 or 4 thrombocytopenia and grade 4 neutropenia. Therefore, 70 mCi/m^2 was determined to be the maximal tolerated dose. Re-treatment with 30 mCi/m^2 was well tolerated. In four patients within this trial, a PSA decline of more than 50% was measured, and in 16 patients, a stabilization of the PSA levels was monitored [59].

Myelosuppression was the most common and severe side effect in these studies. Whereas for ^{90}Y-huJ591 no clear correlation between myelotoxicity and applicated radioactive dose was seen, for ^{177}Lu-huJ591 myelotoxicity and especially thrombocytopenia correlated well with both administered radioactive dose and bone marrow dose [60].

For a proof-of-principle evaluation of PSMA as a target for an antiangiogenesis therapy, ^{111}In-huJ591 was used for the targeting of known metastases in 27 patients with advanced solid tumors of types previously shown to express PSMA in their neovasculature (kidney, colon, lung, bladder, pancreas, breast, melanoma). Tumor imaging was observed in 7/10 kidney cancer patients, 4/4 colorectal cancer patients, 3/3 lung cancer patients, 1/3 bladder cancer patients, 3/3 pancreatic cancer patients, 2/3 breast cancer patients, and 1/1 melanoma patient [43].

Taken together, first preclinical and clinical trials give evidence that anti-PSMA radioimmunoconjugates are well tolerated and demonstrate antitumor activity.

Therefore, targeted radiotherapy against PSMA could be a promising alternative for patients with advanced prostate cancer. Moreover, due to successful in vivo targeting of the neovasculature of different solid tumors, there is also evidence that radiolabeled anti-PSMA mAbs could also serve for antiangiogenesis therapy in future.

Anti-PSMA Immunotoxins

PSMA was also used as target for the construction of immunotoxins, where plant toxins, chemotherapeutic agents, zootoxins, and bacterial toxins were linked to anti-PSMA mAbs or antibody fragments.

First anti-PSMA immunotoxins were generated by Fracasso and colleagues, who linked anti-PSMA mAbs to the ricin A-chain [61]. The plant toxin ricin from *Ricinus communis* is formed by two subunits held together by a disulfide bridge. The ricin A-chain is the catalytically active subunit, which is able to inactivate the protein biosynthesis machinery of the target cell by attacking ribosomal RNA. The B-chain binds ubiquitous cell surface structures and facilitates intracellular trafficking and membrane translocation of ricin [62].

For the construction of the ricin-A-based immunotoxins, the ricin B-chain was exchanged by the anti-PSMA mAbs J591, PEQ226.5, or PM2P079.1 for specific targeting. Linkage of the mAbs to the ricin A-chain was performed using the *N*-succinimidyl-3-(2-pyridyldithio)-propionate (SPDP) or 4-succinimidyloxycarbonyl-alpha-methyl-alpha(2-pyridyldithio)-toluene (SMPT) cross-linkers [61]. Both linkers are heterobifunctional and contain one reactivity toward amines, through the succinimide group, and one reactivity toward sulfhydryls, through the pyridylthiol group. Moreover, both were shown to have a high in vivo stability in former studies with different ricin-A-based immunotoxins [63, 64].

In vitro studies with the anti-PSMA immunotoxins revealed that the choice of both cross-linkers had no influence on the overall activity. All immunotoxins elicited a specific and concentration-dependent cytotoxicity against PSMA-expressing LNCaP cells in the nanomolar range with up to 5,200-fold potentiation of cytotoxicity compared to the unconjugated ricin A-chain. Interestingly, J591-smpt-nRTA showed a 6.3- or 61.8-fold higher potency compared to PEQ226.5-spdp-nRTA or PM2P079.1-spdp-nRNA, respectively. This difference was ascribed to several factors: the derivatization with the cross-linker, steric hindrance by cross-linked ricin A-chain, different PSMA epitopes recognized by the mAbs, and different affinities of the mAbs. Additionally, the immunotoxins induced a growth inhibition of LNCaP multicellular tumor spheroids with 150–200 μm in size, which corresponded to approximately 1,000 cells [61].

Differences in the cytotoxic activity of the immunotoxins containing the native (nRTA) or the recombinant (rRTA) ricin A-chain were also examined. nRTA is endowed with high mannose residues that might interact in vivo with cells bearing mannose receptors, contributing to higher nonspecific toxicity and side effects [65, 66].

Therefore, rRTA would be preferable. However, no differences in the cytotoxicity of nRTA- or rRTA-based anti-PSMA immunotoxins with or without inhibition of mannose receptors were measured in LNCaP cells [61].

A similar immunotoxin was generated by chemically linking the deglycosylated ricin A-chain (dgA) via the SMPT linker to the rat anti-PSMA mAb E6. With this construct, an IC_{50} value of 60 pM, corresponding to the immunotoxin's concentration inducing a 50% reduction in cell viability, was measured for LNCaP cells. Additionally, a significant growth inhibition of subcutaneous LNCaP xenografts of approximately 150 mm^3 in size was reached. Histological examinations indicated that the antitumor effects were mediated through direct cytotoxic effects on the tumor cells [67].

Kuroda and colleagues used the plant toxin saporin for the construction of a further anti-PSMA immunotoxin [69]. Saporin is found in seeds and leaves of the plant *Saponaria officinalis* and belongs to class I ribosome-inactivating proteins [68]. It is an RNA *N*-glycosidase and inhibits protein biosynthesis by cleaving one specific adenine base from ribosomal RNA, which is followed by irreversible ribosomal change. For the construction of the immunotoxin, called hJ591-SAZAP, the humanized mAb J591 was biotinylated for the linkage of a streptavidin–saporin conjugate. Testing cytotoxicity, IC_{50} values of 0.14 and 1.99 nM on PSMA-expressing LNCaP and CWR22Rv1 cells, respectively, were determined for hJ591-SAZAP after 72 h. At the same time, percentages of apoptotic cells of 60.3% in LNCaP cells and of 40.7% in CWR22Rv1 cells were measured. Furthermore, the immunotoxin induced a growth inhibition of LNCaP tumor xenografts in the mouse model. With a molecular weight of approximately 280 kDa, this immunotoxin is relatively large and, due to diffusion limitations in tissues, is thought to be less desirable for the treatment of solid tumors. Further work is therefore focused on the construction of saporin-based conjugates of smaller size and less inherent immunogenicity [69].

Another immunotoxin was constructed by conjugation of a fully human anti-PSMA mAb from transgenic mice with monomethylauristatin E (MMAE) through a valine–citrulline (Val–Cit) linker. This linker was designed to maintain serum stability while maximizing intracellular drug release by human cathepsin B [70]. Auristatins are potent inhibitors of tubulin polymerization, are related to the natural product dolastatin 10, and are about 200 times more potent in vitro than conventional chemotherapeutic agents [71]. With the MMAE-based immunotoxin, a cytotoxicity with IC_{50} values of 83 pM on LNCaP and of 65 pM on the androgen-independent LNCaP subline C4-2, with more than 800-fold selectivity compared to an isotype-control immunotoxin, was determined. In the C4-2 mouse xenograft model, the immunotoxin significantly improved the median survival ninefold relative to the control without signs of toxicity. Treatment effects were manifested by a significant reduction of PSA serum levels. Importantly, 2/5 of animals treated with a dose of 6 mg/kg immunotoxin had no detectable tumor or measurable PSA at day 500 and could be considered cure [70].

The anti-PSMA immunotoxin MLN2704 consists of the mAb huJ591 linked to the chemotherapeutic drug maytansinoid 1 (DM1) by a disulfide bond [72]. DM1, a potent microtubule-depolymerizing drug, is an analogue of maytansine, a naturally occurring ansa macrolide [73]. Maytansine was evaluated as a chemotherapeutic agent in the 1970s and 1980s, but has not developed further because of dose-limiting gastrointestinal and central neurological toxicity [74].

In toxicity studies, MLN2704 was nontoxic in mice up to the highest dose of 60 mg/kg body weight, whereas an equivalent dose of maytansine was toxic. Moreover, the immunotoxin showed an about fivefold higher efficacy in a CWR22 SCID mouse xenograft model than an equivalent amount of DM-1 administered on the same dosage schedule. Hence, MLN2704 fulfilled the criteria for an ideal immunotoxin in this preclinical model, possessing significantly enhanced antitumor activity through antigen-dependent targeting and reduced toxicity by limited systemic exposure of the cytotoxic moiety.

MLN2704 was also tested in a first clinical trial. It was not immunogenic and was safe for a repetitive application in patients with advanced prostate cancer. 2/9 patients treated with a dose of 264 or 343 mg/m^2 sustained a more than 50% decrease in serum PSA versus baseline, accompanied by measurable tumor regression in the patient treated with 264 mg/m^2 [75].

Russell and colleagues cross-linked the mAb J591 to the melittin-like peptide 101 using SPDP [76]. Peptide 101 consists of the first 22 amino acids of melittin, which is a potent zootoxin from honey bee (*Apis mellifera*) venom and which was successfully tested in vitro to selectively kill tumor cells in tumor-specific antibody conjugates [77]. The immunotoxin inhibited the growth of PSMA-positive LNCaP-LN3 but not of PSMA-negative DU145 tumor xenografts after systemic or intratumoral injection. Additionally, the conjugate led to a slight survival improvement of the treated mice. However, a disadvantage of this immunotoxin was the high affinity of the peptide 101 for lipid bilayer membranes, inducing a nonspecific binding followed by nonspecific cytotoxicity. Therefore, this immunoconjugate requires refinement to maximize its potential [76].

To overcome the limitations of chemically coupled mAb-based immunotoxins, such as large size or inhomogeneous preparations, recombinant immunotoxins containing antibody fragments were generated.

The first recombinant immunotoxins against PSMA were called A5-PE40 and D7-PE40 [78, 79]. They contained the single-chain antibody fragments (scFvs) A5 and D7 as binding domains, which were generated by phage display from the anti-PSMA mAbs 3/A12 and 3/F11, respectively. ScFvs, the smallest antigen-binding subunits of antibodies, consist of the variable domain of the heavy chain (V_H) and the variable domain of the light chain (V_L), connected by a flexible peptide linker and retain the full antigen specificity of the parental mAbs. As of their smaller size, scFvs allow a better penetration of tumor tissues, improved pharmacokinetics, and a reduction in immunogenicity compared to mAbs or Fab fragments [80, 81].

Like their parental mAbs, the scFvs A5 and D7 showed a specific binding to PSMA-expressing cancer cells. However, the binding affinity was lower, which can be explained by the scFvs' monovalent binding and the absence of stabilizing constant regions. Additionally, the complete inhibition of the antigen binding of A5 and D7 by an excess of the parental mAbs proved that the scFvs bound to the same extracellular PSMA epitopes.

For the construction of the recombinant anti-PSMA immunotoxins, PE40, the truncated form of *Pseudomonas* exotoxin A, produced by the human pathogenic bacterium *Pseudomonas aeruginosa*, was chosen. PE40 lacks the natural occurring cell binding domain Ia of the exotoxin and only consists of the domains II, Ib, and III. Whereas domain II serves as a membrane translocation domain for cytosolic delivery, the domains Ib and III contain ADP-ribosylation activity that inactivates the eukaryotic elongation factor 2 and leads to cell death [82, 83].

The immunotoxins A5-PE40 and D7-PE40 showed a specific but yet weaker binding to C4-2 cells or PSMA-transfectants compared to the scFvs. This indicated that the PE40 domain partially led to a steric inhibition of the scFv binding domain. Nevertheless, binding affinity was sufficient to induce a high and specific cytotoxicity with IC_{50} values in the low picomolar range in different PSMA-expressing prostate cancer lines representing different tumor stages. In in vivo experiments, D7-PE40 induced no deaths of mice at single doses up to 20 μg and was therefore about three-fold better tolerated than A5-PE40 [79, 84]. Increased ALT and AST serum levels and histopathological examination of livers from animals treated with D7-PE40 indicated that high concentrations of the immunotoxin caused liver toxicity, which was followed by the death of the animals [79]. Onda et al. found that TNF-alpha released by Kupffer cells plays an important role in the indirect hepatocyte damage in mice treated with a PE-based immunotoxin [85]. Lowering the isoelectric point of this immunotoxin led to a decrease of hepatotoxicity, suggesting that macrophages find fewer negatively charged immunotoxin molecules than positively charged ones and consequently release less TNF-alpha that is toxic to the hepatocytes [86].

At nontoxic doses A5-PE40 and D7-PE40 evoked a significant growth inhibition of C4-2 SCID mouse xenografts, whereas PSMA-negative tumors remained totally unaffected [79, 84]. With regard to future clinical applications, further development of A5-PE40 and D7-PE40 is focused on the humanization of the scFvs to reduce the expected immunogenicity in humans. This could be done by grafting the PSMA-binding CDR regions of the scFvs directly to a human framework. In addition, the expected generation of neutralizing antibodies against the PE40 domain in patients could be avoided by elimination of immunodominant epitopes that were detected in a study by Onda et al. [87].

Anti-PSMA Virotherapeutic Agents

In a recent study, measles viruses (MV) of a live attenuated strain were used as an active drug component for the construction of a new anti-PSMA ADC [88]. Oncolytic measles virus is very effective against a variety of tumor types, including prostate cancer [89]. Normally, the virus enters the host cell via one or two measles receptors, CD46 and SLAM. CD46 is ubiquitously expressed on human cells, whereas SLAM is expressed on immune cells. After infection, the virus induces extensive intracellular fusion between the infected cell and neighboring cells to form nonviable multinucleated structures (syncytia), generating a large bystander killing. To generate a tumor-specific virus, the scFv of the anti-PSMA mAb huJ591 was fused to the coat protein of measles virus, in which alanine substitutions of specific residues ablated the viral interaction with CD46 and SLAM. After propagation of the PSMA retargeted virus, called MVG-αPSMA, efficient virus infection and cytopathic killing of PSMA-positive LNCaP and PC3/PIP cells were monitored. Furthermore, MVG-αPSMA induced regression or growth inhibition of LNCaP and PC3/PIP tumor xenografts. After immunostaining, extensive areas of measles virus infection and apoptosis were seen in virus-treated tumors [88].

Preexisting antiviral antibodies in patients, who have been vaccinated or infected by the wild-type measles virus, could form a crucial obstacle for a systemic use of MVG-αPSMA in clinical trials because they can quickly neutralize the virus domain after intravascular administration. Therefore, strategies are under investigation to more effectively deliver the virus to the tumor site. Such strategies could include the intratumoral application of the ADC, hiding the virus in cell carriers [90, 91], shielding the virus using polymers [92, 93], or the use of immunosuppressive drugs to dampen the innate immunity [94].

Conclusions

PSMA features many characteristics as target for prostate cancer ADCs such as a strong and specific expression in the prostate and upregulation in advanced stages of the disease. Radioimmunoconjugates with mAbs binding to the extracellular domain of PSMA demonstrated an efficient targeting of bone- and soft-tissue lesions, which resulted in an objective antitumor response in a subset of prostate cancer patients. Moreover, in preclinical models with small tumors, high cytotoxicity in vitro and specific antitumor activities in vivo could be demonstrated with anti-PSMA immunotoxins and virotherapeutic agents. The best clinical settings for anti-PSMA ADCs are therefore seen to be presented by a situation in which the tumor cell burden is low, i.e., after tumor excision, in the occurrence of a small residual disease, or in the presence of micrometastases.

References

1. Jemal A, Siegel R, Ward E, Hao Y, Xu J, Thun MJ (2009) Cancer statistics, 2009. CA Cancer J Clin 59(4):225–249
2. Meulenbeld HJ, Hamberg P, de Wit R (2009) Chemotherapy in patients with castration-resistant prostate cancer. Eur J Cancer 45(Suppl 1):161–171
3. O'Keefe DS, Su SL, Bacich DJ, Horiguchi Y, Luo Y, Powell CT, Zandvliet D, Russell PJ, Molloy PL, Nowak NJ, Shows TB, Mullins C, Vonder Haar RA, Fair WR, Heston WD (1998) Mapping, genomic organization and promoter analysis of the human prostate-specific membrane antigen gene. Biochim Biophys Acta 1443(1–2):113–127
4. Rajasekaran SA, Anilkumar G, Oshima E, Bowie JU, Liu H, Heston W, Bander NH, Rajasekaran AK (2003) A novel cytoplasmic tail MXXXL motif mediates the internalization of prostate-specific membrane antigen. Mol Biol Cell 14(12):4835–4845

5. Mesters JR, Barinka C, Li W, Tsukamoto T, Majer P, Slusher BS, Konvalinka J, Hilgenfeld R (2006) Structure of glutamate carboxypeptidase II, a drug target in neuronal damage and prostate cancer. EMBO J 25(6):1375–1384
6. Davis MI, Bennett MJ, Thomas LM, Bjorkman PJ (2005) Crystal structure of prostate-specific membrane antigen, a tumor marker and peptidase. Proc Natl Acad Sci USA 102(17):5981–5986
7. Carter RE, Feldman AR, Coyle JT (1996) Prostate-specific membrane antigen is a hydrolase with substrate and pharmacologic characteristics of a neuropeptidase. Proc Natl Acad Sci USA 93(2):749–753
8. Pinto JT, Suffoletto BP, Berzin TM, Qiao CH, Lin S, Tong WP, May F, Mukherjee B, Heston WD (1996) Prostate-specific membrane antigen: a novel folate hydrolase in human prostatic carcinoma cells. Clin Cancer Res 2(9):1445–1451
9. Liu H, Rajasekaran AK, Moy P, Xia Y, Kim S, Navarro V, Rahmati R, Bander NH (1998) Constitutive and antibody-induced internalization of prostate-specific membrane antigen. Cancer Res 58(18):4055–4060
10. Liu J, Kopeckova P, Buhler P, Wolf P, Pan H, Bauer H, Elsasser-Beile U (2009) Kopecek J. Biorecognition and subcellular trafficking of HPMA copolymer-anti-PSMA antibody conjugates by prostate cancer cells, Mol Pharm
11. Bostwick DG, Pacelli A, Blute M, Roche P, Murphy GP (1998) Prostate specific membrane antigen expression in prostatic intraepithelial neoplasia and adenocarcinoma: a study of 184 cases. Cancer 82(11):2256–2261
12. Wolf P, Freudenberg N, Buhler P, Alt K, Schultze-Seemann W, Wetterauer U, Elsasser-Beile U (2010) Three conformational antibodies specific for different PSMA epitopes are promising diagnostic and therapeutic tools for prostate cancer. Prostate 70(5):562–569
13. Silver DA, Pellicer I, Fair WR, Heston WD, Cordon-Cardo C (1997) Prostate-specific membrane antigen expression in normal and malignant human tissues. Clin Cancer Res 3(1):81–85
14. Horoszewicz JS, Kawinski E, Murphy GP (1987) Monoclonal antibodies to a new antigenic marker in epithelial prostatic cells and serum of prostatic cancer patients. Anticancer Res 7(5B):927–935
15. Lopes AD, Davis WL, Rosenstraus MJ, Uveges AJ, Gilman SC (1990) Immunohistochemical and pharmacokinetic characterization of the site-specific immunoconjugate CYT-356 derived from antiprostate monoclonal antibody 7E11-C5. Cancer Res 50(19):6423–6429
16. Wright GLJ, Haley C, Beckett ML, Schellhammer PF (1995) Expression of prostate-specific membrane antigen in normal, benign, and malignant prostate tissues. Urol Oncol 1:18–28
17. Wright GL Jr, Grob BM, Haley C, Grossman K, Newhall K, Petrylak D, Troyer J, Konchuba A, Schellhammer PF, Moriarty R (1996) Upregulation of prostate-specific membrane antigen after androgen-deprivation therapy. Urology 48(2):326–334
18. Sweat SD, Pacelli A, Murphy GP, Bostwick DG (1998) Prostate-specific membrane antigen expression is greatest in prostate adenocarcinoma and lymph node metastases. Urology 52(4):637–640
19. Ross JS, Sheehan CE, Fisher HA, Kaufman RP Jr, Kaur P, Gray K, Webb I, Gray GS, Mosher R, Kallakury BV (2003) Correlation of primary tumor prostate-specific membrane antigen expression with disease recurrence in prostate cancer. Clin Cancer Res 9(17):6357–6362
20. Liu H, Moy P, Kim S, Xia Y, Rajasekaran A, Navarro V, Knudsen B, Bander NH (1997) Monoclonal antibodies to the extracellular domain of prostate-specific membrane antigen also react with tumor vascular endothelium. Cancer Res 57(17):3629–3634
21. Chang SS, Reuter VE, Heston WD, Bander NH, Grauer LS, Gaudin PB (1999) Five different anti-prostate-specific membrane antigen (PSMA) antibodies confirm PSMA expression in tumor-associated neovasculature. Cancer Res 59(13):3192–3198
22. Kinoshita Y, Kuratsukuri K, Landas S, Imaida K, Rovito PM Jr, Wang CY, Haas GP (2006) Expression of prostate-specific membrane antigen in normal and malignant human tissues. World J Surg 30(4):628–636
23. Chang SS, Reuter VE, Heston WD, Gaudin PB (2001) Comparison of anti-prostate-specific membrane antigen antibodies and other immunomarkers in metastatic prostate carcinoma. Urology 57(6):1179–1183

24. Burger MJ, Tebay MA, Keith PA, Samaratunga HM, Clements J, Lavin MF, Gardiner RA (2002) Expression analysis of delta-catenin and prostate-specific membrane antigen: their potential as diagnostic markers for prostate cancer. Int J Cancer 100(2):228–237
25. Colombatti M, Grasso S, Porzia A, Fracasso G, Scupoli MT, Cingarlini S, Poffe O, Naim HY, Heine M, Tridente G, Mainiero F, Ramarli D (2009) The prostate specific membrane antigen regulates the expression of IL-6 and CCL5 in prostate tumour cells by activating the MAPK pathways. PLoS One 4(2):e4608
26. Israeli RS, Powell CT, Corr JG, Fair WR, Heston WD (1994) Expression of the prostate-specific membrane antigen. Cancer Res 54(7):1807–1811
27. Troyer JK, Beckett ML, Wright GL Jr (1995) Detection and characterization of the prostate-specific membrane antigen (PSMA) in tissue extracts and body fluids. Int J Cancer 62(5):552–558
28. Heston WD (1997) Characterization and glutamyl preferring carboxypeptidase function of prostate specific membrane antigen: a novel folate hydrolase. Urology 49(Suppl 3A):104–112
29. O'Keefe DS, Bacich DJ, Heston WD (2004) Comparative analysis of prostate-specific membrane antigen (PSMA) versus a prostate-specific membrane antigen-like gene. Prostate 58(2):200–210
30. Sacha P, Zamecnik J, Barinka C, Hlouchova K, Vicha A, Mlcochova P, Hilgert I, Eckschlager T, Konvalinka J (2007) Expression of glutamate carboxypeptidase II in human brain. Neuroscience 144(4):1361–1372
31. Chang SS, Reuter VE, Heston WD, Gaudin PB (2001) Metastatic renal cell carcinoma neovasculature expresses prostate-specific membrane antigen. Urology 57(4):801–805
32. Baccala A, Sercia L, Li J, Heston W, Zhou M (2007) Expression of prostate-specific membrane antigen in tumor-associated neovasculature of renal neoplasms. Urology 70(2):385–390
33. Conway RE, Petrovic N, Li Z, Heston W, Wu D, Shapiro LH (2006) Prostate-specific membrane antigen regulates angiogenesis by modulating integrin signal transduction. Mol Cell Biol 26(14):5310–5324
34. Troyer J, Feng Q, Beckett M, Wright GJ (1995) Biochemical characterization and mapping of the 7E11-C5.3 epitope of the prostate specific membrane antigen. Urological. Oncology 1:29–37
35. Brown LG, Wegner SK, Wang H, Buhler KR, Arfman EW, Lange PH, Vessella RL (1998) A novel monoclonal antibody 107-1A4 with high prostate specificity: generation, characterization of antigen expression, and targeting of human prostate cancer xenografts. Prostate Cancer Prostatic Dis 1(4):208–215
36. Wang S, Diamond DL, Hass GM, Sokoloff R, Vessella RL (2001) Identification of prostate specific membrane antigen (PSMA) as the target of monoclonal antibody 107-1A4 by proteinchip; array, surface-enhanced laser desorption/ionization (SELDI) technology. Int J Cancer 92(6):871–876
37. Murphy GP, Greene TG, Tino WT, Boynton AL, Holmes EH (1998) Isolation and characterization of monoclonal antibodies specific for the extracellular domain of prostate specific membrane antigen. J Urol 160(6 Pt 2):2396–2401
38. Grauer LS, Lawler KD, Marignac JL, Kumar A, Goel AS, Wolfert RL (1998) Identification, purification, and subcellular localization of prostate-specific membrane antigen PSM′ protein in the LNCaP prostatic carcinoma cell line. Cancer Res 58(21):4787–4789
39. Elsasser-Beile U, Wolf P, Gierschner D, Buhler P, Schultze-Seemann W, Wetterauer U (2006) A new generation of monoclonal and recombinant antibodies against cell-adherent prostate specific membrane antigen for diagnostic and therapeutic targeting of prostate cancer. Prostate 66(13):1359–1370
40. Moffett S, Melancon D, DeCrescenzo G, St-Pierre C, Deschenes F, Saragovi HU, Gold P, Cuello AC (2007) Preparation and characterization of new anti-PSMA monoclonal antibodies with potential clinical use. Hybridoma (Larchmt) 26(6):363–372
41. Regino CA, Wong KJ, Milenic DE, Holmes EH, Garmestani K, Choyke PL, Brechbiel MW (2009) Preclinical evaluation of a monoclonal antibody (3C6) specific for prostate-specific membrane antigen. Curr Radiopharm 2(1):9–17
42. Schulke N, Varlamova OA, Donovan GP, Ma D, Gardner JP, Morrissey DM, Arrigale RR, Zhan C, Chodera AJ, Surowitz KG, Maddon PJ, Heston WD, Olson WC (2003) The homodimer

of prostate-specific membrane antigen is a functional target for cancer therapy. Proc Natl Acad Sci USA 100(22):12590–12595
43. Milowsky MI, Nanus DM, Kostakoglu L, Sheehan CE, Vallabhajosula S, Goldsmith SJ, Ross JS, Bander NH (2007) Vascular targeted therapy with anti-prostate-specific membrane antigen monoclonal antibody J591 in advanced solid tumors. J Clin Oncol 25(5):540–547
44. Kahn D, Williams RD, Manyak MJ, Haseman MK, Seldin DW, Libertino JA, Maguire RT (1998) 111Indium-capromab pendetide in the evaluation of patients with residual or recurrent prostate cancer after radical prostatectomy. The ProstaScint Study Group. J Urol 159(6): 2041–2046
45. Kahn D, Williams RD, Seldin DW, Libertino JA, Hirschhorn M, Dreicer R, Weiner GJ, Bushnell D, Gulfo J (1994) Radioimmunoscintigraphy with 111indium labeled CYT-356 for the detection of occult prostate cancer recurrence. J Urol 152(5 Pt 1):1490–1495
46. Sodee DB, Conant R, Chalfant M, Miron S, Klein E, Bahnson R, Spirnak JP, Carlin B, Bellon EM, Rogers B (1996) Preliminary imaging results using In-111 labeled CYT-356 (Prostascint) in the detection of recurrent prostate cancer. Clin Nucl Med 21(10):759–767
47. Haseman MK, Reed NL, Rosenthal SA (1996) Monoclonal antibody imaging of occult prostate cancer in patients with elevated prostate-specific antigen. Positron emission tomography and biopsy correlation. Clin Nucl Med 21(9):704–713
48. Murphy GP, Elgamal AA, Su SL, Bostwick DG, Holmes EH (1998) Current evaluation of the tissue localization and diagnostic utility of prostate specific membrane antigen. Cancer 83(11): 2259–2269
49. Rosenthal SA, Haseman MK, Polascik TJ (2001) Utility of capromab pendetide (ProstaScint) imaging in the management of prostate cancer. Tech Urol 7(1):27–37
50. Kahn D, Austin JC, Maguire RT, Miller SJ, Gerstbrein J, Williams RD (1999) A phase II study of [90Y] yttrium-capromab pendetide in the treatment of men with prostate cancer recurrence following radical prostatectomy. Cancer Biother Radiopharm 14(2):99–111
51. Deb N, Goris M, Trisler K, Fowler S, Saal J, Ning S, Becker M, Marquez C, Knox S (1996) Treatment of hormone-refractory prostate cancer with 90Y-CYT-356 monoclonal antibody. Clin Cancer Res 2(8):1289–1297
52. Elsasser-Beile U, Reischl G, Wiehr S, Buhler P, Wolf P, Alt K, Shively J, Judenhofer MS, Machulla HJ, Pichler BJ (2009) PET imaging of prostate cancer xenografts with a highly specific antibody against the prostate-specific membrane antigen. J Nucl Med 50(4):606–611
53. Alt K, Wiehr S, Ehrlichmann W, Reischl G, Wolf P, Pichler BJ, Elsasser-Beile U, Buhler P (2010) High-resolution animal PET imaging of prostate cancer xenografts with three different (64)Cu-labeled antibodies against native cell-adherent PSMA. Prostate 70(13):1413–1421
54. Behe M, Alt K, Deininger F, Bühler P, Wetterauer U, Weber WA, Elsässer-Beile U, Wolf P (2011) In vivo testing of 177Lu-labelled anti-PSMA antibody as a new radioimmunotherapeutic agent against prostate cancer. In Vivo 25(1):55–59
55. David KA, Milowsky MI, Kostakoglu L, Vallabhajosula S, Goldsmith SJ, Nanus DM, Bander NH (2006) Clinical utility of radiolabeled monoclonal antibodies in prostate cancer. Clin Genitourin Cancer 4(4):249–256
56. McDevitt MR, Barendswaard E, Ma D, Lai L, Curcio MJ, Sgouros G, Ballangrud AM, Yang WH, Finn RD, Pellegrini V, Geerlings MW Jr, Lee M, Brechbiel MW, Bander NH, Cordon-Cardo C, Scheinberg DA (2000) An alpha-particle emitting antibody ([213Bi]J591) for radioimmunotherapy of prostate cancer. Cancer Res 60(21):6095–6100
57. Vallabhajosula S, Smith-Jones PM, Navarro V, Goldsmith SJ, Bander NH (2004) Radioimmunotherapy of prostate cancer in human xenografts using monoclonal antibodies specific to prostate specific membrane antigen (PSMA): studies in nude mice. Prostate 58(2):145–155
58. Milowsky MI, Nanus DM, Kostakoglu L, Vallabhajosula S, Goldsmith SJ, Bander NH (2004) Phase I trial of yttrium-90-labeled anti-prostate-specific membrane antigen monoclonal antibody J591 for androgen-independent prostate cancer. J Clin Oncol 22(13):2522–2531
59. Bander NH, Milowsky MI, Nanus DM, Kostakoglu L, Vallabhajosula S, Goldsmith SJ (2005) Phase I trial of 177lutetium-labeled J591, a monoclonal antibody to prostate-specific

membrane antigen, in patients with androgen-independent prostate cancer. J Clin Oncol 23(21):4591–4601
60. Vallabhajosula S, Goldsmith SJ, Hamacher KA, Kostakoglu L, Konishi S, Milowski MI, Nanus DM, Bander NH (2005) Prediction of myelotoxicity based on bone marrow radiation-absorbed dose: radioimmunotherapy studies using 90Y- and 177Lu-labeled J591 antibodies specific for prostate-specific membrane antigen. J Nucl Med 46(5):850–858
61. Fracasso G, Bellisola G, Cingarlini S, Castelletti D, Prayer-Galetti T, Pagano F, Tridente G, Colombatti M (2002) Anti-tumor effects of toxins targeted to the prostate specific membrane antigen. Prostate 53(1):9–23
62. Sandvig K, Torgersen ML, Engedal N, Skotland T, Iversen TG (2010) Protein toxins from plants and bacteria: probes for intracellular transport and tools in medicine. FEBS Lett 584(12):2626–2634
63. Knowles PP, Thorpe PE (1987) Purification of immunotoxins containing ricin A-chain and abrin A-chain using blue sepharose CL-6B. Anal Biochem 160(2):440–443
64. Thorpe PE, Wallace PM, Knowles PP, Relf MG, Brown AN, Watson GJ, Blakey DC, Newell DR (1988) Improved antitumor effects of immunotoxins prepared with deglycosylated ricin A-chain and hindered disulfide linkages. Cancer Res 48(22):6396–6403
65. Foxwell BM, Donovan TA, Thorpe PE, Wilson G (1985) The removal of carbohydrates from ricin with endoglycosidases H, F and D and alpha-mannosidase. Biochim Biophys Acta 840(2):193–203
66. Kimura Y, Hase S, Kobayashi Y, Kyogoku Y, Ikenaka T, Funatsu G (1988) Structures of sugar chains of ricin D. J Biochem 103(6):944–949
67. Huang X, Bennett M, Thorpe PE (2004) Anti-tumor effects and lack of side effects in mice of an immunotoxin directed against human and mouse prostate-specific membrane antigen. Prostate 61(1):1–11
68. Stirpe F, Barbieri L, Battelli MG, Soria M, Lappi DA (1992) Ribosome-inactivating proteins from plants: present status and future prospects. Biotechnology (NY) 10(4):405–412
69. Kuroda K, Liu H, Kim S, Guo M, Navarro V, Bander NH (2010) Saporin toxin-conjugated monoclonal antibody targeting prostate-specific membrane antigen has potent anticancer activity. Prostate 70(12):1286–1294
70. Ma D, Hopf CE, Malewicz AD, Donovan GP, Senter PD, Goeckeler WF, Maddon PJ, Olson WC (2006) Potent antitumor activity of an auristatin-conjugated, fully human monoclonal antibody to prostate-specific membrane antigen. Clin Cancer Res 12(8):2591–2596
71. Doronina SO, Toki BE, Torgov MY, Mendelsohn BA, Cerveny CG, Chace DF, DeBlanc RL, Gearing RP, Bovee TD, Siegall CB, Francisco JA, Wahl AF, Meyer DL, Senter PD (2003) Development of potent monoclonal antibody auristatin conjugates for cancer therapy. Nat Biotechnol 21(7):778–784
72. Henry MD, Wen S, Silva MD, Chandra S, Milton M, Worland PJ (2004) A prostate-specific membrane antigen-targeted monoclonal antibody-chemotherapeutic conjugate designed for the treatment of prostate cancer. Cancer Res 64(21):7995–8001
73. Chari RV, Martell BA, Gross JL, Cook SB, Shah SA, Blattler WA, McKenzie SJ, Goldmacher VS (1992) Immunoconjugates containing novel maytansinoids: promising anticancer drugs. Cancer Res 52(1):127–131
74. Blum RH, Wittenberg BK, Canellos GP, Mayer RJ, Skarin AT, Henderson IC, Parker LM, Frei E 3rd (1978) A therapeutic trial of maytansine. Cancer Clin Trials 1(2):113–117
75. Galsky MD, Eisenberger M, Moore-Cooper S, Kelly WK, Slovin SF, DeLaCruz A, Lee Y, Webb IJ, Scher HI (2008) Phase I trial of the prostate-specific membrane antigen-directed immunoconjugate MLN2704 in patients with progressive metastatic castration-resistant prostate cancer. J Clin Oncol 26(13):2147–2154
76. Russell PJ, Hewish D, Carter T, Sterling-Levis K, Ow K, Hattarki M, Doughty L, Guthrie R, Shapira D, Molloy PL, Werkmeister JA, Kortt AA (2004) Cytotoxic properties of immunoconjugates containing melittin-like peptide 101 against prostate cancer: in vitro and in vivo studies. Cancer Immunol Immunother 53(5):411–421

77. Dunn RD, Weston KM, Longhurst TJ, Lilley GG, Rivett DE, Hudson PJ, Raison RL (1996) Antigen binding and cytotoxic properties of a recombinant immunotoxin incorporating the lytic peptide, melittin. Immunotechnology 2(3):229–240
78. Wolf P, Gierschner D, Buhler P, Wetterauer U, Elsasser-Beile U (2006) A recombinant PSMA-specific single-chain immunotoxin has potent and selective toxicity against prostate cancer cells. Cancer Immunol Immunother 55(11):1367–1373
79. Wolf P, Alt K, Wetterauer D, Buhler P, Gierschner D, Katzenwadel A, Wetterauer U, Elsasser-Beile U (2010) Preclinical evaluation of a recombinant anti-prostate specific membrane antigen single-chain immunotoxin against prostate cancer. J Immunother 33(3):262–271
80. Allen TM (2002) Ligand-targeted therapeutics in anticancer therapy. Nat Rev Cancer 2(10):750–763
81. Adams GP, McCartney JE, Tai MS, Oppermann H, Huston JS, Stafford WF 3rd, Bookman MA, Fand I, Houston LL, Weiner LM (1993) Highly specific in vivo tumor targeting by monovalent and divalent forms of 741F8 anti-c-erbB-2 single-chain Fv. Cancer Res 53(17):4026–4034
82. Allured VS, Collier RJ, Carroll SF, McKay DB (1986) Structure of exotoxin A of Pseudomonas aeruginosa at 3.0-Angstrom resolution. Proc Natl Acad Sci USA 83(5):1320–1324
83. Wedekind JE, Trame CB, Dorywalska M, Koehl P, Raschke TM, McKee M, FitzGerald D, Collier RJ, McKay DB (2001) Refined crystallographic structure of Pseudomonas aeruginosa exotoxin A and its implications for the molecular mechanism of toxicity. J Mol Biol 314(4):823–837
84. Wolf P, Alt K, Buhler P, Katzenwadel A, Wetterauer U, Tacke M, Elsasser-Beile U (2008) Anti-PSMA immunotoxin as novel treatment for prostate cancer? High and specific antitumor activity on human prostate xenograft tumors in SCID mice. Prostate 68(2):129–138
85. Onda M, Kreitman RJ, Vasmatzis G, Lee B, Pastan I (1999) Reduction of the nonspecific animal toxicity of anti-Tac(Fv)-PE38 by mutations in the framework regions of the Fv which lower the isoelectric point. J Immunol 163(11):6072–6077
86. Onda M, Nagata S, Tsutsumi Y, Vincent JJ, Wang Q, Kreitman RJ, Lee B, Pastan I (2001) Lowering the isoelectric point of the Fv portion of recombinant immunotoxins leads to decreased nonspecific animal toxicity without affecting antitumor activity. Cancer Res 61(13):5070–5077
87. Onda M, Nagata S, FitzGerald DJ, Beers R, Fisher RJ, Vincent JJ, Lee B, Nakamura M, Hwang J, Kreitman RJ, Hassan R, Pastan I (2006) Characterization of the B cell epitopes associated with a truncated form of Pseudomonas exotoxin (PE38) used to make immunotoxins for the treatment of cancer patients. J Immunol 177(12):8822–8834
88. Liu C, Hasegawa K, Russell SJ, Sadelain M, Peng KW (2009) Prostate-specific membrane antigen retargeted measles virotherapy for the treatment of prostate cancer. Prostate 69(10):1128–1141
89. Msaouel P, Iankov ID, Allen C, Morris JC, von Messling V, Cattaneo R, Koutsilieris M, Russell SJ, Galanis E (2009) Engineered measles virus as a novel oncolytic therapy against prostate cancer. Prostate 69(1):82–91
90. Munguia A, Ota T, Miest T, Russell SJ (2008) Cell carriers to deliver oncolytic viruses to sites of myeloma tumor growth. Gene Ther 15(10):797–806
91. Power AT, Bell JC (2008) Taming the Trojan horse: optimizing dynamic carrier cell/oncolytic virus systems for cancer biotherapy. Gene Ther 15(10):772–779
92. O'Riordan CR, Lachapelle A, Delgado C, Parkes V, Wadsworth SC, Smith AE, Francis GE (1999) PEGylation of adenovirus with retention of infectivity and protection from neutralizing antibody in vitro and in vivo. Hum Gene Ther 10(8):1349–1358
93. Carlisle RC, Benjamin R, Briggs SS, Sumner-Jones S, McIntosh J, Gill D, Hyde S, Nathwani A, Subr V, Ulbrich K, Seymour LW, Fisher KD (2008) Coating of adeno-associated virus with reactive polymers can ablate virus tropism, enable retargeting and provide resistance to neutralising antisera. J Gene Med 10(4):400–411
94. Fulci G, Breymann L, Gianni D, Kurozomi K, Rhee SS, Yu J, Kaur B, Louis DN, Weissleder R, Caligiuri MA, Chiocca EA (2006) Cyclophosphamide enhances glioma virotherapy by inhibiting innate immune responses. Proc Natl Acad Sci USA 103(34):12873–12878

Chapter 16
Targeting CD56 (NCAM)-Expressing Neoplasms with Lorvotuzumab Mertansine

John M. Lambert, James O'Leary, Kathleen R. Whiteman, and Victor S. Goldmacher

Introduction

CD56, also known as NCAM (neural cell adhesion molecule), is a type I plasma membrane glycoprotein of the immunoglobulin (Ig) superfamily [1–3] that is expressed on neuronal tissue, skeletal muscle, and various cell types of neuroendocrine origin [2–8]. CD56/NCAM (hereafter called CD56 in this chapter) is also a characteristic marker for natural killer (NK) cells and is present on a subset of T cells [1, 9, 10]. The extracellular domain comprises five Ig-like domains followed by two fibronectin type III domains [2, 3]. CD56 is thought to play a role in cell–cell adhesion via homophilic binding between the Ig-domains of the molecule and in cell–extracellular matrix interactions and cell signaling [3, 11–14]. CD56 appears to interact with fibroblast growth factor (FGF) receptors, modulating response to its FGF ligands [15–18]. Through these interactions, CD56 it thought to play a key role in the biology of neuronal cells in nerve tissue, mediating neuronal differentiation, migration, and axon growth [12, 15, 19, 20], and it may also play a significant role in cell–cell adhesion and cell migration of some nonneuronal cell types [17, 18]. CD56 expression on NK cells and some T cells may be associated with modulation of maturation, cytokine production, and cytolytic effector functions of these cells [9, 10, 21–27]. In the case of expression on cancer cells, CD56 has been associated with cell migration and invasion, influencing metastatic spread [18, 28, 29].

The complexity of functional properties of CD56 is associated with a multiplicity of structural forms. There are three main isoforms produced by alternative splicing that vary in their cytoplasmic domain, a 180-kDa molecule with a long cytoplasmic domain, a 140-kDa molecule with a short cytoplasmic domain, and a 120-kDa molecule that lacks a transmembrane/cytoplasmic domain and is anchored to the plasma membrane via a glycosyl phosphatidylinositol anchor [2, 3, 30, 31].

J.M. Lambert (✉) • J. O'Leary • K.R. Whiteman • V.S. Goldmacher
ImmunoGen, Inc., 830 Winter Street, Waltham, MA 02451, USA
e-mail: john.lambert@immunogen.com

G.L. Phillips (ed.), *Antibody-Drug Conjugates and Immunotoxins: From Pre-Clinical Development to Therapeutic Applications*, Cancer Drug Discovery and Development, DOI 10.1007/978-1-4614-5456-4_16, © Springer Science+Business Media New York 2013

Further complexity in isoforms is created by the insertion of minor exons such as VASE [19, 32], or MSD1 [33, 34], as well an exon that introduces an in-frame stop codon that results in a secreted 115-kDa isoform [35]. Indeed, at least 27 alternatively spliced mRNA species have been reported present in some tissues [31]. Such alternative splicing of CD56 can result in tissue-specific or developmental stage-specific expression of particular isoforms, allowing fine control of its functional properties [9, 18, 19, 31–36].

Posttranslational addition of complex *N*- and *O*-linked glycans adds another layer of complexity to the isoforms of CD56 expressed on cell surfaces [37–40]. *N*-linked glycans attached to the two *N*-glycosylation sites in the fifth Ig-like domain can also carry linear polysialic acid chains that may be up to 200 sialic acid residues in length [41–43]. The polysialic acid, which is found on CD56 expressed in embryonal tissue and tumor tissue [6, 44], may attenuate the homophilic binding of CD56, reducing cell–cell adhesion and promoting cell migration, and in the context of tumor cell expression, may promote invasion and metastasis [6, 44, 45]. The highly diverse patterns of glycosylation that can vary spatially in tissues, and vary with developmental stage, may provide additional mechanisms for another layer of control of the biological activities of CD56 [6, 37–45].

A variety of cancers express CD56, both hematologic malignancies and tumors of cell types of neuroendocrine origin [4–7, 29, 46, 47]. Expression of the 140-kDa isoform is the dominant species in tumors or cancer cell lines [29, 48], although multiple isoforms also can be found in many cancers [56, 128]. In small cell lung cancer (SCLC), homogeneous expression of CD56 was documented on virtually all samples, including tumor biopsies and SCLC cell lines and xenografts [51–55]. It is occasionally expressed on other lung cancer types associated with neuroendocrine phenotype [4, 5, 53]. Other small cell cancers derived from other organs or tissues such as Merkel cell carcinoma (small cell cancer of skin) also exhibit virtually uniform expression of CD56 [49, 57]. The antigen is also expressed on a variety of other solid tumors such as 50–60% of cases of ovarian cancer [50] and the majority of cases of a variety of neuroendocrine tumors including pancreatic and gastrointestinal neuroendocrine tumors, carcinoid tumors, neuroblastoma, Wilms' tumor, and a subset of renal cell carcinoma [5, 6, 44, 47, 58]. CD56 is expressed by several hematologic neoplasms, including CD56-positive leukemias and lymphomas [59–62], and by 75–80% of cases of multiple myeloma [29, 46, 63, 64]. Expression of CD56 in tumors, especially the polysialic acid-containing glycoform, has been associated with poor prognosis [6, 29, 43, 44, 53, 60, 64, 65].

CD56 makes an attractive target for antibody-mediated therapy. It is highly expressed on a wide variety of aggressive neoplasms with significant unmet medical need. Furthermore, in cancers where the antigen is expressed, the pattern of expression is generally uniform [5, 49, 50, 55–57]. This review briefly describes early attempts to exploit CD56 as a therapeutic target for antibody-based therapeutic agents and then will focus on a promising CD56-targeting immunoconjugate, lorvotuzumab mertansine, which is in clinical evaluation for the treatment of SCLC and multiple myeloma.

Early Immunoconjugates Targeting CD56

Attempts to develop antibody-based therapeutics that target CD56 have concentrated on utilizing such antibodies to deliver a cell-killing payload, either a radionuclide, a protein toxin, or a small molecular weight cytotoxic agent [47]. Studies with several anti-CD56 radioimmunoconjugates have met with little success as therapeutic agents in clinical trials thus far [47] and are not further discussed in this review. However, it is instructive to examine briefly the results of the early studies evaluating the potential of conjugates of anti-CD56 antibodies with various cytotoxic agents for treatment of CD56-expressing malignancies because the results of these studies laid the groundwork for the development of lorvotuzumab mertansine.

An early attempt at targeting a cytotoxic agent to CD56 by conjugating doxorubicin to two anti-CD56 antibodies, SEN7 and MOC31, met with only limited success. The conjugates could kill CD56-expressing cell lines only at high concentrations, 0.5 μM or higher [66]. This result was consistent with the insufficient cytotoxic potency of early conjugates of antibodies with conventional anticancer drugs (reviewed in Refs. [67, 68]).

A solution to the poor potency of these early antibody-cytotoxic agent conjugates was to attempt to target CD56 with immunotoxins, conjugates of antibodies with highly cytotoxic proteins. Six anti-CD56 immunotoxins have been explored. The anti-CD56 murine monoclonal antibodies, MOC-31 and SEN7, were conjugated to the bacterial toxin, *Pseudomonas* exotoxin A, to form conjugates that displayed varying levels of CD56-specific cell-killing activity [69, 70]. A conjugate of an anti-CD56 monoclonal antibody with a streptavidin-protein A fusion protein, complexed with biotinylated glucose oxidase as a cytotoxic moiety, was tested on several SCLC cell lines in vitro and displayed some activity [71]. Three CD56-targeting immunoconjugates of ricin, a potent protein toxin isolated from castor beans [72], were reported. A recombinant fusion protein consisting of the heavy chain of the humanized anti-CD56 antibody N901 coupled with ricin B-chain, to which ricin A-chain was associated, was found to be selectively cytotoxic against the CD56-expressing SCLC cell line SW2 [73]. Conjugates of the SEN7 and N901 antibodies with blocked ricin (bR), a chemically altered form of ricin [74], were also studied [5, 70, 74–79]. Both demonstrated exceptionally high CD56-selective potency in vitro towards CD56-expressing SCLC cell lines [5, 70, 79].

Of all these earlier conjugates, only the N901–bR conjugate went into clinical testing. It was evaluated in a phase I trial and a phase II trial in SCLC patients [75–78]. In the phase I trial (21 patients), one patient with refractory disease had a partial response, and six patients had stable disease [76]. In this study, evidence of tumor targeting was also obtained, despite the relatively low maximum tolerated dose (30 μg/kg/d given by continuous intravenous infusion for 7 days). In the phase II study in patients ($n=9$) that were in complete or near complete response following chemotherapy and/or radiation (≥90% reduction in measurable disease), one patient had stable disease for 4 months, one patient converted from near complete response to a complete response of 3 months duration, and one patient with limited-stage disease that entered the study in complete remission remained so for more than 6 years after completion therapy [75].

Despite these indications of antitumor activity, the studies with N901–bR showed two major obstacles in the development of this agent. One was the nonspecific toxicity exhibited by N901–bR [75, 76], in particular the capillary leak syndrome that has often been seen with protein toxin-based immunotoxins [80–82], likely due to direct damage to vascular endothelial cells. Importantly however, despite CD56 expression in cardiac muscle and peripheral nerve tissue, no significant cardiac toxicity attributable to the immunotoxin was observed, and neither central nor peripheral nervous system toxicity was noted by serial neurologic examinations, electromyography, or nerve conduction studies [75–78]. Thus, the major toxicities of N901–bR were of a nonantigen-related nature suggesting that the CD56 antigen could be targeted if one were to design a conjugate with an appropriate cytotoxic effector that would exhibit less nontarget toxicity. The second obstacle was the development of anti-murine Ig antibodies and anti-ricin antibodies in every patient, severely limiting the period of circulation of active immunotoxin and limiting the number of administered cycles to one [75, 76].

Because of these limitations, further clinical development of N901–bR was abandoned, and, in general, these experiences suggested that targeting CD56 (or other antigens) with protein toxins held little promise [83]. On the other hand, N901–bR demonstrated signals of clinical activity and absence of any major CD56-targeted systemic toxicity. With this in mind, our attention turned to cytotoxic effectors of a different nature with which to arm an anti-CD56 antibody.

Design of an ADC Targeting CD56 Utilizing a Potent Cytotoxic Payload

The next generation of antibody-drug conjugates targeting CD56 aimed to combine non-immunogenic antibodies, humanized or fully human, with small molecular weight cytotoxic agents having the high potency of the potent protein toxin effector molecules used in early immunoconjugates. This research led to the development of lorvotuzumab mertansine, an ADC in clinical development for the treatment of SCLC and multiple myeloma [67, 83].

Lorvotuzumab mertansine is composed of a humanized monoclonal IgG1 antibody (lorvotuzumab) attached to the potent microtubule-targeting agent, the thiol-containing maytansinoid, DM1 (*N2′*-deacetyl-*N2′*-(3-mercapto-1-oxopropyl) maytansine) [46, 67, 84, 85], through reaction of its thiol group with the disulfide-containing linker, *N*-succinimidyl 4-(2-pyridyldithio)pentanoate (SPP). Figure 16.1a shows the chemical structure of the linked maytansinoid in the CD56-targeting ADC.

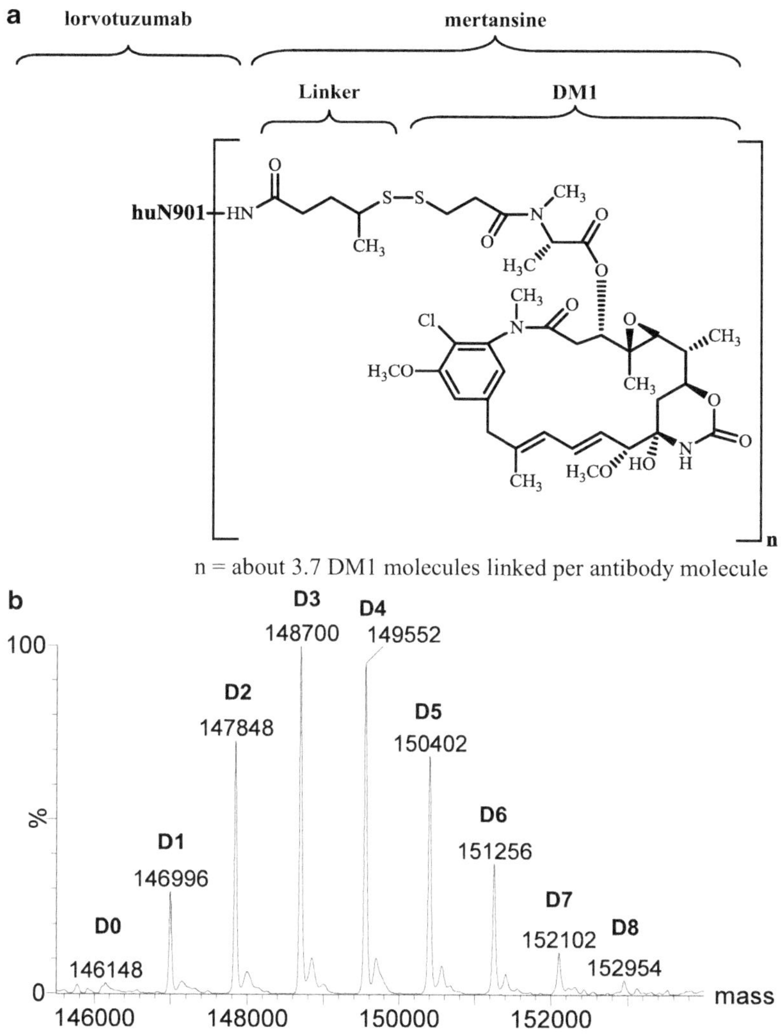

Fig. 16.1 The structure of lorvotuzumab mertansine. (**a**) The chemistry of the linker-DM1 moiety attached to lorvotuzumab via an amide bond to amino groups of lysine residues. n = about 3.7 DM1 molecules linked per antibody molecule. (**b**) Analysis of a research sample of deglycosylated lorvotuzumab mertansine by mass spectroscopy showing the mass distribution profile [98]. The average maytansinoid load was 3.9 per antibody molecule for this experimental test material. The label *D1*, *D2*, etc., identifies the mass peaks of antibody linked to one DM1, two DM1s, etc.

The Antibody Component of Lorvotuzumab Mertansine

The murine monoclonal antibody, N901, is an immunoglobulin of the IgG1 kappa subclass that was generated at the Dana–Farber Cancer Institute (Boston, Massachusetts) by Griffin and colleagues, by immunizing mice with human chronic myeloid leukemia cells [10]. The antibody was found to bind to an antigen known as CD56 identified to be expressed on all NK cells and a minority of T cells [1, 10], an antigen that was later determined to be identical to NCAM [1, 9]. The N901 antibody, which has an apparent equilibrium dissociation constant of 1.1×10^{-10} M as measured by indirect immunofluorescence assays utilizing FACS on an SCLC cell line [86], and 2×10^{-12} M as measured under equilibrium conditions by ELISA methods utilizing isolated plasma membranes from CD56-positive cells [87], was humanized by complementarity determining region grafting [88]. The binding properties of the humanized antibody, lorvotuzumab (also known as huN901), were indistinguishable from those of the "parent" N901 antibody as measured in a variety of binding assays [88].

The Cytotoxic "Payload" Component of Lorvotuzumab Mertansine

Initial studies examined two potent cell-killing agents, DM1 [85] and DC1 [89], created for the purpose of conjugation to antibodies, as the cytotoxic effectors for constructing an ADC targeting CD56. DM1 is a derivative of maytansine, a natural product that targets microtubules that was originally isolated from the Ethiopian shrub, *Maytenus serrata* [90–92]. DM1 induces mitotic arrest, ultimately resulting in cell death, at concentrations as low as 10 pM, likely by suppression of microtubule dynamic instability [93–96]. DC1 is a derivative of adozelesin 2, which is similar in its structure to CC1065 [89]. CC1065 and its analogues, including adozelesin and duocarmycins, bind with high affinity to the DNA minor groove and then alkylate DNA at adenine bases, enabling the cytotoxin to kill cells at sub-nanomolar to picomolar concentrations (reviewed in [89]).

DC1 was conjugated to either murine or humanized N901 via a disulfide-containing linker and tested in vitro using the CD56-expressing SCLC cell line, SW2 [89]. The conjugates were potent in killing SW2 cells (IC_{50} ~0.1 nM after a 24 h exposure), and this activity was CD56-selective, being 200- to 400-fold less cytotoxic for antigen-negative cells. However, evaluation of the therapeutic window of a number of DC1-containing ADCs in vivo suggested that the window was not wide enough for development of effective clinical compounds [67, 68, 89], and so research focused on the maytansinoid payload for creating an ADC for clinical development against CD56-expressing cancers.

The Linker Moiety and Final Design of Lorvotuzumab Mertansine

Lorvotuzumab was modified by reaction of the *N*-hydroxysuccinimide ester group of the SPP linker with lysine amino groups of the antibody to form stable amide bonds. The pyridyldithio groups so attached provide the site of linkage to DMI via thiol-disulfide exchange reactions resulting in a hindered disulfide-containing bond between the attached linker and the DM1 [46, 67, 83–85]. The SPP linker/DM1 combination was selected based on optimal activity in preclinical in vivo models of antitumor activity [84, 97]. The linker reaction is controlled so that about 3.7 DM1 molecules are linked per antibody molecule. Analysis of deglycosylated conjugate by mass spectroscopy indicates that at this average DM1 per antibody load, the distribution of conjugated species is very consistent and approximates a binomial distribution of masses as shown in Fig. 16.1b [98], with the predominant peaks corresponding to 2, 3, and 4 molecules of DM1 linked per antibody and very low amounts of species with either 0 or with 6 (or more) linked DM1/antibody [98]. Peptide mapping studies indicate that about half of the 86 lysine residues in lorvotuzumab participate in the reaction with SPP; thus, each is only partially modified at the average modification level of 3.7 linker-DM1 moieties per antibody molecule [98]. The overall average molecular weight of lorvotuzumab mertansine is about 152,000 Da (including the endogenous glycosylation of the CHO cell-produced antibody), and linked maytansinoid comprises approximately 1.8% by weight.

Mechanism of Action of Lorvotuzumab Mertansine

The maytansinoid payload of lorvotuzumab mertansine is a mitotic inhibitor that interferes with the formation of microtubules likely by suppression of microtubule dynamic instability [93–96]. Proliferating cells treated with this agent arrest in the G2/M phase of the cell cycle and eventually die by apoptosis [91]. Maytansine competes with *vinca* alkaloids for the same binding site on tubulin [93], although it is 100–1,000-fold more potent, and its activity pattern does not cluster with other tubulin-acting agents across the NCI 60 panel of human cancer cell lines [99].

Lorvotuzumab mertansine displays potent in vitro cytotoxicity toward CD56-positive cells [100]. For example, the IC_{50} on the neuroblastoma cell line, IMR32, is about 60 pM, while there was no inhibition of cell growth at 1.5 nM when tested on the antigen-negative colon cancer cell line, COLO 205 (both cell lines were equally sensitive to maytansine). When cells of a multiple myeloma cell line were exposed to lorvotuzumab mertansine, the proportion of cells in the G2/M phase of the cell cycle was significantly increased after 48 h of exposure [46], consistent with the mechanism of action of agents that interfere with microtubule dynamics resulting in cell cycle arrest [91]. This is then followed by increased apoptotic cell death [96, 101].

Internalization appears to be an obligatory step for cell killing by ADCs [96, 102]. CD56 is endocytosed via a clathrin-dependent pathway [103, 104], indicating that the immunoconjugate molecules bound to CD56 on the cell surface are able to be delivered inside the cell. Experiments with lorvotuzumab mertansine in which the DM1 moiety was radiolabeled, which are analogous to those conducted with other maytansinoid conjugates [105, 106], confirm that the ADC binds to the cell surface antigen and is internalized and routed into the lysosomal degradation pathway. There the antibody moiety is completely degraded to its constituent amino acids, yielding lysine-SPP-DM1 as the initial intracellular maytansinoid metabolite.

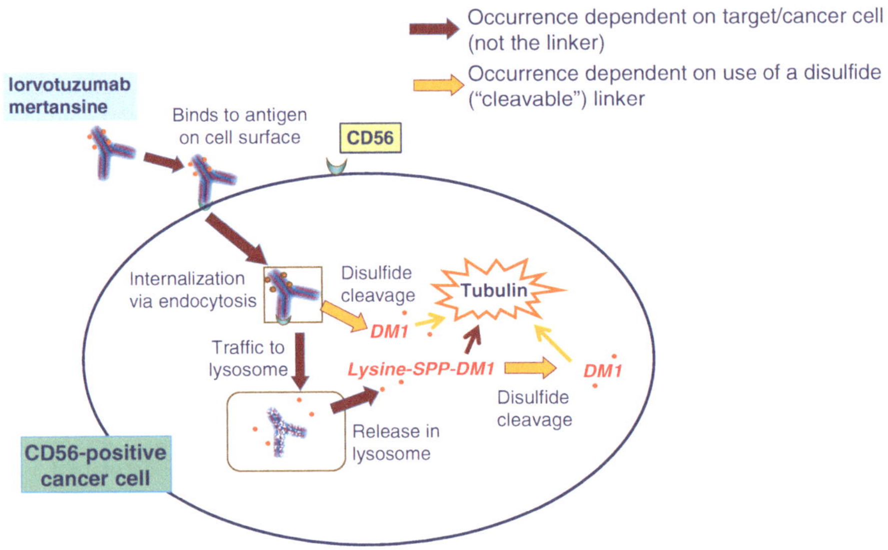

Fig. 16.2 Schematic representation of the mechanism of action of lorvotuzumab mertansine. The drawing is based on studies by Erickson and colleagues [105–108] that established the mechanisms of release of active maytansinoid metabolites within tumor cells

In the reducing environment of the cytoplasm of the cell, the disulfide in the lysine-SPP-DM1 metabolite is subject to further cleavage by thiol-disulfide exchange reactions to release the free thiol, DM1 [107, 108]. It is possible that some DM1 also is released intracellularly from pre-lysosomal compartments by thiol-disulfide exchange reactions within the cell, as has been shown in experimental systems utilizing cell lines with poor lysosomal processing rates [109]. Such evidence suggests that in the case of lorvotuzumab mertansine, both mechanisms of intracellular release of active maytansinoid may be operative, as illustrated in Fig. 16.2. Examining elimination of metabolites from the body in preclinical studies, Erickson and colleagues have shown that DM1 is readily *S*-methylated in the liver by an endogenous *S*-methyl-transferase to form *S*-methyl-DM1, which is then subject to oxidation by liver enzymes to form the less cytotoxic sulfoxide and sulfone derivatives which are eliminated in the bile [107, 110].

Lorvotuzumab induces NK-cell-mediated antibody-dependent cellular cytotoxicity (ADCC) in a dose-dependent manner on target cells expressing high levels of CD56 (estimated at ≥150,000 antibody-binding sites per cell), an activity that was conserved following conjugation to DM1 [111]. While the antibody and its DM1-conjugate also bind to CD56 on the surface of the NK cells, as well as to the target tumor cells, neither the antibody nor its conjugate have any effect on NK cell function [10, 111]. The lack of activity of the ADC on NK cells is related, at least in part, to the relatively low surface expression of CD56 molecules on NK cells, which have an average of only about 2,500 anti-CD56 antibody-binding sites per cell (range 950–9,000; ImmunoGen Inc., internal data). Noteworthy in this regard is the relatively poor activity of AVE9633, an anti-CD33 antibody-maytansinoid conjugate evaluated for treatment of acute myeloid leukemia (AML). While CD33 is a specific marker for myeloid cells and AML, nearly 90% of patient AML cells expressed less than 10,000 CD33 antigens/cell, with the majority having <5,000 antigens/cell; the poor activity of the conjugate was attributed to the relatively low antigen expression [112]. Neither the "naked" lorvotuzumab antibody nor its conjugate shows any complement-dependent cytotoxicity on tumor target cells [111]. "Naked" lorvotuzumab has not been shown to exhibit any direct antiproliferative or proapoptotic activity on cell lines in vitro, or any antitumor activity in vivo, prior to its conjugation with maytansinoids [46, 67, 84].

Activity of Lorvotuzumab Mertansine in Preclinical Models

Studies evaluating the in vivo efficacy of lorvotuzumab mertansine were conducted in immunodeficient mice bearing subcutaneous xenografts of human CD56-positive tumor cell lines derived from SCLC, multiple myeloma, and ovarian cancer. Significant antitumor activity, including complete regressions, were observed with lorvotuzumab mertansine as a single agent. For example, treatment of mice bearing bulky subcutaneous xenografts (~300 mm^3) of the NCI-H929 multiple myeloma cell line with a *single* intravenous dose of about 13 mg/kg of the ADC resulted in complete regressions in 6/6 tumors, with 5 of 6 mice remaining tumor-free until the end of study, as shown in Fig. 16.3. These results are similar to the results of Tassone and colleagues obtained with the OPM2 multiple myeloma xenograft model [46]. Lorvotuzumab mertansine shows a similar high level of antitumor activity in a variety of SCLC models [67, 84, 100], and in addition, antitumor activity has been demonstrated in two CD56-positive xenograft models of ovarian cancer [50]. Mixtures of lorvotuzumab and free maytansine, as well as a nonbinding irrelevant DM1 conjugate, were shown to have no effect on tumor growth in several of these models (e.g., Refs. [46, 67]), indicating that the complete lorvotuzumab mertansine conjugate was required for activity and confirming the lack of antitumor activity of the "naked" antibody. Lorvotuzumab mertansine also showed strong antitumor activity in vivo toward a number of CD56-positive pediatric cancer cell line xenografts (neuroblastoma, rhabdomyosarcoma, Wilms' tumor), evaluated under the Pediatric Preclinical Testing Program of the National Cancer Institute [113], and was active against malignant NK/T cells [114]. The preclinical results provide a strong rationale for the development of lorvotuzumab mertansine for clinical use, the activity of the immunoconjugate comparing very favorably with standard chemotherapeutic treatments in a variety of xenograft models [67, 84, 100].

The activity of lorvotuzumab mertansine combined with standard-of-care chemotherapeutic regimens was assessed in SCLC, multiple myeloma, and ovarian cancer xenograft models [84, 100, 115, 116]. In a model of resistant SCLC using NCI-H69 xenografts, where treatment with a standard doublet of carboplatin (80 mg/kg on day 1) and etoposide (5 mg/kg on days 1–5) or with lorvotuzumab

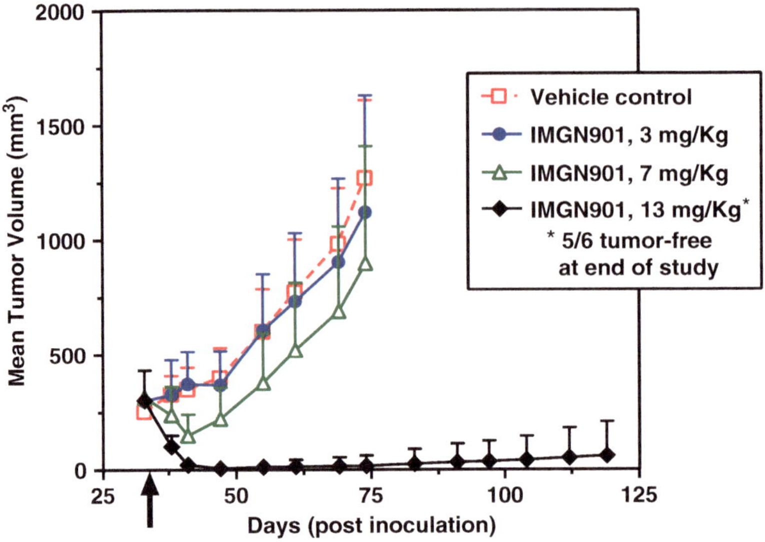

Fig. 16.3 Dose-dependent activity of lorvotuzumab mertansine against established CD56/NCAM—positive multiple myeloma tumor xenografts in SCID mice. SCID mice were inoculated subcutaneously with cells of the NCI-H929 multiple myeloma cell line. Groups of mice (6 per group) were treated with a *single* intravenous injection of lorvotuzumab mertansine (average maytansinoid load of 3.0 per antibody molecule for this experimental test material) at the doses indicated (given as mg of antibody in the conjugate), when the xenografts were large, approximately 300 mm^3 in size. One group received vehicle (buffered saline). Mean tumor volume of each group versus day postinoculation is plotted in the graph. At the highest dose tested, 5 of 6 mice were tumor-free at the end of the study

mertansine (18 mg/kg on days 1 and 8) was inactive or only marginally active at the doses tested, the triple combination treatment showed significant antitumor activity with partial regressions observed [84]. These doses of lorvotuzumab mertansine were well tolerated by the SCID mice, with no weight loss observed as a consequence of dosing. Lorvotuzumab mertansine in combination with bortezomib or lenalidomide demonstrated additive or greater-than-additive antitumor activity, as compared to treatment with each single agent in several multiple myeloma xenograft models [115, 117]. Combination activity of the conjugate with a paclitaxel/carboplatin doublet, liposomal doxorubicin, topotecan, and gemcitabine was also explored in an ovarian xenograft mouse model using the COLO 720E cell line [116]. The combinations were highly active, more so than the individual therapeutic regimens with an increase in the incidence of partial and complete responses in these models over single-agent treatments. The favorable toxicity profile of lorvotuzumab mertansine, similar to that of other maytansinoid immunoconjugates investigated to date [83], and the preclinical results showing increased activity and more durable responses in combination regimens suggest that lorvotuzumab mertansine combinations with approved agents should be well tolerated and could provide significant therapeutic benefit to cancer patients.

Early Clinical Development of Lorvotuzumab Mertansine

Lorvotuzumab mertansine has been evaluated clinically in three phase I dose-escalation studies exploring three different schedules of administration, in both solid tumors and a hematologic cancer. In SCLC and other CD56-expressing solid tumors, the dosing regimens of weekly for 4 weeks on a 6-week cycle [118–120] and daily for 3 consecutive days given every 3 weeks [121] were evaluated in clinical trials. In multiple myeloma, a regimen of dosing weekly for 2 weeks given on a 3-week cycle was studied [122, 123]. Currently, lorvotuzumab mertansine is being studied in combination with lenalidomide plus dexamethasone in multiple myeloma and in combination with carboplatin and etoposide in SCLC. Table 16.1 summarizes the number and type of patients enrolled in each of these five clinical studies, a safety database of over 260 patients treated.

A phase I trial in CD56-positive solid tumors established 75 mg/m^2 (~2.0 mg/kg) as the maximum tolerated dose (MTD), when lorvotuzumab mertansine was administered daily for 3 consecutive days every 3 weeks, and the recommended phase II dose from this schedule was 60 mg/m^2 [121]. In multiple myeloma, a phase I dose-escalation trial established 112 mg/m^2 (~3.0 mg/kg) as the MTD when lorvotuzumab mertansine was administered weekly for 2 consecutive weeks every 3 weeks [122]. The dose intensity at the MTD was similar for the two regimens (224–225 mg/m^2 over 3 weeks). The half-life of the conjugate was about 1–1.5 days at doses ≥60 mg/m^2 across all studies. This is relatively short for an antibody-based therapeutic, likely due to antigen-mediated clearance via the normal tissue antigen sink of CD56-expressing NK cells [118]. The most common side effects were grade 1 or grade 2 including headache, fatigue, neuropathy, elevated transaminases, nausea/vomiting, and myalgia. Dose-limiting toxicities (DLTs) in patients dosed at 140 mg/m^2 weekly for 2 weeks every 3 weeks in the multiple myeloma trial were grade 3 fatigue in two of six patients and grade 3 acute renal failure in one of these two patient [122]. Grade 3 toxicities of myalgia (one patient) and headache and back and shoulder pain (one patient) were the DLTs seen in the two patients dosed at 94 mg/m^2 given daily for 3 days on a 3-week cycle in the solid tumor trial [121, 124]. Earlier findings of dose-limiting headache, with an onset within about 8 h and largely resolved by about 48 h seen in the first lorvotuzumab mertansine phase I clinical trial [118], were not seen in later studies once routine low-dose steroid prophylaxis was utilized prior to treatment [121, 122, 124]. Such prophylaxis was not utilized in study 001 (Table 16.1), likely leading to an overall lower estimate of MTD in the study (60 mg/m^2). Overall, there were no clinically significant changes in hematologic parameters with no evidence of clinically significant myelosuppression. Manageable minimal to mild peripheral neuropathy, a commonly seen side effect of tubulin-acting cytotoxic agents, was observed across all the phase I studies, with grade 1 or grade 2 neuropathy seen in about 30% of patients (most patients had been heavily pretreated with multiple chemotherapy regimens, including agents known to induce neuropathies). There were few observations of grade 3 neuropathy (2.5% of patients) and no grade 4 observations in the phase I studies [118–122, 124].

Table 16.1 Summary of clinical trials conducted with lorvotuzumab mertansine

	Study 001 Phase 1/2 Wkly × 4, Q6wk Enrollment completed	Study 002 Phase 1 D1, 2, 3, Q3wk Enrollment completed	Study 0007 Phase 1/2 Combo LM-Wkly × 2, Q3wk (carboplatin/etoposide) Recruiting	Study 003 Phase 1 Wkly × 2, Q3wk Enrollment completed	Study 0005 Phase 1 Combo LM-Wkly × 3, Q4wk (len/dex) Recruiting	Total number treated
MTD	60 mg/m^2	75 mg/m^2		112 mg/m^2		
Patient type	Number of patients treated with lorvotuzumab mertansine					
SCLC	48	35	13			96
MCC		23	2			25
Ovarian		12	2			14
MM				37	32	69
Other	16	27	16			59
Totals	64	97	33	37	32	263

LM lorvotuzumab mertansine; *SCLC* small cell lung cancer; *MCC* Merkel cell carcinoma; *MM* multiple myeloma
Source: ImmunoGen Clinical Study Reports, May 2012

Encouraging signals of antitumor activity were reported in these three phase I studies of single-agent lorvotuzumab mertansine. In multiple myeloma, of the 37 patients treated at doses ranging from 40 mg/m^2 to 140 mg/m^2 (25 patients treated at ≥112 mg/m^2), there were three objective partial responses and three objective minimal responses, while 15 patients had stable disease for ≥3 months for an overall clinical benefit rate of 41% [122, 125]. The responses in this heavily pretreated phase I patient population were quite durable, with five of six lasting from about 30 weeks to about 75 weeks [125]. In the two trials of CD56-positive solid tumors, study 001 which was a phase I/II trial (32 patients in each part) and study 002 which was a phase I trial with an expanded cohort at MTD (Table 16.1), there were two partial responses (one unconfirmed) and 15 patients with clinically meaningful disease noted from the 68 patients with SCLC from among the 113 total patients treated in these two clinical studies [119–121, 124]. Among the eight patients with Merkel cell carcinoma (MCC) among the 45 evaluable patients on the trial evaluating daily × three dosing every 3 weeks [121], there were two complete responses and three patients with clinically meaningful stable disease (4 to 7+ cycles of treatment). While numbers are small, these are remarkable findings in this rare, aggressive small cell cancer of the skin—the median survival of metastatic MCC is only about 7 months [126]. The findings of activity in MCC support the observations of activity in SCLC since these aggressive cancers are similar in both cell morphology and in the dismal outcome of their clinical course and are both treated with similar chemotherapy regimens (*cis*- or carboplatin plus etoposide).

Based on these promising signals of clinical activity in these difficult-to-treat cancers and on the preclinical results reporting improved antitumor activity of lorvotuzumab mertansine in combination with chemotherapeutic regimens as described above [100, 115–117], coupled with the acceptable tolerability profile of lorvotuzumab mertansine, in particular the lack of clinically meaningful myelosuppression [121, 122, 124], development is now focused on combination treatment regimens. Table 16.1 lists two such studies now under way. One (study 0005) is a clinical trial of lorvotuzumab mertansine given weekly for 3 weeks every 4 weeks in combination with lenalidomide and low-dose dexamethasone in multiple myeloma patients [125, 127], and the second (study 0007) is a study of the conjugate given weekly for 2 weeks every 3 weeks in combination with carboplatin and etoposide in patients with SCLC (http://clinicaltrials.gov). The early experience reported with the lorvotuzumab mertansine plus lenalidomide/dexamethasone combination in a single arm study (first 13 evaluable patients) demonstrates encouraging activity for this regimen in this heavily pretreated population (most patients had received ≥3 prior therapies including an immunomodulatory agent), with 9 of 13 evaluable patients demonstrating clinical benefit including five patients with a very good partial response, three with partial response, and one with minor response [125, 127]. Additionally, the combination showed activity in four patients whose cancers had mutations associated with poor outcomes. In the SCLC trial, the combination study with carboplatin/etoposide was planned as a randomized phase II trial in the setting of previously untreated SCLC patients with extensive-stage disease, after an initial dose-escalation phase (not restricted to SCLC patients) to establish the combination regimen. In the phase II part of the study, patients will be randomized 2:1 to receive up to six cycles of carboplatin/etoposide plus lorvotuzumab mertansine followed by maintenance with the ADC until progression or to receive up to six cycles of the standard of care only. The phase II portion began in March 2012; however, results have not yet been reported for this study (see http://clinicaltrials.gov).

Conclusion

In summary, single-agent lorvotuzumab mertansine has shown promising preliminary evidence of clinical activity in advanced stage SCLC, MCC, and multiple myeloma. The conjugate has demonstrated a favorable safety profile with manageable side effects and no evidence of clinically significant myelosuppression. Its tolerability profile and encouraging single-agent activity provide a sound rationale for exploration of lorvotuzumab mertansine in combination with standard treatment regimens for patients with CD56-positive tumors. Additionally, the single-agent safety profile supports the potential to utilize this conjugate in a maintenance setting. Ongoing clinical development is focused on assessing combination treatment for SCLC with the potential to expand to treatment of other CD56-positive tumor indications such as multiple myeloma, ovarian cancer, a variety of neuroendocrine tumors, and pediatric tumors including neuroblastoma.

References

1. Schubert J, Lanier LL, Schmidt RE (1989) Cluster report: CD56. In: Knapp W, Dorken B, Gilks WR, Rieber EP, Schmidt RE, Stein H, von dem Borne AEG (eds) Leucocyte Typing IV: white cell differentiation antigens. Oxford University Press, New York, pp 699–702
2. Cunningham BA, Hemperly JJ, Murray BA, Prediger EA, Brackenbury R, Edelman GM (1987) Neural cell adhesion molecule: structure, immunoglobulin-like domains, cell surface modulation, and alternative RNA splicing. Science 236:799–806
3. Edelman GM, Crossin KL (1991) Cell adhesion molecules: Implications for a molecular histology. Annu Rev Biochem 60:155–190
4. Carbone DP, Koros AM, Linnoila RI, Jewett P, Gazdar AF (1991) Neural cell adhesion molecule expression and messenger RNA splicing patterns in lung cancer cell lines are correlated with neuroendocrine phenotype and growth morphology. Cancer Res 51:6142–6149
5. Roy DC, Ouellet S, Le Houillier C, Ariniello PD, Perreault C, Lambert JM (1996) Elimination of neuroblastoma and small cell lung cancer cells with an anti-neural cell adhesion molecule immunotoxin. J Natl Cancer Inst 88:1136–1145
6. Roth J, Zuber C, Wagner P, Blaha I, Bitter-Suermann D, Heitz PU (1988) Presence of the long chain form of polysialic acid of the neural cell adhesion molecule in Wilms' tumor. Identification of a cell adhesion molecule as an oncodevelopmental antigen and implications for tumor histogenesis. Am J Pathol 133:227–240
7. Jin L, Hemperly JJ, Lloyd RV (1991) Expression of neural cell adhesion molecule in normal and neoplastic human neuroendocrine tissues. Am J Pathol 138:961–969

8. Prieto AL, Crossin KL, Cunningham BA, Edelman GM (1989) Localization of mRNA for neural cell adhesion molecule (N-CAM) polypeptides in neural and nonneural tissues by *in situ* hybridization. Proc Natl Acad Sci USA 86:9579–9583
9. Lanier LL, Chang C, Azuma M, Ruitenberg JJ, Hemperly JJ, Phillips JH (1991) Molecular and functional analysis of human natural killer cell-associated neural cell adhesion molecule (N-CAM/CD56). J Immunol 146:4421–4426
10. Griffin JD, Hercend T, Beveridge R, Schlossman SF (1983) Characterization of an antigen expressed by human natural killer cells. J Immunol 130:2947–2951
11. Ranheim TS, Edelman GM, Cunningham BA (1996) Homophilic adhesion mediated by the neural cell adhesion molecule involves multiple immunoglobulin domains. Proc Natl Acad Sci USA 93:4071–4075
12. Crossin KL, Krushel LA (2000) Cellular signaling by neural cell adhesion molecules of the immunoglobulin superfamily. Dev Dyn 218:260–279
13. Atkins AR, Gallin WJ, Owens GC, Edelman GM, Cunningham BA (2004) Neural cell adhesion molecule (N-CAM) homophilic binding mediated by the two N-terminal Ig domains is influenced by intramolecular domain-domain interactions. J Biol Chem 279:49633–49643
14. Paratcha G, Ledda F, Ibanez CF (2003) The neural cell adhesion molecule NCAM is an alternative signaling receptor for GNDF family ligands. Cell 113:867–879
15. Walsh FS, Doherty P (1997) Neural cell adhesion molecules of the immunoglobulin superfamily: role in axon growth and guidance. Annu Rev Cell Dev Biol 13:425–456
16. Saffell JL, Williams EJ, Mason IJ, Walsh FS, Doherty P (1997) Expression of a dominant negative FGF receptor inhibits axonal growth and FGF receptor phosphorylation stimulated by CAMs. Neuron 18:231–242, Erratum: Neuron 1998; 20:619
17. Francavilla C, Loeffler S, Piccini D, Kren A, Christofori G, Cavallaro U (2007) Neural cell adhesion molecule regulates the cellular response to fibroblast growth factor. J Cell Sci 120:4388–4394
18. Lehembre F, Yilmaz M, Wicki A, Schomber T, Strittmatter K, Ziegler D et al (2008) NCAM-induced focal adhesion assembly: a functional switch upon loss of E-cadherin. EMBO J 27:2603–2615
19. Liu L, Haines S, Shew R, Akeson RA (1993) Axon growth is enhanced by NCAM lacking the VASE exon when expressed in either the growth substrate or the growing axon. J Neurosci Res 15:327–345
20. Chernyshova Y, Leshchyns'ka I, Hsu S-C, Schachner M, Sytnyk V (2011) The neural cell adhesion molecule promotes FGFR-dependent phosphorylation and membrane targeting of the exocyst complex to induce exocytosis in growth cones. J Neurosci 31:3522–3535
21. Pittet MJ, Speiser DE, Valmori D, Cerottini J-C, Romero P (2000) Cutting edge: cytolytic effector function in human circulating CD8+ T cells closely correlates with CD56 surface expression. J Immunol 164:1148–1152
22. Mavilio D, Lombardo G, Benjamin J, Kim D, Follman D, Marcenaro E et al (2005) Characterization of CD56-/CD16+ natural killer (NK) cells: a highly dysfunctional NK subset expanded in HIV-infected viremic individuals. Proc Natl Acad Sci USA 102:2886–2891
23. Ahn JK, Chung H, Lee D, Yu YS, Yu HG (2005) $CD8^{bright}$CD56+ T cells are cytotoxic effectors in patients with active Behcet's uveitis. J Immunol 175:6133–6142
24. Kelly-Rogers J, Madrigal-Estebas L, O'Connor T, Doherty DG (2006) Activation-induced expression of CD56 by T cells is associated with a reprogramming of cytolytic activity and cytokine secretion profile *in vitro*. Human Immunol 67:863–873
25. Chan A, Hong D-L, Atzberger A, Kollnberger S, Filer AD, Buckley CD et al (2007) $CD56^{bright}$ human NK cells differentiate into $CD56^{dim}$ cells: role of contact with peripheral fibroblasts. J Immunol 179:89–94
26. Lemster BH, Michel JJ, Montag DT, Paat JJ, Studenski SA, Newman AB, Vallejo AN (2008) Induction of CD56 and TCR-independent activation of T cells with aging. J Immunol 180:1979–1990
27. Moretta L (2010) Dissecting $CD56^{dim}$ human NK cells. Blood 116:3689–3691

28. Johnson JP (1991) Cell adhesion molecules of the immunoglobulin supergene family and their role in malignant transformation and progression to metastatic disease. Cancer Metastasis Rev 10:11–22
29. Gattenlohner S, Stuhmer T, Leich E, Reinhard M, Etschmann B, Volker HU et al (2009) Specific detection of CD56 (NCAM) isoforms for the identification of aggressive malignant neoplasms with progressive development. Am J Pathol 174:1160–1171
30. Hemperly JJ, Edelman GM, Cunningham BA (1986) cDNA clones of the neural cell adhesion molecule (N-CAM) lacking a membrane-spanning region consistent with evidence for membrane attachment *via* a phosphatidylinositol intermediate. Proc Natl Acad Sci USA 83:9822–9826
31. Reyes AA, Small SJ, Akeson R (1991) At least 27 alternatively spliced forms of the neural cell adhesion molecule mRNA are expressed during rat heart development. Mol Cell Biol 11:1654–1661
32. Small SJ, Akeson R (1990) Expression of the unique NCAM VASE exon is independently regulated in distinct tissues during development. J Cell Biol 111:2089–2096
33. Dickson G, Gower HJ, Barton CH, Prentice HM, Elsom VL, Moore SE et al (1987) Human muscle neural cell adhesion molecule (N-CAM): identification of a muscle-specific sequence in the extracellular domain. Cell 50:1119–1130
34. Barton CH, Dickson G, Gower HJ, Rowett LH, Putt W, Elsom V et al (1988) Complete sequence and *in vitro* expression of a tissue-specific phosphatidylinositol-linked N-CAM isoform from skeletal muscle. Development 104:165–173
35. Gower HJ, Barton CH, Elsom VL, Thompson J, Moore SE, Dickson G, Walsh FS et al (1988) Alternative splicing generates a secreted form of N-CAM in muscle and brain. Cell 55:955–964
36. Murray BA, Owens GC, Prediger EA, Crossin KL, Cunningham BA, Edelman GM (1986) Cell surface modulation of the neural cell adhesion molecule resulting from alternative mRNA splicing in a tissue-specific developmental sequence. J Cell Biol 103:1431–1439
37. Liedtke S, Geyer H, Wuhrer M, Geyer R, Frank G, Gerardy-Schahn R et al (2001) Characterization on N-glycans from mouse brain neural cell adhesion molecule. Glycobiology 11:373–384
38. Ong E, Suzuki M, Belot F, Yeh J-C, Franceschini I, Angata K et al (2002) Biosynthesis of the HNK-1 glycans on O-linked oligosaccharides attached to the neural cell adhesion molecule (NCAM). J Biol Chem 277:18182–18190
39. Albach C, Damoc E, Denzinger T, Schachner M, Przybylski M, Schmitz B (2004) Identification of N-glycosylation sites of the murine neural cell adhesion molecule NCAM by MALDI-TOF and MALDI-FTICR mass spectrometry. Anal Bioanal Chem 378:1129–1135
40. Kleene R, Schachner M (2004) Glycans and neural cell interactions. Nat Rev Neurosci 5:195–08
41. Finne J, Finne U, Deagostini-Bazin H, Goridis C (1983) Occurrence of alpha 2–8 linked polysialosyl units in a neural cell adhesion molecule. Biochem Biophys Res Commun 112:482–487
42. Foley DA, Swartzentruber KG, Lavie A, Colley KJ (2010) Structure and mutagenesis of neural cell adhesion molecule domains: evidence for flexibility in the placement of polysialic acid attachment sites. J Biol Chem 285:27360–27371
43. Hemperly JJ, Murray BA, Edelman GM, Cunningham BA (1986) Sequence of a cDNA clone encoding the polysialic acid-rich and cytoplasmic domains of the neural cell adhesion molecule N-CAM. Proc Natl Acad Sci USA 83:3037–3041
44. Roth J, Zuber C, Wagner P, Taatjes DJ, Weisgerber C, Heitz PU et al (1988) Reexpression of poly(sialic acid) units of the neural cell adhesion molecule in Wilms tumor. Proc Natl Acad Sci USA 85:2999–3003
45. Johnson CP, Fujimoto I, Rutishauser U, Leckband DE (2005) Direct evidence that neural cell adhesion molecule (NCAM) polysialylation increases intermembrane repulsion and abrogates adhesion. J Biol Chem 280:137–145
46. Tassone P, Gozzini A, Goldmacher V, Shammas MA, Whiteman KR, Carrasco DR et al (2004) In vitro and in vivo activity of the maytansinoid immunoconjugate

huN901-N2′-deacetyl-N2′-(3-mercapto-1-oxopropyl)-maytansine against CD56+ multiple myeloma cells. Cancer Res 64:4629–4636
47. Jensen M, Berthold F (2007) Targeting the neural cell adhesion molecule in cancer. Cancer Lett 258:9–21
48. Saito S, Tanio Y, Tachibana I, Hayashi S, Kishimoto T, Kawase I (1994) Complementary DNA sequence encoding the major neural cell adhesion molecule isoform in a human small cell lung cancer cell line. Lung Cancer 10:307–318
49. McNiff JM, Cowper SE, Lazova R, Subtil A, Glusac EJ (2005) CD56 staining in Merkel cell carcinoma and natural killer-cell lymphoma: magic bullet, diagnostic pitfall, or both? J Cutan Pathol 32:541–545
50. Whiteman KR, Murphy MF, Cohane KP, Sun W, Carrigan CN, Mayo MF et al (2008) Preclinical evaluation of IMGN901 (huN901-DM1) as a potential therapeutic for ovarian cancer. Proc Am Assoc Cancer Res 49:Abstr 2135
51. Aletsee-Ufrecht M, Langley K, Rotsch M, Havemann K, Gratzl M (1990) NCAM: a surface marker for human small cell lung cancer cells. FEBS Lett 267:295–300
52. Rygaard K, Moller C, Bock E, Spang-Thomsen M (1992) Expression of cadherin and NCAM in human small cell lung cancer cell lines and xenografts. Br J Cancer 65:573–577
53. Kibbelaar RE, Moolenaar KE, Michalides RJ, Bitter-Suermann D, Addis BJ, Mooi WJ (1989) Expression of the embryonal neural cell adhesion molecule N-CAM in lung carcinoma. Diagnostic usefulness of monoclonal antibody 735 for the distinction between small cell lung cancer and non-small cell lung cancer. J Pathol 159:23–28
54. Zangemeister-Wittke U, Stahel RA (1999) Novel approaches to the treatment of small-cell lung cancer. Cell Mol Life Sci 55:1585–1598
55. Kontogianni K, Nicholson AG, Butcher D, Sheppard MN (2005) CD56: a useful tool for the diagnosis of small cell lung carcinomas on biopsies with extensive crush artifact. J Clin Pathol 58:978–980
56. Moolenaar CE, Pieneman C, Walsh FS, Mooi WJ, Michalides RJ (1992) Alternative splicing of neural-cell-adhesion molecule mRNA in human small-cell lung cancer cell line H69. Int J Cancer 51:238–243
57. Carrigan CN, Xu S, Zhao Y,Testa N, Gabriel R, O'Keefe J et al (2010) The antigen target of lorvotuzumab mertansine (IMGN901), CD56, is expressed at significant levels in Merkel cell carcinoma (MCC). Proc Am Assoc Cancer Res 51:Abstr 5335
58. Daniel L, Bouvier C, Chetaille B, Gouvernet J, Luccioni A, Rossi D et al (2003) Neural cell adhesion molecule expression in renal cell carcinomas: relation to metastatic behavior. Hum Pathol 34:528–532
59. Ikushima S, Yoshihara T, Matsumura T, Misawa S, Morioka Y, Hibi S, Imashuku S (1991) Expression of CD56/NCAM on hematopoietic malignant cells. A useful marker for acute monocytic and megakaryocytic leukemias. Int J Hematol 54:395–403
60. Baer MR, Stewart CC, Lawrence D, Authur DC, Byrd JC, Davey FR et al (1997) Expression of the neural cell adhesion molecule CD56 is associated with short remission duration and survival in acute myeloid leukemia with t(8;21) (q22; q22). Blood 90:1643–1648
61. Lanza F, Bi S, Castoldi G, Goldman JM (1993) Abnormal expression of N-CAM (CD56) adhesion molecule on myeloid and progenitor cells from chronic myeloid leukemia. Leukemia 7:1570–1575
62. Feuillard J, Jacob M-C, Valensi F, Maynadie M, Gressin R, Chaperot L et al (2002) Clinical and biologic features of CD4+ CD56+ malignancies. Blood 99:1556–1563
63. van Camp B, Durie BGM, Spier C, de Waele M, Riet IV, Vela E et al (1990) Plasma cells in multiple myeloma express a natural killer associated antigen CD56 (NKH-1; Leu 10). Blood 76:377–382
64. Kaiser U, Auerbach B, Oldenburg M (1996) The neural cell adhesion molecule NCAM in multiple myeloma. Leuk Lymphoma 20:389–395
65. Amoureux M-C, Coulibaly B, Chinot O, Loundou A, Metellus P, Pougon G, Figarella-Branger D (2010) Polysialic acid neural cell adhesion molecule (PSA-NCAM) is an adverse prognosis factor in glioblastoma, and regulates olig2 expression in glioma cells. BMC Cancer 10:91

66. Froesch BA, Stahel RA, Zangemeister-Wittke U (1996) Preparation and functional evaluation of new doxorubicin immunoconjugates containing an acid-sensitive linker on small-cell lung cancer cells. Cancer Immunol Immunother 42:55–63
67. Blättler WA, Chari RVJ (2001) Drugs to enhance the therapeutic potency of anticancer antibodies: antibody-drug conjugates as tumor-activated prodrugs. In: Ojima I, Vite GD, Altmann K-H (eds) Anticancer agents: frontiers in cancer chemotherapy. ASC Symp Ser 796:317–338
68. Lambert JM (2005) Drug-conjugated monoclonal antibodies for the treatment of cancer. Curr Opin Pharmacol 5:543–549
69. Myklebust AT, Godal A, Fodstad O (1994) Targeted therapy with immunotoxins in a nude rat model for leptomeningeal growth of human small cell lung cancer. Cancer Res 54:2146–2150
70. Zangemeister-Wittke U, Collinson AR, Frosch B, Waibel R, Schenker T, Stahel RA (1994) Immunotoxins recognising a new epitope on the neural cell adhesion molecule have potent cytotoxic effects against small cell lung cancer. Br J Cancer 69:32–39
71. Yu A, Choi J, Ohno K, Levin B, Rom WN, Meruelo D (2000) Specific cell targeting for delivery of toxins into small-cell lung cancer using a streptavidin fusion protein complex. DNA Cell Biol 19:383–388
72. Robertus J (1991) The structure and action of ricin, a cytotoxic N-glycosidase. Semin Cell Biol 2:23–30
73. Krek CE, Ladino CA, Goldmacher VS, Blättler WA, Guild BC (1995) Expression and secretion of a recombinant ricin immunotoxin from murine myeloma cells. Protein Eng 8:481–489
74. Lambert JM, Goldmacher VS, Collinson AR, Nadler LM, Blättler WA (1991) An immunotoxin prepared with blocked ricin: a natural plant toxin adapted for therapeutic use. Cancer Res 51:6236–6242
75. Fidias P, Grossbard M, Lynch TJ Jr (2002) A phase II study of the immunotoxin N901-blocked ricin in small-cell lung cancer. Clin Lung Cancer 3:219–222
76. Lynch TJ Jr, Lambert JM, Coral F, Shefner J, Wen P, Blättler WA, Collinson AR et al (1997) Immunotoxin therapy of small-cell lung cancer: a phase I study of N901-blocked ricin. J Clin Oncol 15:723–734
77. Epstein C, Lynch T, Shefner J, Wen P, Maxted D, Braman V et al (1994) Use of the immunotoxin N901-blocked ricin in patients with small-cell lung cancer. Int J Cancer Suppl 8:57–59
78. Lynch TJ Jr (1993) Immunotoxin therapy of small-cell lung cancer. N901-blocked ricin for relapsed small-cell lung cancer. Chest 103:436S–439S
79. Goldmacher VS, Lambert JM, Blättler WA (1992) The specific cytotoxicity of immunoconjugates containing blocked ricin is dependent on the residual binding capacity of blocked ricin: evidence that the membrane binding and A-chain translocation activities of ricin cannot be separated. Biochem Biophys Res Commun 183:758–766
80. Siegall CB, Liggitt D, Chace D, Mixan B, Sugai J, Davidson T, Steinitz M (1997) Characterization of vascular leak syndrome induced by the toxin component of *Pseudomonas* exotoxin-based immunotoxins and its potential inhibition with nonsteroidal anti-inflammatory drugs. Clin Cancer Res 3:339–345
81. Smallshaw JE, Ghetie V, Rizo J, Fulmer JR, Trahan LL, Ghetie MA, Vitetta ES (2003) Genetic engineering of an immunotoxin to eliminate pulmonary vascular leak in mice. Nat Biotechnol 21:387–391
82. Grossbard ML, Gribben JG, Freedman AS, Lambert JM, Kinsella J, Rabinowe SN et al (1993) Adjuvant immunotoxin therapy with anti-B4-blocked ricin after autologous bone marrow transplantation for patients with B-cell non-Hodgkin's lymphoma. Blood 81:2263–2271
83. Lambert JM (2010) Antibody-maytansinoid conjugates: a new strategy for the treatment of cancer. Drugs Fut 35:471–480
84. Whiteman KR, Xie H, Mayo MF, Audette CA, Steeves RM, Glickman JN et al (2012) Lorvotuzumab mertansine, a CD56-targeting antibody-maytansinoid conjugate with potent antitumor activity against CD56-positive small cell lung cancer models. (submitted for publication)
85. Chari RVJ, Martell BA, Gross JL, Cook SB, Shah SA, Blättler WA et al (1992) Immunoconjugates containing novel maytansinoids: promising anticancer drugs. Cancer Res 52:127–131

86. Roguska MA, Pedersen JT, Keddy CA, Henry AH, Searle SJ, Lambert JM et al (1994) Humanization of murine monoclonal antibodies through variable domain resurfacing. Proc Natl Acad Sci USA 91:969–973
87. Vater CA, Reid K, Bartle LM, Goldmacher VS (1995) Characterization of antibody binding to cell surface antigens using a plasma membrane-bound plate assay. Anal Biochem 224:39–50
88. Roguska MA, Pedersen JT, Henry AH, Searle SMJ, Roja CM, Avery B et al (1996) A comparison of two murine monoclonal antibodies humanized by CDR-grafting and variable domain resurfacing. Protein Eng 9:895–904, Erratum: Protein Eng. 1997; 10:181
89. Chari RVJ, Jackel KA, Bourret LA, Derr SM, Tadayoni BM, Mattocks KM et al (1995) Enhancement of the selectivity and antitumor efficacy of a CC-1065 analogue through immunoconjugate formation. Cancer Res 55:4079–4084
90. Kupchan SM, Komoda Y, Court WA, Thomas GT, Smith RM, Karim A et al (1972) Maytansine, a novel antileukemic ansa macrolide from *Maytenus ovatus*. J Am Chem Soc 94:1354–1356
91. Remillard S, Rebhun LI, Howie GA, Kupchan SM (1975) Antimitotic activity of the potent tumor inhibitor maytansine. Science 189:1002–1005
92. Widdison WC, Wilhelm SD, Cavanagh EE, Whiteman KR, Leece BA, Kovtun Y et al (2006) Semisynthetic maytansine analogues for the targeted treatment of cancer. J Med Chem 49:4392–4408
93. Mandelbaum-Shavit F, Wolpert-DeFilippes MK, Johns DG (1976) Binding of maytansine to rat brain tubulin. Biochem Biophys Res Commun 72(1):47–54
94. Wolpert-DeFilippes MK, Bono VH Jr, Dion RL, Johns DG (1975) Initial studies on maytansine-induced metaphase arrest in L1210 murine leukemia cells. Biochem Pharmacol 24:1735–1738
95. Rao PN, Freireich EJ, Smith ML, Loo TL (1979) Cell cycle phase-specific cytotoxicity of the antitumor agent maytansine. Cancer Res 39:3152–3155
96. Lopus M, Oroudjev E, Wilson L, Wilhelm S, Widdison W, Chari R, Jordan MA (2010) Maytansine and cellular metabolites of antibody-maytansinoid conjugates strongly suppress microtubule dynamics by binding to microtubules. Mol Cancer Ther 9:2689–2699
97. Kellogg BA, Garrett L, Kovtun Y, Lai KC, Leece B, Miller M et al (2011) Disulfide-linked antibody-maytansinoid conjugates: optimization of *in vivo* activity by varying the steric hindrance at carbon atoms adjacent to the disulfide linkage. Bioconjugate Chem 22:717–727
98. Wang L, Amphlett G, Blättler WA, Lambert JM, Zhang W (2005) Structural characterization of the maytansinoid-monoclonal antibody immunoconjugate, huN901-DM1, by mass spectrometry. Protein Sci 14:2436–2446
99. Scherf U, Ross DT, Waltham M, Smith LH, Lee JK, Tanabe L et al (2000) A gene expression database for the molecular pharmacology of cancer. Nat Genet 24:236–244
100. Chari RVJ, Xie H, Steeves RM, Lambert JM (2005) Additive and synergistic effects of combination treatment with huN901-DM1 (BB-10901) and chemotherapeutic agents in small cell lung cancer xenograft tumor models. Proceedings of AACR-NCI-EORTC international conference: molecular targets and cancer therapeutics, p. 70 (Abstr A58)
101. Oroudjev E, Lopus M, Wilson L, Audette C, Provenzano C, Erickson H et al (2010) Maytansinoid-antibody conjugates induce mitotic arrest by suppressing microtubule dynamic instability. Mol Cancer Ther 9:2700–2713
102. Kovtun YV, Goldmacher VS (2007) Cell killing by antibody-drug conjugates. Cancer Lett 255:232–240
103. Minana R, Duran JM, Tomas M, Renau-Piqueras J, Guerri C (2001) Neural cell adhesion molecule is endocytosed *via* a clathrin-dependent pathway. Eur J Neurosci 13:749–756
104. Diestel S, Schaefer D, Cremer H, Schmitz B (2007) NCAM is ubiquitylated, endocytosed and recycled in neurons. J Cell Sci 120:4035–4049
105. Erickson HK, Park PU, Widdison WC, Kovtun YV, Garrett LM, Hoffman K et al (2006) Antibody-maytansinoid conjugates are activated in targeted cancer cells by lysosomal degradation and linker-dependent intracellular processing. Cancer Res 66:4426–4433

106. Erickson HK, Widdison WC, Mayo MF, Whiteman K, Audette C, Wilhelm SD et al (2010) Tumor delivery and *in vivo* processing of disulfide-linked and thioether linked antibody-maytansinoid conjugates. Bioconjug Chem 21:84–92
107. Erickson H, Wilhelm S, Widdison W, Leece B, Sun X, Kovtun Y et al (2008) Evaluation of the cytotoxic potencies of the major maytansinoid metabolites of antibody-maytansinoid conjugates formed in preclinical mouse models. Proc Am Assoc Cancer Res 49:Abstr 2150
108. Sun X, Clancy L, Ellis M, Whiteman KR, Pinkas J, Lazar A, Erickson HK (2011) Lorvotuzumab mertansine displays favorable pharmacokinetics and tumor delivery in mouse models. Proceedings of AACR-NCI-EORTC International Conference: Molecular Targets and Cancer Therapeutics. Mol Cancer Ther 10(Suppl 11):Abstr B195
109. Maloney E, Fishkin N, Audette C, Clancy L, Sun X, Chari R, Singh R (2009) Designing potent antibody-maytansinoid conjugates (AMCs): the impact of lysosomal processing efficiency and conjugate linker selection on anticancer activity. Proceedings of AACR-NCI-EORTC International Conference: Molecular Targets and Cancer Therapeutics. Mol Cancer Ther; 8(Suppl 12):Abstr B120
110. Sun X, Widdison W, Mayo M, Wilhelm S, Leece B, Chari R et al (2011) Design of antibody-maytansinoid conjugates allows for efficient detoxification via liver metabolism. Bioconjug Chem 22:728–735
111. Skaletskaya A, Setiady YY, Park PU, Lutz RJ (2011) Lorvotuzumab mertansine (IMGN901) immune effector activity and its effect on NK cells. Proc Am Assoc Cancer Res 52:Abstr 770
112. Lapusan S, Vidriales MB, Thomas X, de Botton S, Vekhoff A, Tang R et al (2012) Phase I studies of AVE9633, an anti-CD33 antibody-maytansinoid conjugate, in adult patients with relapsed/refractory acute myeloid leukemia. Invest New Drugs 30(3):1121–1131
113. Houghton PJ, Maris JM, Keir ST, Gorlick R, Kolb EA, Kang M et al (2011) Pediatric preclinical testing program (PPTP) stage 1 evaluation of the CD56-targeting antibody-drug conjugate lorvotuzumab mertansine (IMGN901). Proceedings of AACR-NCI-EORTC international conference: molecular targets and cancer therapeutics. Mol Cancer Ther 10 (Suppl 11):Abstr C105
114. Ishitsuka K, Jimi S, Goldmacher VS, Ab O, Tamura K (2008) Targeting CD56 by the maytansinoid immunoconjugate IMGN901 (huN901-DM1): a potential therapeutic modality implication against natural killer/T cell malignancy. Br J Haematol 141:129–131
115. Whiteman KR, Ab O, Bartle LM, Foley K, Goldmacher VS, Lutz RJ (2008) Efficacy of IMGN901 (huN901-DM1) in combination with bortezomib and lenalidomide against multiple myeloma cells in preclinical studies. Proc Am Assoc Cancer Res 49:Abstr 2146
116. Whiteman KR, Johnson HA, Xu Shanqin, Pinkas J and Lutz RJ (2011) Lorvotuzumab mertansine (IMGN901) in combination with standard-of-care paclitaxel/carboplatin therapy is highly active in a preclinical xenograft model of ovarian cancer. Proc Am Assoc Cancer Res 52:Abstr 1781
117. Whiteman KR, Johnson H, Xu S, Moreland J, Vyas V, Bartle LM et al (2009) Combination therapy with IMGN901 and lenalidomide plus low-dose dexamethasone is highly effective in multiple myeloma xenograft models. Proc Am Assoc Cancer Res 50:Abstr 2799
118. Tolcher AW, Forouzesh B, McCreery H, Hammond L, Patnaik A, Lambert J et al (2002) A phase I and pharmacokinetic study of BB-10901, a maytansinoid immunoconjugate, in CD56 expressing tumors. Eur J Cancer 38(Suppl 7):S152–S153, Abstr 509
119. McCann J, Fossella FV, Villalona-Calero MA, Tolcher AW, Fidias P, Raju R et al (2007) Phase II trial of huN901-DM1 in patients with relapsed small cell lung cancer (SCLC) and CD56-positive small cell carcinoma. J Clin Oncol 25(18S):Abstr 18084
120. Fossella F, Woll PJ, Lorigan P, Tolcher A, O'Brien M, O'Keeffe J et al (2009) Clinical experience of IMGN901 (BB-10901) in patients with small cell lung carcinoma. J Thorac Oncol [13th World Conference on Lung Cancer, 2009] 4(Suppl 9):Abstr 6327 (PD 4.3.5)
121. Woll PJ, O'Brien M, Fossella F, Shah M, Clinch Y, O'Keeffe J et al (2010) Phase I study of lorvotuzumab mertansine (IMGN901) in patients with CD56-positive solid tumors. Ann Oncol 21(Suppl 8):Abstr 536P

122. Chanan-Khan A, Wolf J, Garcia J, Gharibo M, Jagannath S, Manfredi D et al (2010) Efficacy analysis from a phase I study of lorvotuzumab mertansine (IMGN901) used as monotherapy in patients with heavily pre-treated CD56-positive multiple myeloma. Blood 116:Abstr 1962
123. Lutz RJ, Whiteman KR (2009) Antibody-maytansinoid conjugates for the treatment of myeloma. mAbs 1:548–551
124. Woll P, Fossella FV, O'Brien MO, Clinch Y, Donaldson K, O'Keeffe J et al (2008) Phase I study of IMGN901 (BB-10901) in patients with CD56-positive solid tumors. EORTC-NCI-AACR international conference: molecular targets and cancer therapeutics (Abstract 510)
125. Berdeja JG, Ailawadhi S, Weitman SD, Zildjian S, O'Leary JJ, O'Keeffe J et al (2011) Phase I study of lorvotuzumab mertansine (LM, IMGN901) in combination with lenalidomide (Len) and dexamethasone (Dex) in patients with CD56-positive relapsed or relapsed/refractory multiple myeloma (MM). J Clin Oncol 29:(Suppl):Abstr 8013
126. Allen PJ, Bowne WB, Jaques DP, Brennan MF, Busam K, Coit DG (2005) Merkel cell carcinoma: prognosis and treatment of patients from a single institution. J Clin Oncol 23:2300–2309
127. Berdeja JG, Ailawadhi MD, Niesvizky R, Wolf JL, Zildjian SH, O'Leary J, Chanan-Khan A (2010) Phase I study of lorvotuzumab mertansine (IMGN901) in combination with lenalidomide and dexamethasone in patients with CD56-positive relapsed or relapsed/refractory multiple myeloma—a preliminary safety and efficacy analysis of the combination. Blood 116:Abstr 1934
128. Van Duijnhoven HL, Helfrich W, de Leij L, Roebroek AJ, van de Ven WJ, Healey K et al (1992) Splicing of the VASE exon of neural cell adhesion molecule (NCAM) in human small-cell lung carcinoma (SCLC). Int J Cancer 50:118–123

Part VI
Metabolism

Chapter 17
Studies on the Metabolism of Antibody–Drug Conjugates

Xiuxia Sun and Hans Erickson

Antibody–drug conjugates (ADCs) are targeted anticancer agents that utilize the specificity of monoclonal antibodies (Ab) to deliver potent cell-killing agents specifically to cancer cells that express the target antigen [1–3]. The two most advanced ADCs brentuximab vedotin (SGN-35, Adcetris®) and trastuzumab emtansine (trastuzumab-DM1, trastuzumab-SMCC-DM1, trastuzumab-MCC-DM1, T-DM1) have shown favorable efficacy and safety in the clinic. SGN-35 recently received accelerated approval from the FDA for the treatment of patients with Hodgkin lymphoma and anaplastic large-cell lymphoma (ALCL) (see Chap. 10) and T-DM1 is in several advanced clinical trials for the treatment of HER2-positive metastatic breast cancer (see Chap. 11).

Both T-DM1 and SGN-35 are armed with highly potent antimitotic cell-killing agents (Fig. 17.1). SGN-35 is comprised of an average of four auristatin molecules (MMAE) linked to the chimeric anti-CD30 IgG1 antibody via a protease-cleavable dipeptide linker, and T-DM1 is comprised of an average of 3.5 maytansinoid molecules (DM1) linked to the HER2-binding antibody, trastuzumab, via a non-reducible thioether linker. SGN-35 and T-DM1 were both found to be active and well tolerated in several preclinical studies. SGN-35 was shown to be highly cytotoxic toward multiple CD30-expressing cancer cells in vitro and in several mouse xenograft models [4–6]. T-DM1 was found to be highly active toward HER2-positive breast carcinoma cancer cells and displayed antitumor efficacy in several trastuzumab- and lapatinib-resistant breast xenograft models [7, 8]. Both conjugates were found to be well tolerated in rodent models at doses much higher than their minimally effective doses in mouse xenograft models [6, 8]. T-DM1 was also found to retain the antibody-dependant cell-mediated cytotoxicity (ADCC) and the inhibitory mechanisms associated with trastuzumab [7].

X. Sun • H. Erickson (✉)
ImmunoGen, Inc., Waltham, MA 02451, USA
e-mail: xiuxia.sun@immunogen.com, hans.erickson@immunogen.com

G.L. Phillips (ed.), *Antibody-Drug Conjugates and Immunotoxins: From Pre-Clinical Development to Therapeutic Applications*, Cancer Drug Discovery and Development, DOI 10.1007/978-1-4614-5456-4_17, © Springer Science+Business Media New York 2013

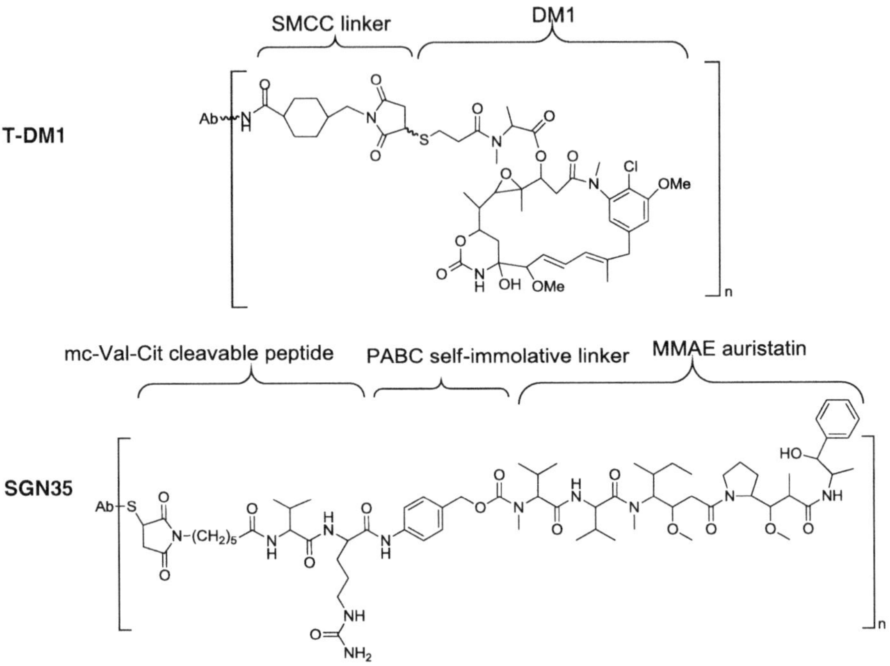

Fig. 17.1 Structures of T-DM1 and SGN-35

Efforts are underway to understand the factors that contribute to the clinical successes of T-DM1 and SGN-35. Maytansinoids and auristatins inhibit tubulin polymerization in vitro, and exposure of cells to low concentrations of each results in rapid arrest in the G2/M phase of the cell cycle. Radioactive and LC/MS-based assays have been developed that can characterize low levels of catabolites [9–13]. Tritium and carbon-14 were incorporated into the DM1 and MMAE portions of T-DM1 and SGN-35, respectively [10, 12, 14]. The radioisotopes were incorporated at stable sites within the molecules where they would not exchange or be readily metabolized Fortunately, maytansinoids and auristatin (MMAE) are highly stable, allowing for their isolation in high yields from organic extracts of cells and tissues.

Activation of T-DM1 In Vitro

Activation of several Ab-SMCC-DM1 conjugates was shown to occur via catabolism of the antibody component within the targeted cancer cells in vitro to yield lysine-SMCC-DM1 [10, 15, 16]. Recently, T-DM1 was specifically shown to be activated by producing the same catabolite (Fig. 17.2) [17]. HER2-positive breast carcinoma cells were exposed in vitro to T-[^{3}H]DM1 for 2–3 h on ice, washed, and then incubated in fresh culture medium. This short exposure format allows for just

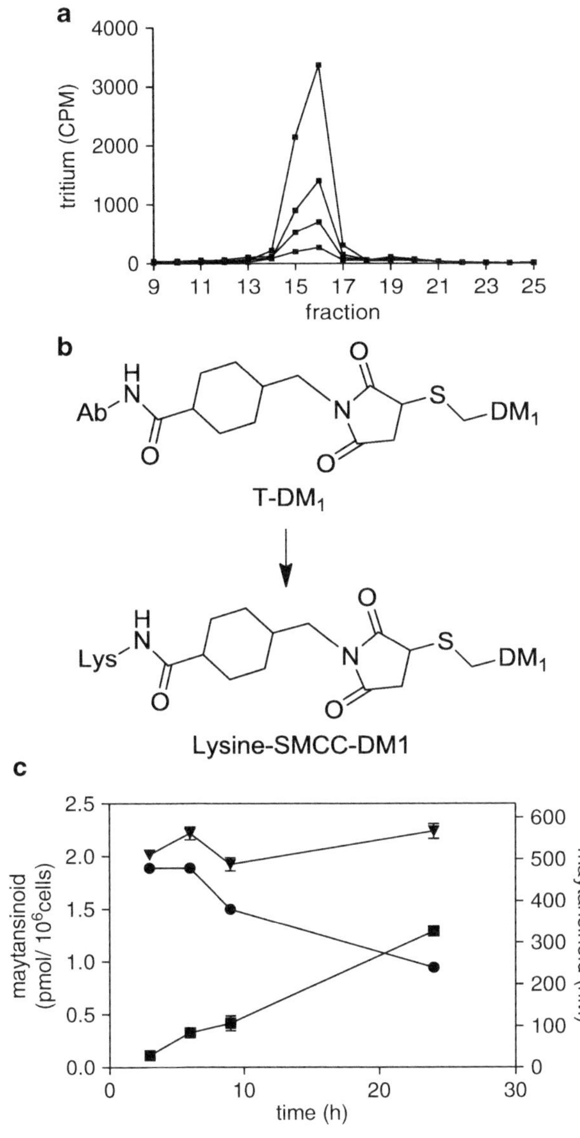

Fig. 17.2 Activation of trastuzumab-DM1 conjugates in HER2-positive breast carcinoma cells BT474EEI. (**a**) HPLC radiograms of the target-cell catabolites following exposure of BT474EEI cells to T-[^{3}H]DM1. Cells were harvested at 3, 6, 9, and 24 h and analyzed for maytansinoids. The chromatograms show the fraction number (abscissa) and the counts per minute (ordinate). (**b**) Scheme for the activation of T-DM1. (**c**) Rates for the catabolism of T-DM1. The concentration lysine-SMCC-DM1 (*filled squares*) was calculated from the radioactivities in A and plotted versus time. The corresponding concentration of intact conjugate still associated with the cells (*filled circles*) was determined from the radioactivity associated with the acetone precipitates. (*filled triangles*) Total maytansinoid levels. Adapted from [17]

a

DMx	In vitro IC_{50} (nM)				
	A375 (mel)	BJAB (B-cell)	COLO205 (colon)	KB (cervix)	MOLT-4 (T-cell)
maytansine	0.05	0.03	0.08	0.05	0.09
lysine-N^{ε}-SMCC-DM1	8	8	17	10	16
S-methyl-DM1	0.02	0.01	0.03	0.02	0.03

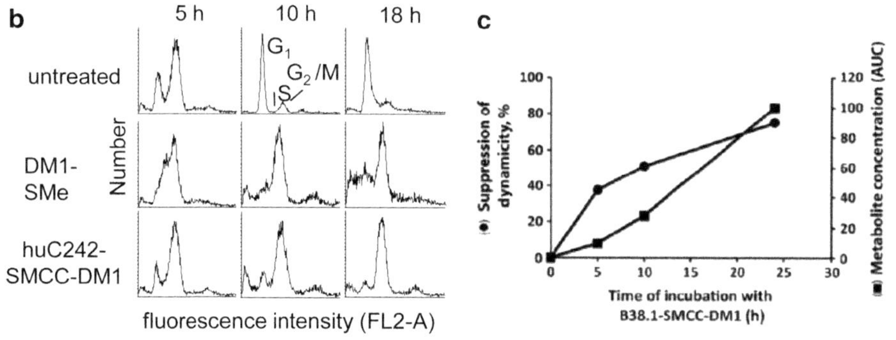

Fig. 17.3 Cytotoxic potency of lysine-SMCC-DM1. (**a**) Cell-killing activities of the maytansinoids were measured after 5 days using a WST-based cell viability assay. Adapted from [34]. (**b**) COLO 205 cells were synchronized in S phase with a 24 h treatment of 2 μg/mL aphidicolin. The cells were released from S phase by the removal of aphidicolin and incubated with 10^{-8} M DM1-SMe (version of DM1 that is stable in culture media), 3×10^{-9} M huC242-SMCC-DM1, or left untreated FACS analysis was performed at 5, 10, and 18 h after aphidicolin release. Adapted from [10]. (**c**) Dynamic instability of microtubules in MCF7 cells following exposure to anti-EpCAM-SMCC-DM1. Cells were exposed to 6.8 nmol/L conjugate (IC_{50} concentration). Time-lapse images of individual microtubules were recorded by epifluorescence microscopy and microtubule ends were tracked over time to determine the dynamic instability of individual microtubules. Lysine-SMCC-DM1 levels (metabolite concentration AUC) were determined using anti-EpCAM-SMCC-[^{3}H]DM1 as described in Fig. 17.2. Adapted from [16]

a single round of antigen-mediated catabolism and provides an accurate measure for the rate of antigen-mediated catabolism [13]. Accumulation of lysine-SMCC-DM1 was observed in several HER2-positive breast cancer cell lines exposed to T-DM1. Catabolism was found to be efficient with about 50% conversion by 19 h in all cell lines tested. Efflux of the lysine-SMCC-DM1 catabolite was observed in cells with high (10^6 antigens/cell) HER2 levels while no efflux could be observed in the BT474EEI cells that have lower (0.25×10^6) HER2 levels [17]. The variable efflux is consistent with the results of a separate study that suggest cellular efflux occurs once a high enough concentration is achieved within the cells to saturate the tubulin-binding sites [11]. The rate for the HER2-mediated lysosomal degradation of ^{125}I-trastuzumab by HER2-positive SKBr3 cells was reported to be similar to the catabolism rate for T-DM1 [18], indicating that conjugation to DM1 does not affect the catabolism kinetics of trastuzumab. This is also consistent with another study that found T-DM1 to retain all the binding and activity properties associated with trastuzumab [7].

Cytotoxic Potency of the Catabolite Derived from T-DM1

Several studies suggest that lysine-SMCC-DM1 is the active catabolite of T-DM1 and other Ab-SMCC-DM1 conjugates. It is the sole catabolite found, and its formation within cancer cells has been found to precede the mitotic arrest of cells in G2/M [10]. In another study, a correlation was observed between the formation of lysine-SMCC-DM1 within EpCAM-positive cancer cells exposed to an anti-EpCAM-SMCC-DM1 conjugate and the suppression of tubulin dynamicity [16]. The lysine-SMCC-DM1 catabolite of T-DM1 displays poor cytotoxic potency (IC_{50} ~7–17 nM) in cell-based viability assays compared to more lipophilic maytansinoids such as maytansine and *S*-methyl-DM1 (Table 17.1). However, this is likely due to its limited cell permeability once released from a cell rather than poor inhibitory activity. Taken together, these studies suggest that lysine-SMCC-DM1 levels may provide a pharmacodynamic marker for T-DM1 activity.

T-DM1 Has No Bystander Killing Activity

Antibody–maytansinoid conjugates prepared with cleavable disulfide linkers, but not the uncleavable thioether linker of SMCC-DM1, were found to display cytotoxic potency toward both antigen-negative and antigen-positive cells when cocultured[15].

Table 17.1 Cytotoxic potencies of maytansinoids toward human carcinoma cell lines in vitro

	In vitro IC_{50} (nM)				
Metabolites	A375 (melanoma)	BJAB (B cell)	COLO205 (colon)	KB (cervix)	MOLT-4 (T cell)
Maytansine	0.045	0.033	0.081	0.047	0.09
Lysine-N^{ε}-SMCC-DM1	8.1	7.5	17	9.7	16
S-methyl-DM1 sulfoxide	9.7	7.1	17	23	19
S-methyl-DM1 sulfone	–	1.7	5.9	3.5	–
S-methyl-DM4 sulfoxide	0.55	0.55	1.3	2.0	1.9
S-methyl-DM4 sulfone	0.075	0.17	0.63	0.80	1.1

All metabolites were chemically synthesized. Cell-killing activities of the metabolites were measured after 5 days using a WST-based cell viability assay. Adapted from [34]

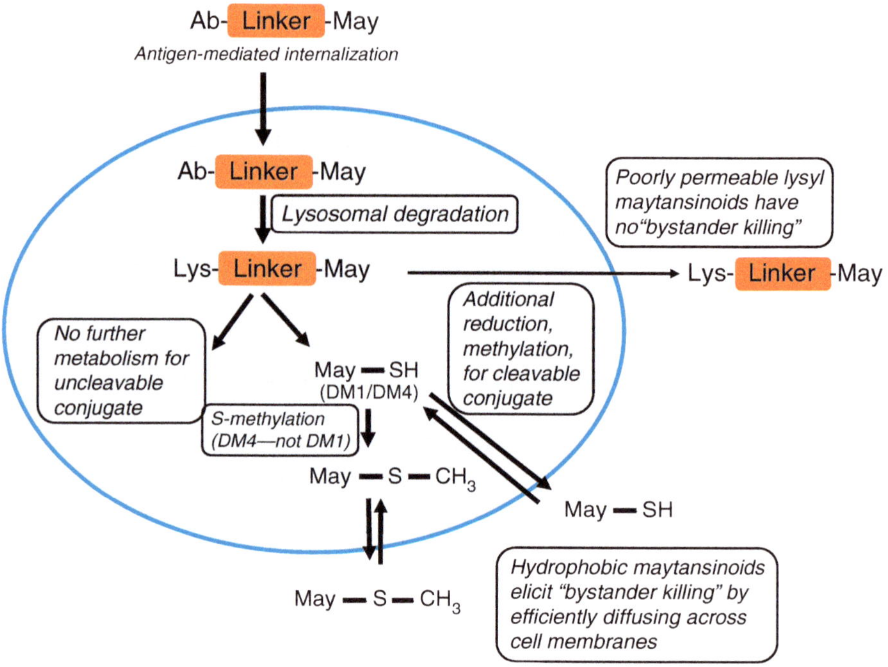

Fig. 17.4 Scheme for the activation and bystander killing of antibody–maytansinoid conjugates. Adapted from [10]

Eradication of the cancer cells that lack the target antigen in the mixture is often referred to as bystander killing. The poor cytotoxic potency of the lysine-SMCC-DM1 catabolite in cell-based assays provides a likely explanation for the lack of bystander killing of antibody–maytansinoid conjugates that utilize uncleavable linkers such as T-DM1 [15, 19]. On the other hand, the generation and subsequent efflux of lipophilic maytansinoid catabolites of the disulfide-linked conjugates provide an explanation for the ability of the disulfide-linked conjugates to eradicate both cell populations (Fig. 17.4) [10]. The identification of these low molecular weight diffusible catabolites in the tumor tissue of mice treated with the disulfide-linked anti-CanAg–maytansinoid conjugates provided additional support for bystander killing mechanisms in solid tumors [11]. Bystander killing mechanisms may overcome the numerous barriers that serve to limit access of antibody-based therapeutics to solid tumor targets [20–22].

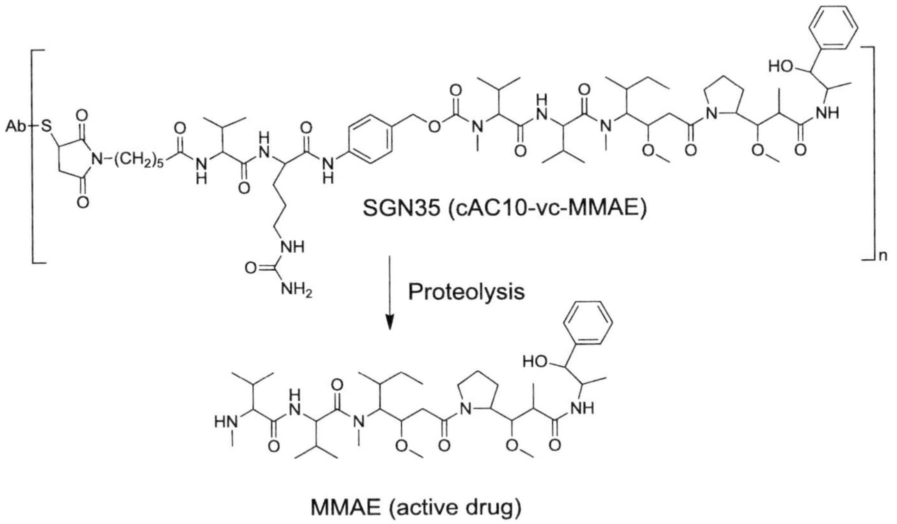

Fig. 17.5 Activation of SGN-35

Activation of SGN-35 In Vitro

MMAE was designed to be released from SGN-35 after cleavage of the amide bond between the citrulline and PABC followed by fragmentation of the PABC spacer. Cell-free studies of SGN-35 [23] and antibody–doxorubicin conjugates utilizing the same linker [24] demonstrated efficient release of the cytotoxic moiety via cleavage of the linker upon treatment with cathepsin B. A short assay format similar to that described for T-DM1 in Fig. 17.2 was used to investigate the activation of ^{14}C-SGN-35 within targeted cancer cells. SGN-35 was found to be converted to MMAE within CD30-positive L540cy Hodgkin lymphoma cells and Karpas299 ALCL cells [16]. The half-life for catabolism of SGN-35 to MMAE was found to be 22 h and 17 h in the L540cy and Karpas299 cells, respectively—similar to the 19 h half-life observed for T-DM1 (Fig. 17.2). Continuous exposure of the CD30-positive cells to SGN-35 resulted in about two- to threefold more MMAE than was observed over the same time frame using the short exposure assays presumably due to new synthesis of CD30 at the cell surface during the course of the incubation [16]. Pretreatment of cells with the lysosomotropic agent chloroquine before exposure to SGN35 greatly diminished the levels of released MMAE, consistent with a MMAE release mechanism that invokes lysosomal cleavage.

SGN-35 Has Bystander Killing

The MMAE catabolite formed within cells exposed to SGN-35 was found to efflux from the cells and accumulate in the medium [12]. Unlike the lysine-SMCC-DM1 catabolite of T-DM1 that has little cytotoxic potency once released from the cell, the MMAE catabolite is cell permeable and able to elicit bystander killing in a manner similar to that described for disulfide-linked antibody–maytansinoid conjugates [15]. The results from an in vitro bystander assay showed effective elimination of antigen-negative Ramos Burkitt's lymphoma cells that were cocultured with CD30-positive cells following treatment of the mixed culture with SGN-35 [12]. Both the CD30-positive cells and Ramos cells are highly sensitive (IC_{50} = 0.04–0.21 nM) to unconjugated MMAE. The observed bystander activity may contribute to the impressive clinical activity of SGN35 in patients with Hodgkin lymphoma where CD30 expression is known to be heterogeneous [12].

ADC Uptake into Solid Tumors

The amount of an antibody that binds to the individual tumor cells in a solid tumor in vivo is limited by several factors such as stromal and epithelial barriers that limit antibody penetration [20, 21, 25]. Antibody localization to tumors varies from 0.003% to 0.008% of the injected dose of antibody per gram (ID/g) of tumor, depending on the tumor type, as measured in human clinical trials [26]. An ID/g of 0.01% reaching the tumor translates to a maximal antibody concentration at the tumor of about 200 nM following an antibody dose of 6 mg/kg. Tumor localization values in a mouse xenograft tend to be in the range of 5–20% ID/g [27, 28] which gives a similar antibody concentration of 50–200 nM in the tumor following a dose of 6 mg/kg. This is a therapeutically efficacious concentration for ADCs like T-DM1 and SGN-35 that exert their cytotoxic effects towards cancer cells in vitro at picomolar concentrations [8, 12]. However, the antibody may not be distributed uniformly within the tumor resulting in areas of very high (lethal) concentrations and areas of low (sublethal) concentrations. Indeed, several studies have reported heterogeneous distribution of the antibody in the tumor tissue at doses in this range [29–31].

Uptake of T-[^{3}H]DM1 and a nonspecific IgG1-SMCC-[^{3}H]-DM1 conjugate was assessed in mouse bearing BT474EEI xenografts following administration of a single bolus i.v. dose of 10 mg/kg (Fig. 17.6) [17]. The total maytansinoid concentration in the tumors (T-DM1 + catabolites) was found to reach a maximum level at about 1–2 days with peak concentration of approximately 9% ID/g (equivalent to 700 nmol/L). The tumor uptake of the nonspecific IgG1-SMCC-[^{3}H]-DM1 conjugate was found to be 2.3-fold lower (3.9% ID/g at 24 h). The concentration of the sole catabolite, lysine-SMCC-DM1, in the tumors was measured and found to steadily increase following administration to a maximal concentration of nearly 150 nM at around 2 day (Fig. 17.7). The concentration of lysine-SMCC-DM1

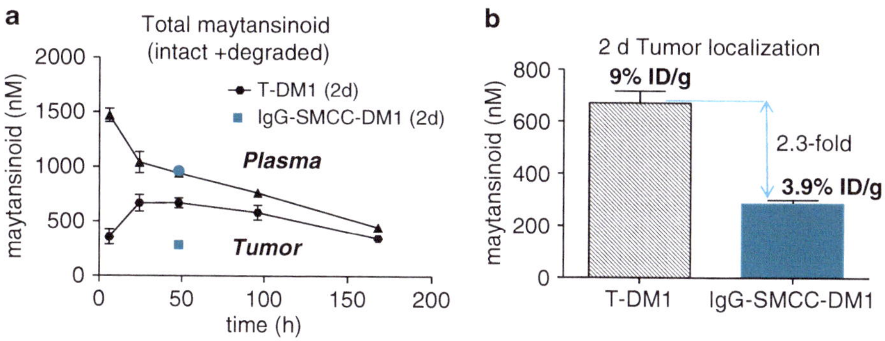

Fig. 17.6 HER2-dependent tumor localization of T-DM1. (**a**) Plasma clearance (*filled triangles*) and accumulation of total maytansinoids (T-DM1 + catabolites) (*filled circles*) following administration of a single i.v. dose of 200 μg/kg (based on DM1 concentration ~10 mg/kg based on Ab concentration) of T-[^{3}H]DM1. Plasma concentration (*filled blue circles*) and total maytansinoid (*filled blue squares*) for non-targeting IgG1-MCC-[^{3}H]DM1 24 h after a single i.v. dose of 200 μg/kg (based on DM1 concentration). Concentrations of conjugate in plasma (DM1 concentration) and total maytansinoid (conjugate + catabolites) in tumor were calculated from the total radioactivity in plasma and tumors samples, respectively. (**b**) The 24 h maytansinoid concentrations at the tumor from (**a**). Adapted from [17]

achieved at the tumor was only twofold lower than the concentration observed in the cells exposed to T-DM1 in vitro shown in Fig. 17.2, suggesting very high tumor delivery and activation of T-DM1 [17]. The concentration of lysine-SMCC-DM1 in the tumors of the mice treated with the IgG-SMCC-DM1 control was fivefold lower. The higher ratio observed for the catabolite levels compared to the total maytansinoid levels shown in Fig. 17.6B reflects an additional targeting benefit that improves the specificity window between the targeting and non-targeting ADCs. Consistent with these findings is the lack of antitumor activity in xenograft mouse models for non-targeting IgG-SMCC-DM1 conjugates [8].

The uptake values for T-DM1 shown in Fig. 17.6 agree well with another study that reported values ranging from 9% ID/g to 23% ID/g for radiolabeled trastuzumab (^{111}In-DTPA-trastuzumab) and 2.7–8.6% for a nonbinding ^{111}In-DTPA-mIgG in several HER2-positive mouse xenograft models [28]. The wide variability in the nonspecific IgG uptake led to a poor correlation between the uptake of trastuzumab and HER2 density. However, when the uptake values of trastuzumab were divided by the values for the nonspecific IgG and replotted versus the antigen density, a strong correlation was observed (Fig. 17.8). The study highlights two important points. First, significant levels of antibody are taken up by tumors irrespective of specific antigen binding. Second, as reported elsewhere [27], large increases in the level of the target antigen result in only modest increases in tumor uptake.

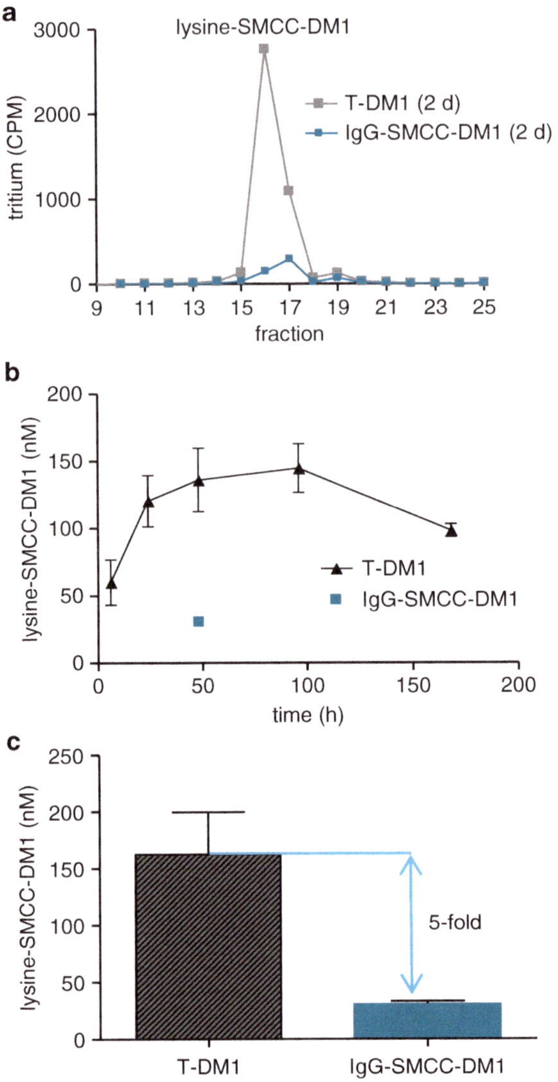

Fig. 17.7 HER2-dependent tumor activation of T-DM1 to lysine-SMCC-DM1. (**a**) HPLC radiograms associated with the 2 d tumor catabolites of T-[^{3}H]DM1 (*filled gray squares*) and non-targeting IgG1-SMCC-[^{3}H]DM1(*filled blue squares*). The radiograms show the fraction number (abscissa) and counts per minute of tritium (*CPM*) (ordinate). (**b**) Concentrations lysine-SMCC-DM1 in the tumor tissue was calculated from the peaks of radioactivity in the radiograms like those shown in (**a**) and tumor weights. (**c**) The concentration of lysine-SMCC-DM1 in the tumors at 24 h from (**a**). Adapted from [17]

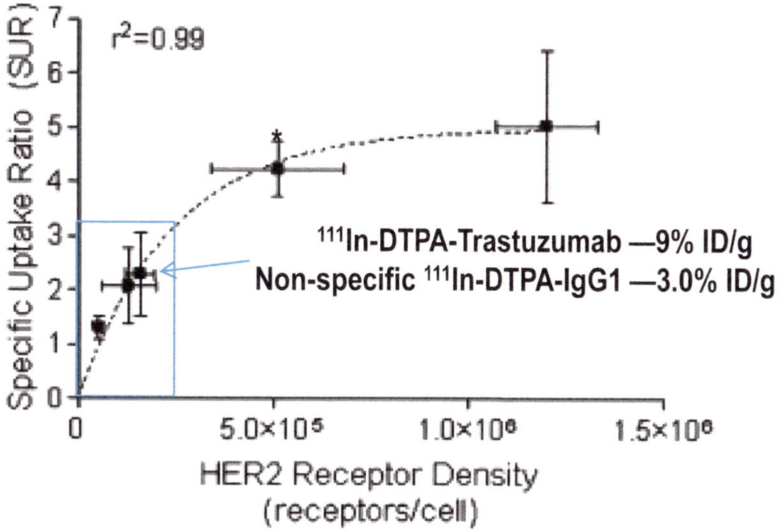

Fig. 17.8 Uptake of ^{111}In-DTPA-trastuzumb and non-targeting ^{111}In-DTPA-IgG1 in a panel of breast cancer xenografts at 72 h post injection. Five breast xenograft models in athymic mice with varying HER2 expression were evaluated for tumor uptake. Groups of three to four mice received a single i.v. dose of 10 μg ^{111}In-DTPA-trastuzumb or non-targeting ^{111}In-DTPA-IgG. Mice were sacrificed, and the tumors were collected, weighed, and counted for radioactivity in a γ-counter. Tumor uptake is expressed as a specific uptake ratio (*SUR*) defined as the uptake (%ID/g) of ^{111}In-DTPA-trastuzumab divided by the non-targeting ^{111}In-DTPA-IgG. For illustration, the arrow points to the data for one of the models where the uptake of ^{111}In-DTPA-trastuzumab was 9.0% and non-targeting ^{111}In-DTPA was 3.9% to give a SUR of 2.3. Adapted from [28]

Impact of Linker on the Tumor Uptake and Catabolism of T-DM1

During the preclinical development of T-DM1, several disulfide-linked trastuzumab–maytansinoid conjugates were found to exhibit similar activity to T-DM1 in mouse xenograft models (Fig. 17.9, [8]). The trastuzumab-SMCC-DM1 was found to be better tolerated in rats and display better pharmacokinetics than the trastuzumab-SPP-DM1 disulfide-linked conjugate tested. Given its superior therapeutic window and favorable pharmacokinetics, trastuzumab-SMCC-DM1 (trastuzumab emtansine) was selected for clinical development [8]. To explore the role of the linker on the tumor delivery, the uptake and catabolism of trastuzumab-SPP-DM1 were compared to trastuzumab-SMCC-DM1. As expected from previous reports [8, 19], trastuzumab-SPP-DM1 had a faster plasma clearance than trastuzumab-SMCC-DM1 (Fig. 17.10). As might be expected, slower trastuzumab-SMCC-DM1 clearance translated to higher overall tumor concentrations (conjugate plus catabolites),

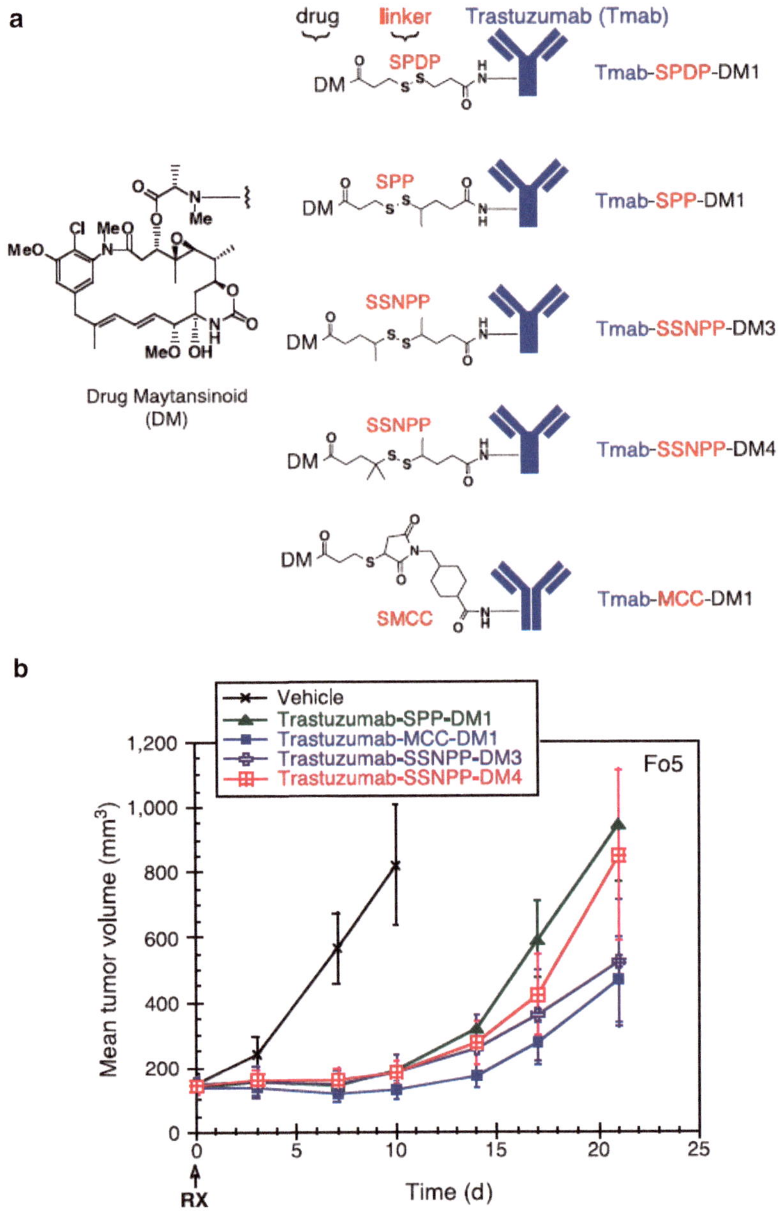

Fig. 17.9 Antitumor activity of 10 mg/kg (based on antibody dose) of trastuzumab–maytansinoid conjugates prepared with SMCC-DM1 and cleavable disulfide-based linkers in mice bearing mammary tumor transplants from the MMTV-HER2 Fo5 line. Adapted from [8]

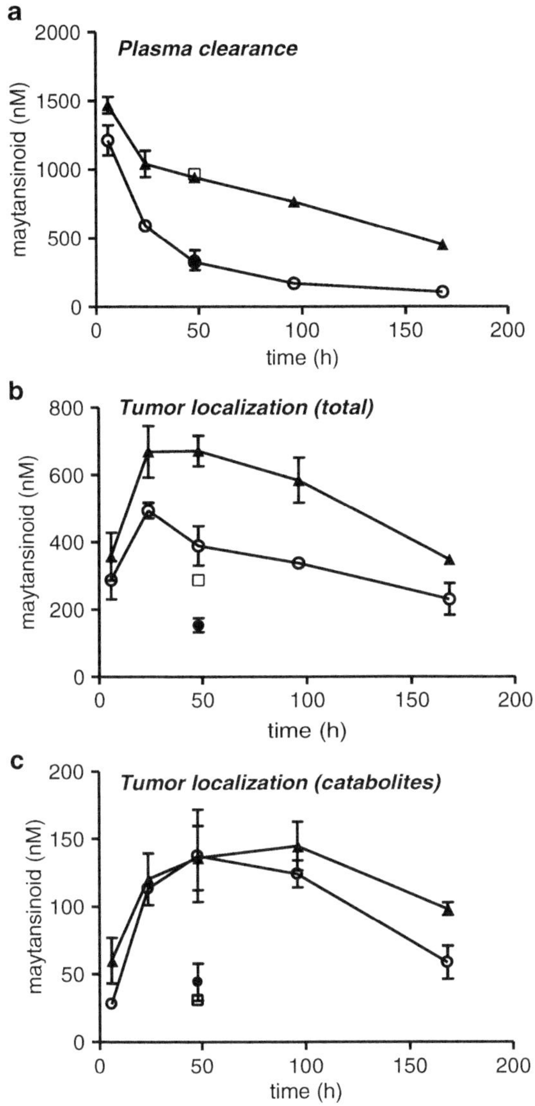

Fig. 17.10 The effect of linker on tumor delivery of trastuzumab-DM1. (**a**) Plasma clearance of conjugate (*top panel*) and accumulation of total maytansinoids (*middle*) and maytansinoid catabolites (*bottom*) in tumors following administration of a single i.v. dose of 200 μg/kg (based on amount of conjugated DM1) of T-[^{3}H]DM1 (*filled triangles*), T-SPP-[^{3}H]DM1 (*open circles*), 5B6-MCC-[^{3}H]DM1 (*open squares*), and 5B6-SPP-[^{3}H]DM1 (*filled circles*) to mice. Concentrations of conjugate in plasma (DM1 dose) and total maytansinoid (conjugate + catabolites) in tumor were calculated from the total radioactivity in plasma and tumors samples, respectively. The maytansinoid catabolite levels in the tumors were determined by the radioactivity associated with HPLC catabolites (lysine-SMCC-DM1 for T-DM1 and lysine-SPP-DM1 + DM1 for T-SPP-DM1). Adapted from [17]

but, unexpectedly, similar levels of tumor catabolite were observed (Fig. 17.8). These results indicate that while these different linkers have clear impact on the PK and the chemical nature of the catabolites formed, both linkers achieve the same active payload delivery to the tumor.

Catabolism and Hepatobiliary Clearance of T-DM1

Most of the administered dose of an antibody-based therapeutic is slowly catabolized by the liver and other tissues of the reticuloendothelial system [32]. In a study in rats, the maytansinoid metabolites of T-DM1 were found to be eliminated predominantly through the feces [33]. Similar studies in mice indicate that the maytansinoid metabolites of disulfide-linked antibody–maytansinoid conjugates are also cleared via hepatobiliary elimination. To investigate the fate during elimination of ADCs that utilize the SMCC-DM1 linker, the liver tissues of CD-1 non-tumor-bearing mice were analyzed for maytansinoid metabolites following a single 15 mg/kg dose of IgG-SMCC-[^{3}H]DM1 [34]. To investigate the role of the linker component, two disulfide-linked ADCs, Ab-SPDB-DM4 and Ab-SPP-DM1, were also evaluated (Fig. 17.11). Shown in Fig. 17.12 are the metabolites isolated from the liver tissues. A stark difference was observed in the complexity of the observed liver metabolites for the three conjugates. Lysine-SMCC-DM1 was the only metabolite of the Ab-SMCC-DM1 conjugate observed, while the two disulfide-linked conjugates had several metabolites observed. No other metabolites of Ab-SMCC-DM1 were detected suggesting little if any metabolic modification of the maytansinoid macrocycle or the thioether linker indicating that lysine-SMCC-DM1 resists chemical alteration in the hepatocytes during clearance. An additional minor peak was identified as N2′-[3-[[1-[[4-(carboxy)cyclohexyl]methyl]-2,5-dioxo-3-pyrrolidinyl]thio]-1-oxopropyl]-N2′-deacetylmaytansine (MCC-DM1, 22.5 min, M+Na=997.4)—an unconjugated maytansinoid species present at low levels in the pre-administration conjugate preparation (less than 5% of the total maytansinoid in the conjugate sample).

The corresponding lysine-linker-maytansinoid species were also observed in the liver extracts of mice treated with the disulfide-linked conjugates. The additional observed metabolites suggest a degradation path for the conjugates shown in Fig. 17.13c where initial lysosomal degradation in the liver and the rest of the tissues of the reticuloendothelial system yields the corresponding lysine-linker-maytansinoid. These disulfide-linked species are further cleaved to yield the corresponding free maytansinoid thiols which in turn are *S*-methylated. All catabolites are ultimately eliminated through the liver where the *S*-methyl-maytansinoid catabolites are oxidized to the corresponding *S*-methyl sulfoxide and *S*-methyl-sulfone metabolites. These oxidized metabolites were found to have relatively low cytotoxic potency in cell-based viability assays (Table 17.1). Efficient *S*-methylation

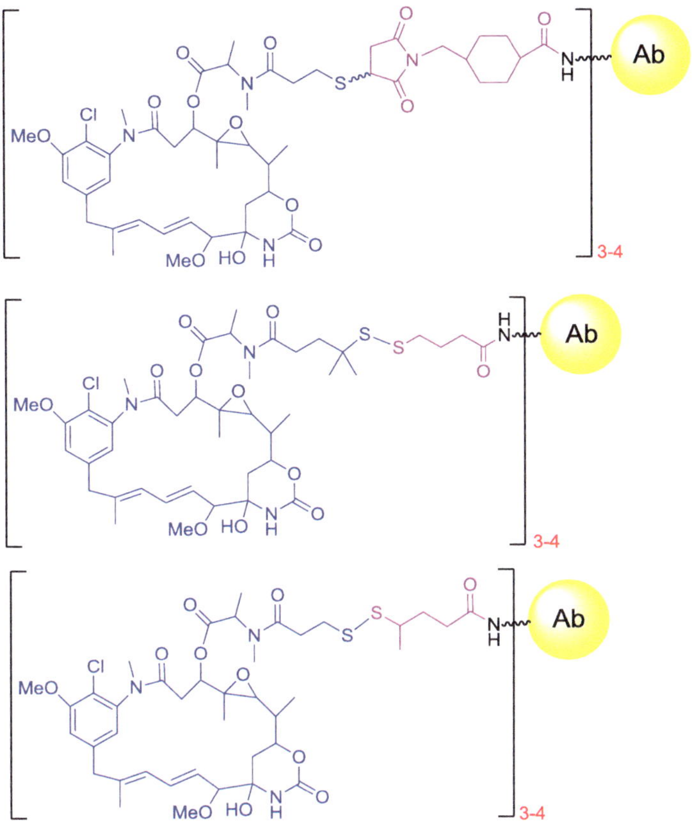

Fig. 17.11 Structural representation of antibody–maytansinoid conjugates evaluated for catabolism and metabolism studies in mice

and oxidation of the catabolites occurs in the liver prior to elimination [34]. Conversion of the antibody–maytansinoid conjugates to their corresponding lower potency metabolites may be important in minimizing GI distress in patients. Severe gastrointestinal toxicity was observed in patients treated with maytansine itself, the "parent" cytotoxic agent of DM1 [35]. However, no significant gastrointestinal toxicity has been observed in patients treated with T-DM1 or disulfide-linked conjugates [2, 36–43]. This is possibly explained by the relatively lower cytotoxic potency of their expected catabolites and metabolites compared to the potency of maytansine (Table 17.1).

Mild and reversible elevation of liver enzymes and minimal degeneration of hepatocytes in both rats and monkeys were noted at high doses of T-DM1 in preclinical studies [7, 8]. The lysine-SMCC-DM1 metabolite that is cytotoxic to cancer

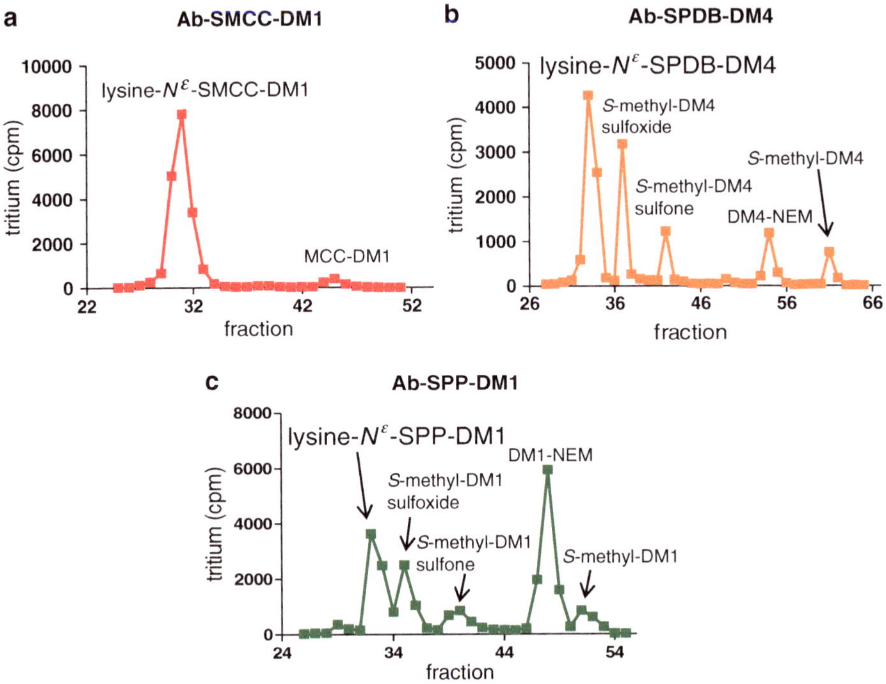

Fig. 17.12 Maytansinoid metabolites of cleavable and uncleavable [^{3}H]AMCs formed in liver. Mice were treated with a single 300 μg/kg dose (based on amount of conjugated DM1 or DM4) of mAb-SMCC-[^{3}H]DM1, mAb-SPP-[^{3}H]DM1, or mAb-SPDB-[^{3}H]DM4 and two mice from each group were sacrificed after 2 h, 6 h, 1 d, 4 d, and 7 d and liver tissues samples were collected. Liver tissues were homogenized and portions of the homogenates were extracted and analyzed for ^{3}H-maytansinoid metabolites by HPLC. The chromatograms show the fraction number on the abscissa and the counts per minute of tritium (*CPM*) on the ordinate. (**a**) The sole metabolite of the uncleavable conjugate is lysine-SMCC-DM1. (**b**) The five metabolites for mAb-SPP-DM1 are lysine-SPP-DM1, DM1, *S*-methyl-DM1, *S*-methyl-DM1 sulfoxide, and *S*-methyl-DM1 sulfone. (**c**) The corresponding five metabolites of mAb-SPDB-DM4 are lysine-SPDB-DM4, DM4, *S*-methyl-DM4, *S*-methyl-DM4 sulfoxide, and *S*-methyl-DM4 sulfone. Catabolites were identified by LC/MS. Adapted from [34]

cells where it is produced following intracellular degradation of T-DM1 may possibly be cytotoxic to liver cells during catabolism and clearance of T-DM1. Thrombocytopenia was the dose-limiting toxicity in patients treated with T-DM1 with only minor increases in liver enzymes observed [36]. These observations suggest that the exposure of liver tissue to lysine-SMCC-DM1 does not induce clinically significant liver toxicity at doses expected to be efficacious [8, 36]. One possible reason is mature, fully differentiated, nondividing cells of organs such as liver may be able to tolerate significant exposure to antimitotic agents.

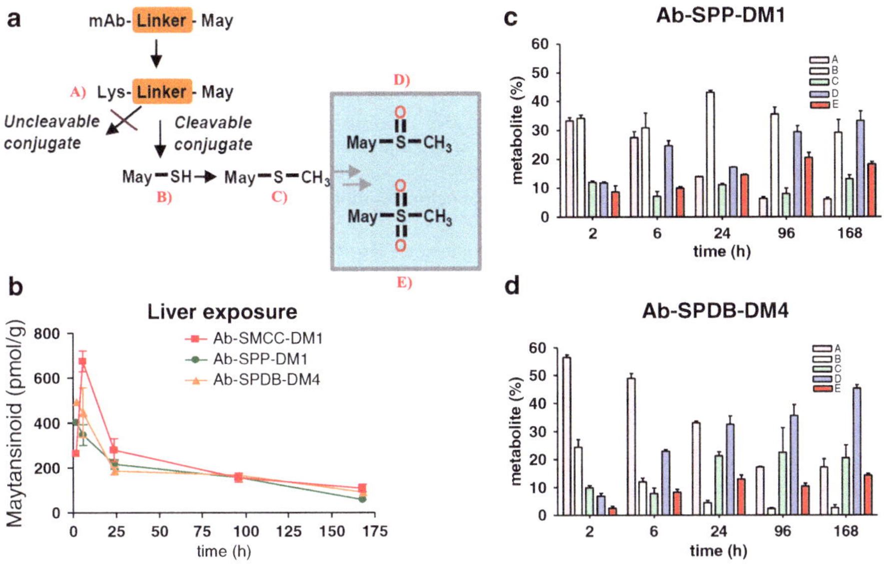

Fig. 17.13 Degradation and elimination of antibody–maytansinoid conjugates. (**a**) Initial catabolism of both cleavable and uncleavable conjugates yields the corresponding lysine-linker-maytansinoid (May) metabolites. For Ab-SMCC-DM1, lysine-SMCC-DM1 is the only observed catabolite. For the cleavable disulfide-linked conjugates Ab-SPDB-DM4 and Ab-SPP-DM1, additional reduction yields DM4 and DM1, respectively. These free maytansinoid thiols are then methylated by an endogenous *S*-methyltransferase to form *S*-methyl-DM1 and *S*-methyl-DM4. Subsequent oxidation steps yield the corresponding sulfoxide and sulfone metabolites. (**b**) The levels for the total maytansinoid metabolites in liver tissue for mAb-SMCC-[^{3}H]DM1 (*filled red squares*), mAb-SPP-[^{3}H]DM1 (*filled green circles*), and mAb-SPDB-[^{3}H]DM4 (*filled yellow triangles*). The radioactivities associated with the metabolites in Fig. 17.12 were converted to pmol/g of metabolite using the specific radioactivities of the DM1 and DM4 and the measured liver weights. (**c**) Amounts of the five observed metabolites of the disulfide-linked conjugates at each time as percentages of total metabolite levels. The percentages for each of the five metabolites of the two disulfide-linked conjugates were calculated by dividing the amount of each metabolite (pmol/g) by the sum of the five metabolites. (**a**–**c**) Adapted from [34]

Conclusions

Optimizations of several parameters have markedly improved the efficacy and tolerability of ADCs in preclinical models. These parameters include the target antigen, the choice of linker chemistry, the nature and potency of the cytotoxic agent, the number of cytotoxic agents linked, and the sites of conjugation [1, 2, 6, 44, 45]. Promising clinical data with T-DM1 and SGN-35 suggests that these improvements are translating to the clinic successes. Understanding how the various parameters contribute to the clinical success of these ADC may allow for further improvements to ADC technologies. The studies provide the first steps. Additional catabolism studies probing the influence of individual parameters on efficacy and safety of T-DM1 and SGN-35 should shed further light on the anatomy of an ideal ADC.

References

1. Chari RV (2008) Targeted cancer therapy: conferring specificity to cytotoxic drugs. Acc Chem Res 41:98–107
2. Lambert JM (2010) Antibody-maytansinoid conjugates: a new strategy for the treatment of cancer. Drugs Fut 35(6):471–480
3. Lambert JM (2005) Drug-conjugated monoclonal antibodies for the treatment of cancer. Curr Opin Pharmacol 5:543–549
4. Doronina SO, Toki BE, Torgov MY, Mendelsohn BA, Cerveny CG, Chace DF, DeBlanc RL, Gearing RP, Bovee TD, Siegall CB, Francisco JA, Wahl AF, Meyer DL, Senter PD (2003) Development of potent monoclonal antibody auristatin conjugates for cancer therapy. Nat Biotechnol 21:778–784
5. Francisco JA, Cerveny CG, Meyer DL, Mixan BJ, Klussman K, Chace DF, Rejniak SX, Gordon KA, DeBlanc R, Toki BE, Law CL, Doronina SO, Siegall CB, Senter PD, Wahl AF (2003) cAC10-vcMMAE, an anti-CD30-monomethyl auristatin E conjugate with potent and selective antitumor activity. Blood 102:1458–1465
6. Hamblett KJ, Senter PD, Chace DF, Sun MM, Lenox J, Cerveny CG, Kissler KM, Bernhardt SX, Kopcha AK, Zabinski RF, Meyer DL, Francisco JA (2004) Effects of drug loading on the antitumor activity of a monoclonal antibody drug conjugate. Clin Cancer Res 10:7063–7070
7. Junttila TT, Li G, Parsons K, Phillips GL, Sliwkowski MX (2011) Trastuzumab-DM1 (T-DM1) retains all the mechanisms of action of trastuzumab and efficiently inhibits growth of lapatinib insensitive breast cancer. Breast Cancer Res Treat 128:347–356
8. Lewis Phillips GD, Li G, Dugger DL, Crocker LM, Parsons KL, Mai E, Blattler WA, Lambert JM, Chari RV, Lutz RJ, Wong WL, Jacobson FS, Koeppen H, Schwall RH, Kenkare-Mitra SR, Spencer SD, Sliwkowski MX (2008) Targeting HER2-positive breast cancer with trastuzumab-DM1, an antibody-cytotoxic drug conjugate. Cancer Res 68:9280–9290
9. Alley SC, Zhang X, Okeley NM, Anderson M, Law CL, Senter PD, Benjamin DR (2009) The pharmacologic basis for antibody-auristatin conjugate activity. J Pharmacol Exp Ther 330:932–938
10. Erickson HK, Park PU, Widdison WC, Kovtun YV, Garrett LM, Hoffman K, Lutz RJ, Goldmacher VS, Blattler WA (2006) Antibody-maytansinoid conjugates are activated in targeted cancer cells by lysosomal degradation and linker-dependent intracellular processing. Cancer Res 66:4426–4433
11. Erickson HK, Widdison WC, Mayo MF, Whiteman K, Audette C, Wilhelm SD, Singh R (2010) Tumor delivery and in vivo processing of disulfide-linked and thioether-linked antibody-maytansinoid conjugates. Bioconjug Chem 21:84–92
12. Okeley NM, Miyamoto JB, Zhang X, Sanderson RJ, Benjamin DR, Sievers EL, Senter PD, Alley SC (2010) Intracellular activation of SGN-35, a potent anti-CD30 antibody-drug conjugate. Clin Cancer Res 16:888–897
13. Singh R, Erickson HK (2009) Antibody-cytotoxic agent conjugates: preparation and characterization. Methods Mol Biol 525:445–467, xiv
14. Xie H, Audette C, Hoffee M, Lambert JM, Blattler WA (2004) Pharmacokinetics and biodistribution of the antitumor immunoconjugate, cantuzumab mertansine (huC242-DM1), and its two components in mice. J Pharmacol Exp Ther 308:1073–1082
15. Kovtun YV, Audette CA, Ye Y, Xie H, Ruberti MF, Phinney SJ, Leece BA, Chittenden T, Blattler WA, Goldmacher VS (2006) Antibody-drug conjugates designed to eradicate tumors with homogeneous and heterogeneous expression of the target antigen. Cancer Res 66:3214–3221
16. Oroudjev E, Lopus M, Wilson L, Audette C, Provenzano C, Erickson H, Kovtun Y, Chari R, Jordan MA (2010) Maytansinoid-antibody conjugates induce mitotic arrest by suppressing microtubule dynamic instability. Mol Cancer Ther 9(10):2700–2713
17. Erickson HK, Lewis Phillips GD, Leipold DD, Provenzuno CA, Mai E, Johnson HA, Gunter B, Audette CA, Gupta M, Pinkas J, Tibbitts J (2012) The effect of different likners on target cell catabolism and pharmacokinetics/pharmacodynamics of transtuzuman maytansinoid consdgates. Mol Cancer Ther 11:1133–1142

18. Austin CD, De Maziere AM, Pisacane PI, van Dijk SM, Eigenbrot C, Sliwkowski MX, Klumperman J, Scheller RH (2004) Endocytosis and sorting of ErbB2 and the site of action of cancer therapeutics trastuzumab and geldanamycin. Mol Biol Cell 15:5268–5282
19. Kellogg BA, Garrett L, Kovtun Y, Lai KC, Leece B, Miller M, Payne G, Steeves R, Whiteman KR, Widdison W, Xie H, Singh R, Chari RV, Lambert JM, Lutz RJ (2011) Disulfide-linked antibody-maytansinoid conjugates: optimization of in vivo activity by varying the steric hindrance at carbon atoms adjacent to the disulfide linkage. Bioconjug Chem 22:717–727
20. Jain RK (1999) Transport of molecules, particles, and cells in solid tumors. Annu Rev Biomed Eng 1:241–263
21. Thurber GM, Schmidt MM, Wittrup KD (2008) Antibody tumor penetration: transport opposed by systemic and antigen-mediated clearance. Adv Drug Deliv Rev 60:1421–1434
22. Beckman RA, Weiner LM, Davis HM (2007) Antibody constructs in cancer therapy: protein engineering strategies to improve exposure in solid tumors. Cancer 109:170–179
23. Sutherland MS, Sanderson RJ, Gordon KA, Andreyka J, Cerveny CG, Yu C, Lewis TS, Meyer DL, Zabinski RF, Doronina SO, Senter PD, Law CL, Wahl AF (2006) Lysosomal trafficking and cysteine protease metabolism confer target-specific cytotoxicity by peptide-linked anti-CD30-auristatin conjugates. J Biol Chem 281:10540–10547
24. Dubowchik GM, Radia S, Mastalerz H, Walker MA, Firestone RA, Dalton King H, Hofstead SJ, Willner D, Lasch SJ, Trail PA (2002) Doxorubicin immunoconjugates containing bivalent, lysosomally-cleavable dipeptide linkages. Bioorg Med Chem Lett 12:1529–1532
25. Christiansen J, Rajasekaran AK (2004) Biological impediments to monoclonal antibody-based cancer immunotherapy. Mol Cancer Ther 3:1493–1501
26. Sedlacek H-H, Seemann G, Hoffmann D, Czech J, Lorenz P, Kolar C, Bosslet K (1992) Antibodies as carriers of cytotoxicity, vol. 43. Karger, Marburg
27. Cai W, Ebrahimnejad A, Chen K, Cao Q, Li ZB, Tice DA, Chen X (2007) Quantitative radioimmunoPET imaging of EphA2 in tumor-bearing mice. Eur J Nucl Med Mol Imaging 34:2024–2036
28. McLarty K, Cornelissen B, Scollard DA, Done SJ, Chun K, Reilly RM (2009) Associations between the uptake of 111In-DTPA-trastuzumab, HER2 density and response to trastuzumab (Herceptin) in athymic mice bearing subcutaneous human tumour xenografts. Eur J Nucl Med Mol Imaging 36:81–93
29. Juweid M, Neumann R, Paik C, Perez-Bacete MJ, Sato J, van Osdol W, Weinstein JN (1992) Micropharmacology of monoclonal antibodies in solid tumors: direct experimental evidence for a binding site barrier. Cancer Res 52:5144–5153
30. Blumenthal RD, Fand I, Sharkey RM, Boerman OC, Kashi R, Goldenberg DM (1991) The effect of antibody protein dose on the uniformity of tumor distribution of radioantibodies: an autoradiographic study. Cancer Immunol Immunother 33:351–358
31. Baker JH, Lindquist KE, Huxham LA, Kyle AH, Sy JT, Minchinton AI (2008) Direct visualization of heterogeneous extravascular distribution of trastuzumab in human epidermal growth factor receptor type 2 overexpressing xenografts. Clin Cancer Res 14:2171–2179
32. Wright A, Sato Y, Okada T, Chang K, Endo T, Morrison S (2000) In vivo trafficking and catabolism of IgG1 antibodies with Fc associated carbohydrates of differing structure. Glycobiology 10:1347–1355
33. Shen BQ, Bumbaca D, Saad O, Yue Q, Pastuskora CV, Khojasteh SC, Tibbitts J, Kaur S, Wang B, Chu YW, Lorusso PM, Girish S (2012) Catabolic fate and Pharmacokinetic Characterization of transtuzoman emtansine (T-DM1): an emphasison preclinical and clinical catabolism. Curr Drug Metab 13:901–910
34. Sun X, Widdison W, Mayo M, Wilhelm S, Leece B, Chari R, Singh R, Erickson H (2011) Design of antibody-maytansinoid conjugates allows for efficient detoxification via liver metabolism. Bioconjug Chem 22:728–735
35. Issell BF, Crooke ST (1978) Maytansine. Cancer Treat Rev 5:199–207
36. Krop IE, Beeram M, Modi S, Jones SF, Holden SN, Yu W, Girish S, Tibbitts J, Yi JH, Sliwkowski MX, Jacobson F, Lutzker SG, Burris HA (2010) Phase I study of trastuzumab-DM1, an HER2 antibody-drug conjugate, given every 3 weeks to patients with HER2-positive metastatic breast cancer. J Clin Oncol 28:2698–2704

37. Chanan-Khan A, Jagannath S, Heffner T, Avigan D, Lee K, Lutz RJ, Haeder T, Ruehle M, Uherek C, Wartenberg-Demand A et al (2009) Phase I Study of BT062 given as repeated single dose once every 3 weeks in patients with relapsed or relapsed/refractory multiple myeloma. Blood (Ash Annual Meeting Abstracts) (abstract 1862)
38. Chanan-Khan A, Wolf J, Gharibo M, Jagannath S, Munshi N, Anderson K, DePaolo D, Lee K, Miller KC, Guild R et al (2009) Phase 1 Study of IMGN901, used as a monotherapy, in patients with heavily pre-treated CD56-positive multiple myeloma. A preliminary safety and efficacy analysis. Blood (Ash Annual Meeting Abstracts) (abstract 2283)
39. Fossella F, Woll PJ, Lorigan P, Tolcher A, O'Brien M, O'Keeffe J, Zildjian S, Qin A, O'Leary J, Villalona-Calero M (2009) Investigation of IMGN901 in CD56+ solid tumors: results from a phase I/II trial (study 001) and a phase I trial (study 002). 13th World Conference on Lung Cancer
40. Smith SV (2005) Technology evaluation: huN901-DM1, ImmunoGen. Curr Opin Mol Ther 7:394–401
41. Tolcher AW, Ochoa L, Hammond LA, Patnaik A, Edwards T, Takimoto C, Smith L, de Bono J, Schwartz G, Mays T, Jonak ZL, Johnson R, DeWitte M, Martino H, Audette C, Maes K, Chari RV, Lambert JM, Rowinsky EK (2003) Cantuzumab mertansine, a maytansinoid immunoconjugate directed to the CanAg antigen: a phase I, pharmacokinetic, and biologic correlative study. J Clin Oncol 21:211–222
42. Younes A, Bartlett NL, Leonard JP, Kennedy DA, Lynch C, Sievers EL, Forero-Torres A (2010) Brentutimah vedotin (S6N-35) for relapsed CD-30 positive lymphomas. N Engl J Med 363:1812–1821
43. Younes A, Kim S, Romaguera J, Copeland A, deCastro Farial S, Kwak LW, Fayad L, Hagemeister F, Fanale M, Neelapu S et al (2012) Phase I Multidose–escalation study of the Anti–CDIT Maytansinoid immunoconjugate SAR3419 administered by intravenous infusion every 3 weeks to patients with relapsed/refractory B-cell lymphomn. J Clin Oncol 22:2776–2782
44. Junutula JR, Raab H, Clark S, Bhakta S, Leipold DD, Weir S, Chen Y, Simpson M, Tsai SP, Dennis MS, Lu Y, Meng YG, Ng C, Yang J, Lee CC, Duenas E, Gorrell J, Katta V, Kim A, McDorman K, Flagella K, Venook R, Ross S, Spencer SD, Lee Wong W, Lowman HB, Vandlen R, Sliwkowski MX, Scheller RH, Polakis P, Mallet W (2008) Site-specific conjugation of a cytotoxic drug to an antibody improves the therapeutic index. Nat Biotechnol 26:925–932
45. Senter PD (2009) Potent antibody drug conjugates for cancer therapy. Curr Opin Chem Biol 13:235–244

Part VII
Immunotoxins

Chapter 18
Design, Development, and Characterization of Recombinant Immunotoxins Targeting HER2/neu

Yu Cao and Michael G. Rosenblum

Background

The human epidermal growth factor receptor 2 (HER2), also known as ErbB2, c-erbB2, or HER2/neu, was initially discovered in 1985 by two independent laboratories [1, 2]. HER2/neu is a 185 kDa (1,255 aa) transmembrane receptor encompassing an intracellular tyrosine kinase domain and an extracellular ligand binding component [3–5]. Extensive clinical studies have shown that overexpression of HER2/neu is found in 20–40% of patients with breast, ovarian, endometrial, gastric, bladder, prostate, and lung cancers. Studies clearly demonstrate that HER2/neu overexpression correlates with the prevalence of metastatic spread of many tumors and is generally considered to be a poor prognostic indicator [6–9].

Since HER2/neu overexpression by tumor cells is quite specific, therapies directed against this receptor have rapidly gained recognition for their selectivity and efficacy in the clinical setting. While targeting of HER2/neu with humanized antibodies such as trastuzumab (Herceptin; Genentech) has proven to be an effective approach for the treatment of HER2/neu-overexpressing breast cancers, there are a significant number of patients with HER2/neu-positive tumors who do not respond or who acquire resistance to this therapy [10–13]. Therefore, there is a need for novel therapeutic approaches using HER2/neu not only as a target for interfering with the growth factor signaling component but also for receptor-mediated delivery of cytotoxic agents.

Immunotoxins are a novel approach for the development of highly specific, targeted agents and which generally employ a powerful class of protein toxins [14, 15]. These include plant toxins such as ricin [16–25], saporin [26–29], and gelonin [30–32], which inactivate ribosomes, and single-chain bacterial toxins

Y. Cao • M.G. Rosenblum (✉)
Immunopharmacology and Targeted Therapy Laboratory, Department of Experimental Therapeutics, MD Anderson Cancer Center, Houston, TX 77030, USA
e-mail: mrosenbl@mdanderson.org

G.L. Phillips (ed.), *Antibody-Drug Conjugates and Immunotoxins: From Pre-Clinical Development to Therapeutic Applications*, Cancer Drug Discovery and Development, DOI 10.1007/978-1-4614-5456-4_18, © Springer Science+Business Media New York 2013

Diphtheria toxin (DT) [33] and *Pseudomonas* exotoxin (PE) [34–43], which ADP ribosylate elongation factor 2 (EIF2). Anti-HER2/neu immunotoxins have been created initially by chemically conjugating an antibody to a whole protein toxin or, for more selective activity, using a protein toxin devoid of its natural binding domain [19, 23, 30, 44]. Technical advances in antibody engineering now enable us to produce various antibodies or antibody fragments in *Escherichia coli*, and as a result, HER2/neu-specific antibodies and engineered fragments thereof have been developed to deliver various toxins to HER2/neu-positive tumor cells [45–51]. Various anti-HER2/neu immunotoxins which have been developed or are currently under evaluation are described in Table 18.1.

Antibody–Drug Conjugates: Promise and Problems

Antibody-based therapeutics is of growing significance for cancer therapy. To date, two of the most promising strategies to enhance the antitumor activity of antibodies are antibody–drug conjugates (ADCs) and antibodies (or fragments) chemically conjugated or genetically fused to various toxins (immunotoxins).

One successful application of the ADC approach is Trastuzumab–DM1. This is a covalent conjugation of trastuzumab with the maytansinoid DM1—a highly toxic derivative of the antimitotic drug maytansine. The therapeutic potential of Trastuzumab–DM1 has been extensively investigated in both in vitro and in vivo models of trastuzumab sensitive and insensitive breast cancers [52–56]. It has demonstrated remarkable activity in phase I and II studies in which it was given to patients harboring trastuzumab-insensitive breast tumors [57, 58]. Furthermore, several other ADCs using anti-HER2/neu antibodies have been developed and have shown potent antitumor activity [59, 60]. Despite successful reports, it is important to note that this strategy has some limitations. The first is the limited reproducibility of chemical conjugation due to the fact that there are numerous coupling sites on an antibody molecule. Secondly, chemically modified antibodies have demonstrated a greater tendency to aggregate, especially when multiple drug molecules are conjugated to a single antibody. Furthermore, it is challenging to remove remaining unconjugated antibodies from the ADC mixture. Finally, the emergence of multidrug resistance (MDR and MRP) mechanisms in tumors from heavily treated patients may engender cross-resistance to ADCs.

With the development of recombinant DNA technology, anti-HER2/neu immunotoxins composed of antibodies (or fragments) and protein toxins have become a promising alternative approach for HER2/neu-positive tumors. Compared to the ADC approach, one attractive advantage of immunotoxins is that the targeting antibody and antitumor toxin can be produced directly as a single molecule, thus avoiding laborious chemical conjugation steps. In addition, the linkage between the toxin and targeting antibody is identical and exactly defined in a given preparation of recombinant immunotoxin, thereby promoting homogeneity of the final product. Compared with chemical conjugates, genetically engineered immunotoxins

Table. 18.1 Immunotoxins developed for HER2/neu targeted therapy

Toxin source	Toxin	Targeting device	Production	Tumor type
Plant	Gelonin	Humanized anti-HER2 mAb	Chemical conjugation	Ovarian cancer [30]
		Human anti-HER2 scFv	Recombinant protein	Ovarian cancer [31], breast cancer [32]
	Saporin	Murine anti-HER2 mAb	Chemical conjugation	Breast cancer [26, 29], Melanoma [27]
		Murine anti-HER2 mAb	Indirect bridge-linking	Ovarian cancer [28]
	Ricin	Murine anti-HER2 mAb	Chemical conjugation	Breast cancer [17, 20, 21, 23, 24], ovarian cancer [16, 18, 19], gastric cancer [22]
		Murine anti-HER2 Fab′	Chemical conjugation	Lung cancer [25]
Bacteria	Pseudomonas exotoxin	Murine anti-HER2 scFv	Recombinant protein	Ovarian cancer [36, 122], epidermoid cancer [40, 183], prostate cancer [34, 184], lung cancer [185–187], gastric cancer [84, 123, 188–190], schwannoma cancer [191], breast cancer [42, 50, 124]
			Recombinant gene delivery	Gastric cancer [152], ovarian cancer [192]
		Murine anti-HER2 disulfide-stabilized Fv fragments (dsFv)	Recombinant protein	Gastric cancer [38, 43], epidermoid cancer [49], breast cancer [48]
		Murine bivalent anti-HER2 dsFv $(dsFv)_2$	Recombinant protein	Epidermoid cancer [41, 51]
		Murine-bispecific scFv (anti-HER2 and anti-EGFR)	Recombinant protein	Epidermoid cancer [37, 46]
		Humanized anti-HER2 Fab′	Liposome-mediated chemical conjugation	Breast cancer [35, 39, 151]
		Humanized anti-HER2 mAb	Indirect bridge-linking	Epidermoid cancer [40, 193]
	Diptheria toxin	Murine-bispecific scFv (anti-HER2 and anti-EpCAM)	Recombinant protein	Colon cancer [33]
	Staphylococcal enterotoxin	Murine anti-HER2 mAb	Chemical conjugation	Colon cancer [44]
		Human anti-HER2 scFv	Recombinant protein	Breast cancer [47]
	Bacillus Cyt2Aa1 toxin	Human anti-HER2 scFv	Recombinant protein	Breast cancer [45]

can be easily designed to enhance antitumor efficacy. Finally, data suggests that the emergence of MDR cellular protection mechanisms in heavily pretreated patients may not impact cytotoxic effects of immunotoxins.

We have provided general principles for development of anti-HER2/neu immunotoxins, and current strategies to employ these molecules for directed cancer therapy are discussed focusing mainly on design optimization to improve antitumor efficacy and off-target toxicity.

Anti-HER2/neu Immunotoxins

Construction of Recombinant Immunotoxins

HER2/neu-overexpressing cancers are a model of disease for the development of rationally designed targeted therapies. The scientific advances in understanding the role of HER2/neu function, the structural aspects of HER2/neu function, and the signaling partners and circuitry underlying tumorigenic HER2/neu signaling have afforded unique opportunities for rational drug design to target these pathways. The development and application of various HER2/neu-targeted therapies has benefited greatly by a more advanced understanding of HER2/neu function and biology [61, 62].

Overall, strategies to enhance anti-HER2/neu immunotoxin potency include improvements to the affinity and specificity of targeting moiety, identification and incorporation of new and better toxins, reengineering known toxins for reduced immunogenicity, and designing novel linkers between toxins and targeting moieties to optimize toxin translocation to the cytosol [63–66]. Numerous excellent reviews have previously compared the advantages and disadvantages of a variety of cytotoxic proteins including bacterial, plant, and mammalian toxins successfully employed for the construction of immunotoxins [67, 68]. This review will address how linker design and antibody affinity affect immunotoxins in tumor-specific targeted therapies.

Peptide Linker Designs

The development of various linkers which bridge disparate molecules such as small drugs conjugated to tumor-targeting carriers has been the subject of numerous studies for the past few years [69, 70]. Based on numerous prior studies, the incorporation and design of linkers is critical to the success of ADCs. Conceptually, an ideal linker must be stable in systemic circulation, while being efficiently cleaved to allow rapid release of an active form of the drug once the construct has been internalized into the tumor cell target. To this end, a variety of linkers have been designed with different chemical structures and stabilities [71, 72]. Selection of an appropriate linker depends on the type of cancer and the required cytotoxic agent. Furin is a

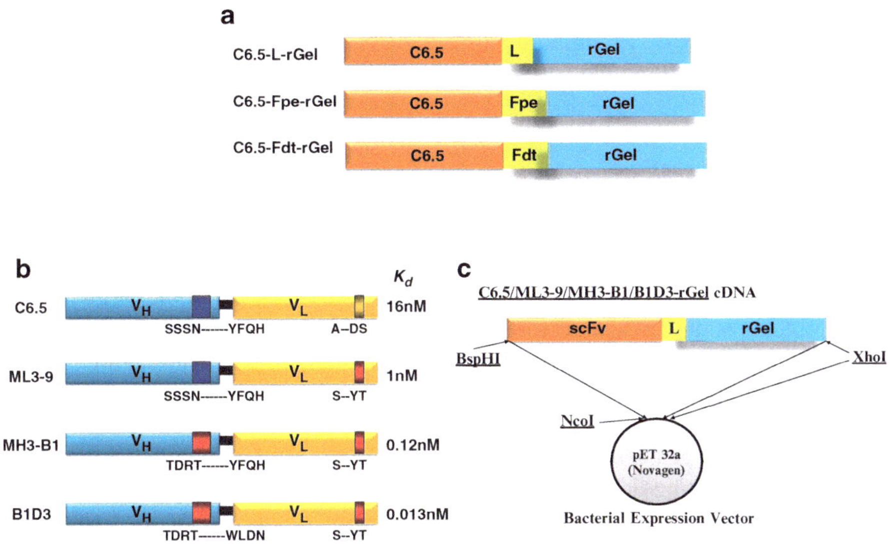

Fig. 18.1 Construction and preparation of scFv/rGel immunotoxins. (**a**) Schematic diagram of immunotoxin constructs containing scFv C6.5, peptide linker (L, Fpe or Fdt), and rGel toxin. (**b**) Amino acid mutations and affinity parameters of the C6.5 and its mutants, ML3-9, MH3-B1, and B1D3. The listed amino acids for each scFv indicate mutations to the sequence and the substituting amino acids. *Dashes* indicate no changes from the original sequence. (**c**) Diagram of immunotoxin constructions containing scFv (C6.5, ML3-9, MH3-B1, or B1D3) and rGel

cellular endoprotease and has been implicated in proteolytically activating large numbers of secreted proteins such as prohormones, growth factors, receptors, and viral glycoproteins. These proteins are synthesized as inactive precursors and must be proteolytically cleaved to become functionally mature. In previous studies, the inclusion of furin-cleavable linkers into fusion constructs containing ribotoxins, caspase3, or granzyme B (GrB) has demonstrated a significant improvement in specific toxicity compared to constructs containing stable linkers [73, 74].

The incorporation of cleavable linkers for immunotoxins is essential since, in general, the toxin components are enzymatically inactive in the construct until intracellular release from their cell-targeting carriers [75, 76]. For recombinant gelonin (rGel)-based constructs, the enzymatic (*N*-glycosidase) activity of the toxin is preserved in the intact fusion constructs, eliminating the absolute necessity for intracellular release of the rGel component. Nevertheless, we explored a variety of different linker strategies to determine whether intentionally cleavable linkers offered an advantage over linkers which were designed for flexibility only. Illustrations of various immunotoxin constructs are shown in Fig. 18.1a. The initial rGel-based immunotoxins consisted of a flexible linker (GGGGS, "L") tethering the C-terminus of the human anti-HER2/neu single-chain antibody (scFv) C6.5 to the native rGel N-terminus. The C6.5/rGel construct was further engineered by incorporating two different enzymatically sensitive furin cleavage linkers between scFv and toxin components. The two furin-sensitive sequences designated "Fpe" (TRHRQPRGWEQL, 12 amino acid residues to PE273-284 sequence) and "Fdt" (AGNRVRRSVG, 10 amino acid residues to DT187-196 sequence), respectively.

Tumor-Targeting scFv

Previous studies identified a recombinant murine anti-HER2/neu scFv designated e23, and fusion constructs containing catalytic toxins such as PE and DT were shown to specifically kill HER2/neu-expressing cells [33, 43]. A major drawback of such proteins is their potential for immune response after repeated administration. Repeated doses may cause hypersensitive reactions and lead to neutralization of the immunotoxins by antibodies directed against the nonhuman domains [77, 78]. The development of immunotoxins containing human or humanized components may circumvent these problems. Such immunotoxins may display reduced immunogenicity although antibodies to the toxin components may still limit prolonged therapy [79, 80]. We previously reported in vitro characterization and in vivo antitumor efficacy studies of an immunotoxin composed of the human chimeric anti-HER2/neu antibody (BACH-250) chemically conjugated to rGel. The BACH-250/rGel conjugate demonstrated potent and specific cytotoxicity against HER2/neu-overexpressing human tumor cells in culture and against ovarian SKOV3 tumor xenografts [30]. However, the potential problems of diffusion of relatively large molecules such as full-length antibodies into solid tumors have been extensively addressed by Jain et al. [81]. The treatment of solid tumors presents a significant challenge since therapeutic antibodies must diffuse into the tumor against a hydrostatic pressure gradient and into disordered vasculature. These theoretical issues may not limit clinical response with antibodies alone since higher applied doses may circumvent these effects [81–83], but it may not be possible to overcome these limitations with higher doses of antibody–drug conjugates or immunotoxins because these agents frequently have a much narrower therapeutic window.

Over the past decade, a variety of different anti-HER2/neu recombinant antibody formats have been engineered which are suitable for diverse therapeutic applications and include monovalent, bivalent, and multivalent derivatives; single- or double-chain formats; and covalently or noncovalently linked assemblies of antibody heavy (V_H) and light chain variable domains (V_L) [84–89]. Among these, human scFv appear to be effective when utilized as targeting domains incorporated into chimeric fusion proteins. They consist of antibody V_H and V_L sequences genetically linked via a flexible linker, and they lack constant regions and Fc domains, thereby preventing possible binding to normal tissues and cells via interaction with Fc receptors. We previously engineered a series of novel fusion proteins created from various human anti-HER2/neu scFv designated C6.5 and various affinity mutants (designated ML3-9, MH3-B1, and B1D3, created by site-directed amino acid substitutions in the CDR3s). The affinities of the scFvs ranged from 10^{-8} to 10^{-11} M (Fig. 18.1b) [90, 91]. Recombinant immunotoxins containing each scFv and rGel were constructed by overlapping PCR and were designated C6.5/rGel, ML3-9/rGel, MH3-B1/rGel, and B1D3/rGel, respectively (Fig. 18.1c).

Functional Activity Analysis of Immunotoxins

Tumor-antigen affinity and specificity of scFvs are important variables which may impact off-target tissue distribution and toxicity in vivo. These attributes have led to the commonly held concept that scFv must have high affinity in order to be therapeutically relevant. However, studies by Adams et al. suggested that high-affinity scFv may be suboptimal vehicles and that lower-affinity scFv appear to diffuse more uniformly throughout the tumor interior [92, 93]. In addition, since the presence of shed tumor antigen has the potential to misdirect the targeted constructs through immune complex formation [64, 94], higher-affinity scFv could potentially be less effective compared to lower-affinity constructs. Therefore, applying a series of rGel-containing fusion constructs composed of various linkers and scFv mutants with varying affinity to HER2/neu, we will examine the impact of construct design on in vitro cytotoxicity, pharmacodynamics, and antitumor efficacy. Further investigations included the effect of antibody affinity on behavior in the presence of soluble antigen, formation of immune complexes, and the coincident development of off-target toxicity.

In Vitro Studies: Impact of Various Design Modifications on In Vitro Immunotoxin Cytotoxic Activity

Effects of Linker Design on Immunotoxin Potency and Functional Stability

Based on C6.5/rGel containing the universal flexible GGGGS linker, we introduced proteolytically cleavable linkers (Fpe and Fdt) and to examine whether this change would improve killing efficiency. To investigate the susceptibility of various chimeric toxins to proteolytic cleavage, purified fusions were subjected to proteolysis with recombinant furin. As indicated in Fig. 18.2a, the Fdt linker was the most sensitive to cleavage among all constructs tested. In contrast, cleavage of the molecule containing the Fpe linker was highly dependent on pH. As expected, the L linker was found to be comparatively resistant to intracellular protease action without regard to the pH.

The intracellular release of rGel after endocytosis of various C6.5/rGel fusion constructs was next assessed in SKOV3 cells (Fig. 18.2b). Although the maximal rGel release of different fusions was achieved at different time points, the absolute amounts of delivered rGel found in the cytosol were virtually identical. Therefore, this data confirms the observation that introduction of an unstable furin cleavage linker does not improve the intracellular rGel release of the constructs.

The linkers tethering the C6.5 scFv and the rGel toxin demonstrated a differential sensitivity to protease action which may result in different clearance and metabolic kinetics in vivo [95, 96]. We next performed a stability study of the constructs in human plasma (Fig. 18.2c, d). The binding activity and cytotoxicity

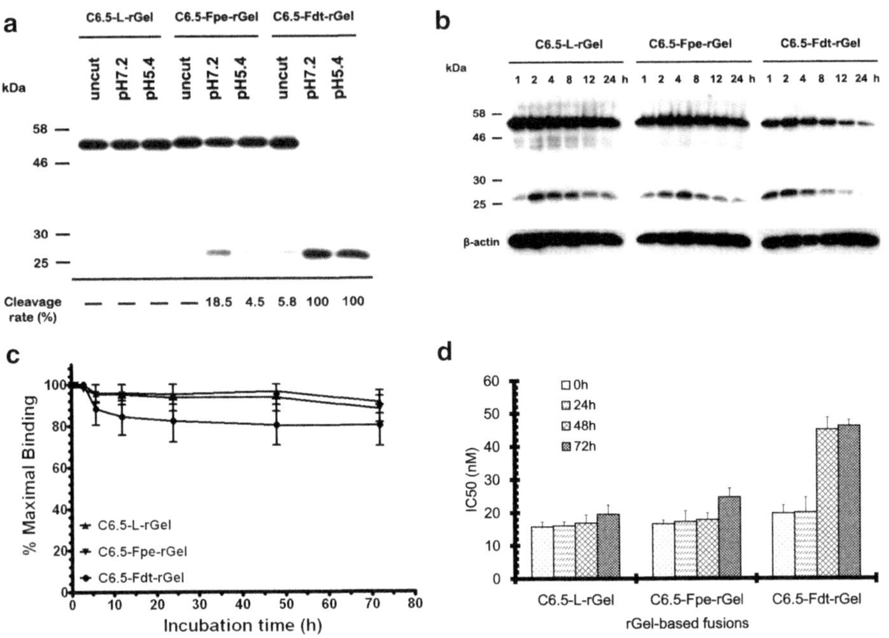

Fig. 18.2 Functional analysis of C6.5/rGel series immunotoxins in vitro. (**a**) Western blot analysis of furin cleavage of purified C6.5/rGel fusion constructs. (**b**) Western blot analysis of intracellular rGel release of C6.5/rGel fusions in SKOV3 cells. (**c**, **d**) Functional stability analysis of the fusions by whole-cell ELISA and cytotoxicity on SKOV3 cells. The proteins were incubated in human plasma at 37 °C for up to 72 h before test

of the C6.5–Fdt–rGel construct was shown to be the least stable after incubation because of the instability of the Fdt linker. On the other hand, of all molecules tested, the C6.5–L–rGel demonstrated the highest degree of stability after plasma incubation. The two companion molecules with the furin-cleavable linkers Fpe or Fdt demonstrated significantly less stability in vitro.

Based on our studies, introduction of a furin-cleavable linker between C6.5 and rGel did not result in improved intracellular rGel release and cytotoxic effects *in vitro*, despite showing more sensitivity to protease cleavage and greater intracellular release of the rGel component. On the other hand, the rGel-based molecules with the furin-cleavable linkers demonstrated significantly less functional stability *in vitro*. The enzymatic stability of the linker can seriously affect the pharmacokinetics of immunotoxins and can apparently impact loss of targeting function and in vivo efficacy. Therefore, we clearly demonstrated the highly individualized nature of some payloads and targeted constructs and that observations regarding rGel may not necessarily translate to other payloads.

The Impact of scFv Affinity on Immunotoxin Activity

Although previous studies suggested that the binding affinity for antigen plays a pivotal role in the total concentration and penetration of scFv into tumors [92, 93], few companion studies have been conducted to determine whether scFv-based immunotoxins display the same behavior with regard to the relationship between affinity, tumor penetration, tumor residence, and efficacy. Therefore, based on the flexible GGGGS linker, we created a series of rGel-based immunotoxins from affinity mutants of the human anti-HER2/neu scFv C6.5.

To ensure that immunotoxins retained antigen binding ability, the fusion proteins were compared in an ELISA-based binding assay using HER2/neu-positive (SKBR3, BT474 M1) and HER2/neu-negative (MCF7) cells. All the scFv/rGel constructs demonstrated specific and significant ELISA binding to HER2/neu-positive cells with negligible binding to negative cells (Fig. 18.3a). The equilibrium dissociation constants (K_d) were calculated, and the affinities of immunotoxins for BT474 M1 cells were found to be 53.13 nM (C6.5/rGel), 1.45 nM (ML3-9/rGel), 0.18 nM (MH3-B1/rGel), and 0.027 nM (B1D3/rGel). The correlation between the K_d values of the scFvs and fusion constructs was found to be significant with a correlation coefficient of 0.939 ($p<0.01$), indicating that introduction of the rGel component did not affect the binding affinity of the scFv.

We next examine the ability of various affinity scFv/rGel fusions to specifically internalize into target cells. Immunofluorescence staining was performed on HER2/neu-positive and HER2/neu-negative cells after exposure to the constructs (Fig. 18.3b). As quantified by relative fluorescence (Fig. 18.3c), the internalization efficiency into HER2/neu-positive cells was shown to increase with increasing antibody affinity. For BT474 M1 cells, the relative fluorescence intensities were 56.30 (C6.5/rGel), 73.69 (ML3-9/rGel), 86.29 (MH3-B1/rGel), and 90.41 (B1D3/rGel). There was a good correlation between increases in apparent affinity and internalization efficiency ($r^2=0.8289$; $p<0.01$), indicating that efficient binding to the cell surface appears to be primarily responsible for rapid internalization after cell exposure.

The cytotoxicity of the various scFv/rGel constructs was then tested against a panel of different tumor cell lines (Table 18.2). As expected, there appeared to be a good correlation ($r^2=0.7812$; $p<0.01$) between apparent affinity and IC_{50} values. The highest targeting indices were found for the highest-affinity construct (B1D3/rGel). Therefore, in vitro, binding affinity appeared to mediate internalization efficiency, and this appeared to directly impact the overall cytotoxic effects observed. Furthermore, against HER2/neu-negative cells, there was little or no specific cytotoxicity of the constructs compared to rGel itself.

Based on scFv/rGel immunotoxins, we demonstrated that increasing affinity could improve cell binding ability, internalization efficiency, and cytotoxic activity on HER2/neu-positive cells. However, fusion toxins with a tenfold increase in affinity did not show a corresponding improvement in either internalization or a concomitant improvement in cytotoxic effects. This suggests that the internalization rate of the construct may primarily be associated with HER2/neu receptor recycling and the rate of antigen endocytosis and this may primarily be unaffected by the

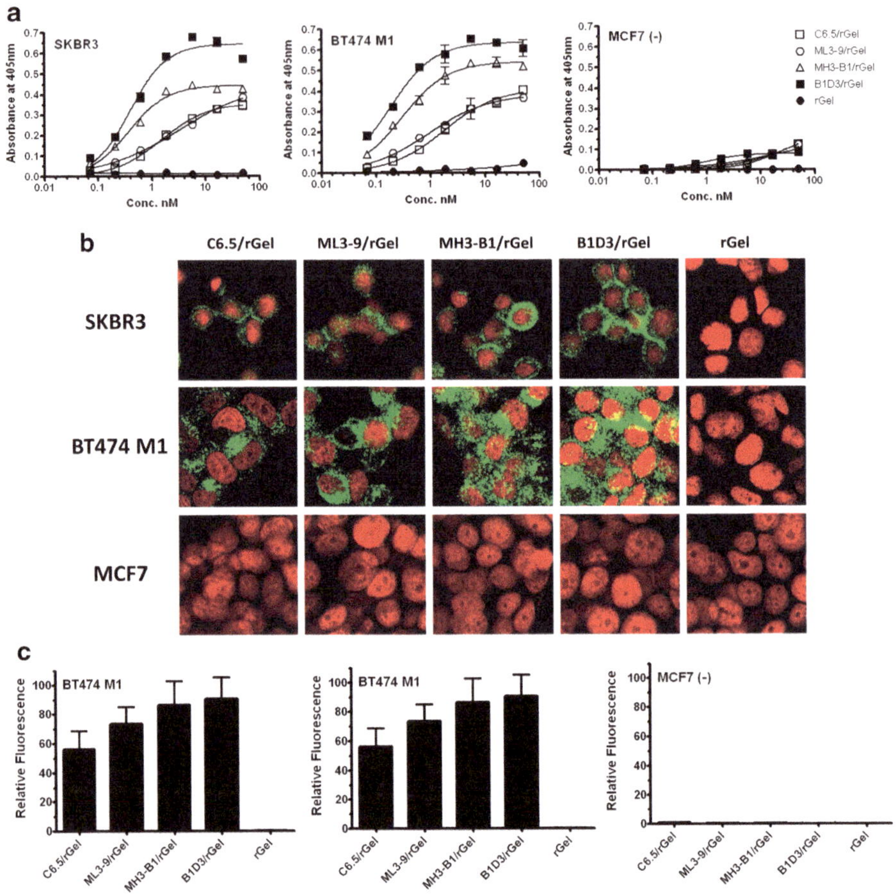

Fig. 18.3 Characterization and comparison of different scFv/rGel immunotoxins. (**a**) Evaluation binding activity of the fusion constructs to HER2/neu-positive (SKBR3 and BT474 M1) and HER2/neu-negative (MCF7) cells by whole-cell ELISA. (**b**) Internalization of the immunotoxins on HER2/neu-positive and HER2/neu-negative cells. Cells were subjected to immunofluorescent staining with anti-rGel antibody (FITC-conjugated secondary), with propidium iodine nuclear counterstaining. (**c**) Quantification of internalization rate of the immunotoxins. The bar graphs were calculated from relative fluorescence estimation, and the values are expressed as mean ± S.D ($n > 50$)

affinity of immunotoxin binding [97, 98]. Moreover, intracellular trafficking and distribution of the toxin component to the ribosomal compartment may be additional critical factors which can define immunotoxin sensitivity [99].

Mechanistic Studies of Immunotoxin Cytotoxic Activity

Studies of bacterial and plant immunotoxins have provided us with essential information regarding intracellular routing and translocation events [100, 101], and this

Table 18.2 Comparative cytotoxicity of rGel-based fusion constructs against various tumor cell lines

Cell line	Tumor type	HER2/neu Expression level	IC_{50} (nM) (TI)* C6.5/rGel	ML3-9/rGel	MH3-B1/rGel	B1D3/rGel	rGel
SKBR3	Breast	****	6.4 (165)	5.0 (211)	2.7 (387)	1.9 (567)	1061
BT474 M1	Breast	****	18.9 (12)	10.9 (20)	3.9 (56)	1.2 (177)	219.8
NCI-N87	Gastric	****	30.1 (32)	20.4 (47)	9.1 (106)	4.9 199)	965.6
Calu3	Lung	****	24.3 (22)	18.1 (29)	13.0 (41)	10.0 (53)	531.1
MDA MB231	Breast	*	145.8 (2)	149.9 (2)	155 (2)	204.8 (1)	297.3
MCF7	Breast	*	246.9 (1)	246.7 (1)	260.6 (1)	266.9 (1)	247.4
A375m	Melanoma	*	61.4 (3)	126.9 (2)	153.9 (1)	173.9 (1)	207.3
Me180	Cervical	*	160.8 (1)	185.4 (1)	194.6 (1)	213.1 (1)	222.5

*Targeting index (TI) represents IC_{50} of rGel/IC_{50} of immunotoxin

information can be employed in the design of optimized constructs. The mechanism of cytotoxicity of anti-HER2/neu immunotoxins generally involves inhibition of cellular protein synthesis, although the point of attack in this pathway can vary slightly depending on the toxin [102, 103].

The plant-derived toxins are primarily ribosome-inactivating proteins (RIPs) and are enzymes which depurinate rRNA, thus inhibiting protein synthesis. They may also depurinate other polynucleotide substrates [104–106]. rGel is an *N*-glycosidase generating cytotoxic effects which are the direct result of protein synthesis inhibition (Fig. 18.4a). Although there have been numerous preclinical studies of rGel-based immunotoxins for the treatment of both solid and hematological tumors, the actual mechanisms behind the induction of cell death appear to vary depending on the cell type targeted [107–109]. This occurs because the basic mechanism of protein synthesis inhibition due to the rGel component causes the loss of different high-turnover proteins in cells derived from different tumor types. This finally results in cytotoxic patterns and mechanisms which can vary widely based on the proteins critical for survival of different cell types targeted.

The cytotoxic effects mediated by our rGel-based immunotoxins were analyzed including apoptosis, necrosis, and autophagy in BT474 M1 cells. As shown in Fig. 18.4b, scFv/rGel fusions did not activate caspase-dependent apoptosis in target cells, showing no cleavage of the caspase substrate PARP. We next assessed lactate dehydrogenase (LDH) release, a marker of abrupt membrane lysis, and found that exposure of BT474 M1 cells to immunotoxins did not induce necrotic cell death using this parameter (Fig. 18.4c).

We next examined whether the cytotoxic effects of these immunotoxins activate autophagic signaling. As shown in Fig. 18.4d, the ratio of LC3-II formation to the β-actin control was shown to be increased after treatment with the fusion constructs, demonstrating that autophagic flux was induced by rGel-based immunotoxins in BT474 M1 cells. In addition, autophagic induction by fusion constructs was further validated by the observed selective release of cellular high mobility group box 1

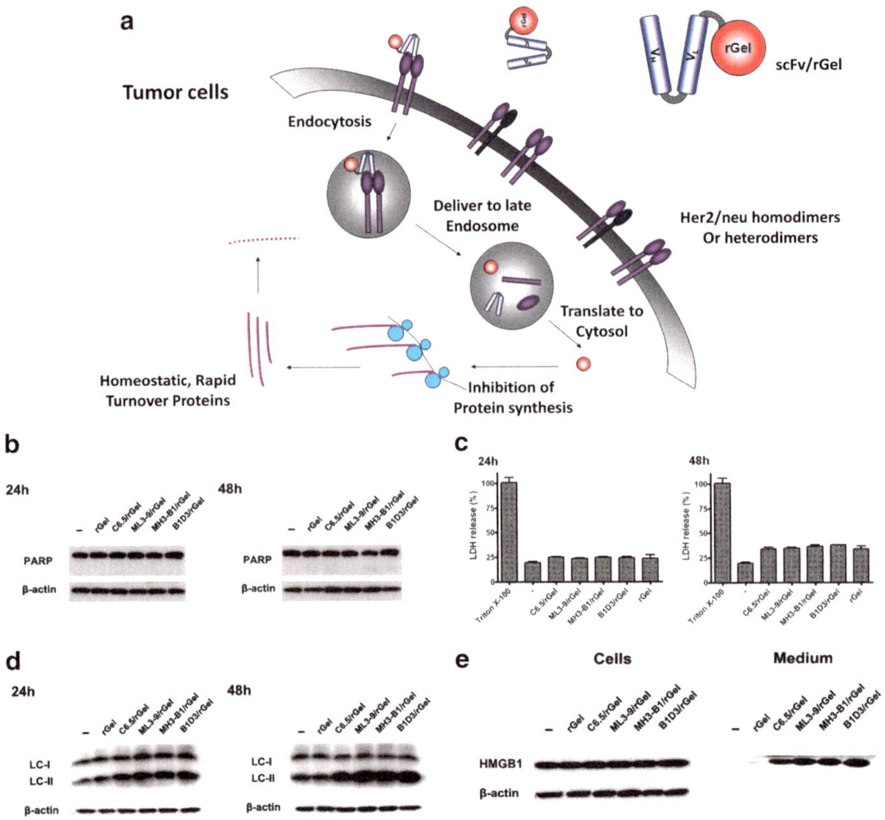

Fig. 18.4 Cell-killing mechanism analysis of the immunotoxins on BT474 M1 cells. (**a**) A generalized view of cytotoxic mechanism of anti-HER2/neu scFv/rGel fusions in targeted cells. (**b**) Western blot analysis of PARP cleavage after 24 and 48 h of scFv/rGel fusions treatment. (**c**) Evaluation of necrosis by LDH release after treatment with fusion proteins or Triton X-100 (mean ± S.D. from three replicates). (**d**) Analysis of LC3 after treated with scFv/rGel fusions for 24 and 48h. (**e**) Analysis of cell extract and medium for HMGB1 protein after immunotoxins treatment for 48 h

(HMGB1) (Fig. 18.4e). Tumor cells undergoing autophagy can selectively release the nuclear high mobility group box 1 (HMGB1) protein without displaying characteristics of necrosis [110]. These data indicated that the observed cytotoxic effects of fusion toxins in BT474 M1 cells appeared to be mediated not through an apoptotic or necrotic mechanisms but by the efficient induction of autophagic cell death.

There are numerous mechanistic connections between apoptosis, necrosis, and autophagy suggesting that the different death mechanisms are intimately related [111, 112]. A spectrum of characteristics can be displayed by a dying cell, and this appears to be regulated, in part, by the amount of autophagy that occurs as cells die. When autophagy is not activated, caspase activation occurs more readily, and dying cells undergo apoptosis. Conversely, when autophagy is high, caspase activation is blocked, but cells destined to die can release HMGB1 without membrane lysis and true necrosis. Thus, characteristics associated with rGel-intoxicated cells may contain elements of multiple cell death mechanisms.

Influence of Soluble HER2/neu Antigen on Immunotoxin Activity

In addition to the characteristics of the targeting moiety, the presence of soluble antigen levels is clearly another factor in the potential therapeutic application of targeted agents [113]. Pharmacokinetic studies of anti-HER2/neu antibodies in patients have demonstrated an inverse association between serum concentrations of antibody and the levels of shed HER2/neu antigen [114, 115]. This observation may be explained, in part, by formation of soluble antigen: antibody complexes leading to a more rapid clearance by the reticuloendothelial system (RES). Clinical studies of Herceptin have shown that HER2/neu plasma concentrations greater than 500 ng/mL (~10 nM) were associated with shorter serum half-life and subtherapeutic trough levels of the antibody [116, 117].

To investigate the impact of soluble antigen on HER2/neu targeted immunotoxins, we evaluated the internalization of the immunotoxins in the presence of added soluble, purified HER2/neu extracellular domain (ECD) in BT474 M1 cells (Fig. 18.5a, b). The addition of ECD was shown to reduce the cellular internalization of all the constructs. The highest-affinity B1D3/rGel construct showed a significant reduction in activity in the presence of antigen, whereas the lower-affinity fusions exhibited a lesser impact of added ECD.

We next utilized a coimmunoprecipitation method to examine whether the decreased cellular internalization observed was due to formation of immune complexes between immunotoxins and ECD. As shown in Fig. 18.5c, the highest-affinity construct (B1D3/rGel) and the lowest-affinity construct (C6.5/rGel) formed the highest and lowest (respectively) amounts of immune complex with added ECD. Intermediate-affinity molecules (ML3-9/rGel and MH3-B1/rGel) generated intermediate levels of immune complexes. Therefore, the reduction in cell internalization observed with the high-affinity B1D3/rGel fusion was the result of immune complex formation with soluble ECD, and this competed for binding and internalization of the immunotoxin to the cell-associated antigen.

A competitive cytotoxicity assay was next performed on SKBR3 and BT474 M1 cells by adding HER2/neu ECD to various concentrations of each fusion construct (Fig. 18.5d). All the fusion constructs showed an increase in IC_{50} in the presence of ECD. Constructs with low and medium affinity showed the least impact of ECD on cytotoxic effects, while high-affinity B1D3/rGel showed the greatest reduction in cytotoxic effects. The addition of various concentration of ECD to a fixed dose of each of the immunotoxins demonstrated similar effects (Fig. 18.5e). The high-affinity B1D3/rGel was impacted to the greatest extent in the presence of ECD, while the constructs with low or medium affinity showed less impact on cytotoxicity. Therefore, immunotoxins with relatively high association constant rate but a lower dissociation rate than other constructs appear to have the greatest propensity to be mis-targeted in the presence of soluble antigens.

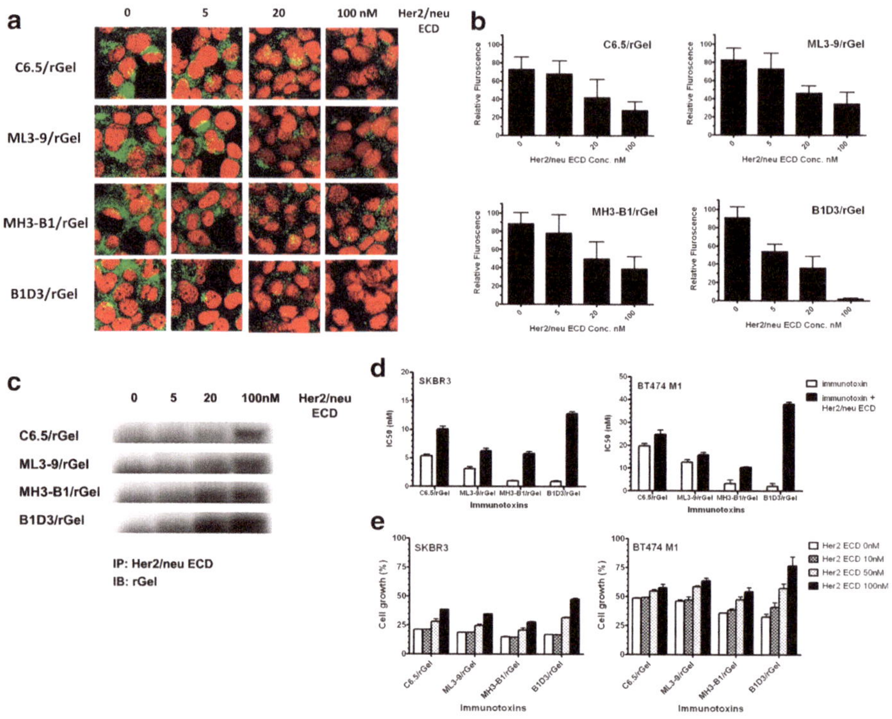

Fig. 18.5 Competitive analysis of the scFv/rGel in the presence of free HER2/neu ECD. (**a**) Competitive internalization assay of 20 nM immunotoxins with different concentration of the HER2/neu ECD on BT474 M1 cells. (**b**) Quantification of competitive internalization rate of the fusion proteins. Values are expressed as mean ± S.D ($n > 50$). (**c**) Coimmunoprecipitation of scFv/rGel and HER2/neu ECD complex. The supernatant was subjected to HER2/neu immunoprecipitation, followed by Western blot for rGel. (**d**) Competitive activity of the immunotoxins in the presence of 20 nM ECD. Values are presented as IC_{50}. (**e**) Competitive cytotoxicity of 20 nM immunotoxins with different concentration of the ECD on HER2/neu-positive cells

In Vivo Studies of Immunotoxins: Antitumor Efficacy and Off-Target Toxicity

Antitumor Activity of scFv/rGel

Antibody-mediated therapy has been much more successful for hematological malignancies than for solid tumors, likely reflecting their overall greater physical accessibility to targeted therapeutics [118, 119]. The treatment of solid tumors presents a much greater challenge since the therapeutic antibodies must diffuse into the tumor against hydrostatic pressure and into a disordered intratumoral vasculature [83]. Low-molecular weight immunotoxins have better diffusion properties and are more successful at penetrating solid tumors [120, 121]. In addition to the properties of the tumor tissue itself and general antibody pharmacology, other relationships also exist between an antibody and its antigen that can shape penetration, catabolism, specificity, and efficacy [92].

Potent antitumor activity in animal models has been described for immunotoxins derived from the murine HER2/neu-specific scFv e23 and FRP5 both fused to the PE toxin [14, 122–124]. These two immunotoxins were studied in phase I clinical trials where the primary toxicity with the e23 construct was hepatotoxicity observed in all the patients. Immunohistochemistry showed the presence of HER2/neu on normal hepatocytes thus explaining the liver toxicity [49, 125]. The immunotoxins targeting HER2/neu may result in unexpected organ toxicities due to expression of low levels of HER2/neu on normal cells. Another HER2/neu immunotoxin designated scFv (FRP5)-ETA was well tolerated by the majority of patients, with adverse reactions mainly restricted to fully reversible symptoms such as pain and inflammation at the injection sites, which might be partly due to differences in administration route [14, 36, 126, 127].

An anti-HER2/neu immunotoxin containing a diabody linked to PE was first described by Pastan et al. [41, 51]. These divalent immunotoxins were found to be ~tenfold more cytotoxic in vitro than their monovalent counterparts but, surprisingly, were only about twofold more active against tumors in vivo. The reasons for this remain unclear, but Pastan et al. suggest that the high functional affinity of the diabodies results in the formation of a binding-site barrier at the tumor periphery which impedes immunotoxin penetration into the tumor mass and suggests that bivalent fusion toxins containing PE may have limited value compared to their monovalent counterparts.

To assess the impact of antibody affinity of immunotoxins we performed *in vivo* efficacy studies using anti-HER2/neu fusion constructs in mice bearing well-established BT474 M1 xenografts. As shown in Fig. 18.6a, treatment with the scFv/rGel fusions all demonstrated antitumor effects after i.v. administration, with the intermediate-affinity MH3-B1/rGel showing more enhanced and long-lasting tumor inhibition effects compared to lower-affinity C6.5/rGel and ML3-9/rGel. Administration of the immunotoxins resulted in little obvious toxicity with the exception of the highest-affinity B1D3/rGel. As shown in Fig. 18.6b, mice treated with this agent showed considerable body weight loss (~27%), and all the mice in this group died after the fourth injection. On-target toxicity, or the toxicity of the construct to liver as a result of expression of HER2/neu on hepatocytes, is a common problem found in clinical studies. However, antibody C6.5 and its mutant scFv do not cross-react with the murine HER2/neu analog [90, 91]. Therefore, the toxicity of the high-affinity B1D3/rGel construct may be associated with mis-targeting through the formation of immune complexes with shed, tumor-derived HER2/neu antigen, leading to significant off-target toxicity.

Off-Target Toxicity of Immunotoxins: Impact of Affinity

The emergence of clinically relevant, nonspecific toxicity has limited the therapeutic potential of numerous immunotoxins [79, 128, 129] and is a significant limitation to the clinical development of this class of molecules in general. Therefore, it is

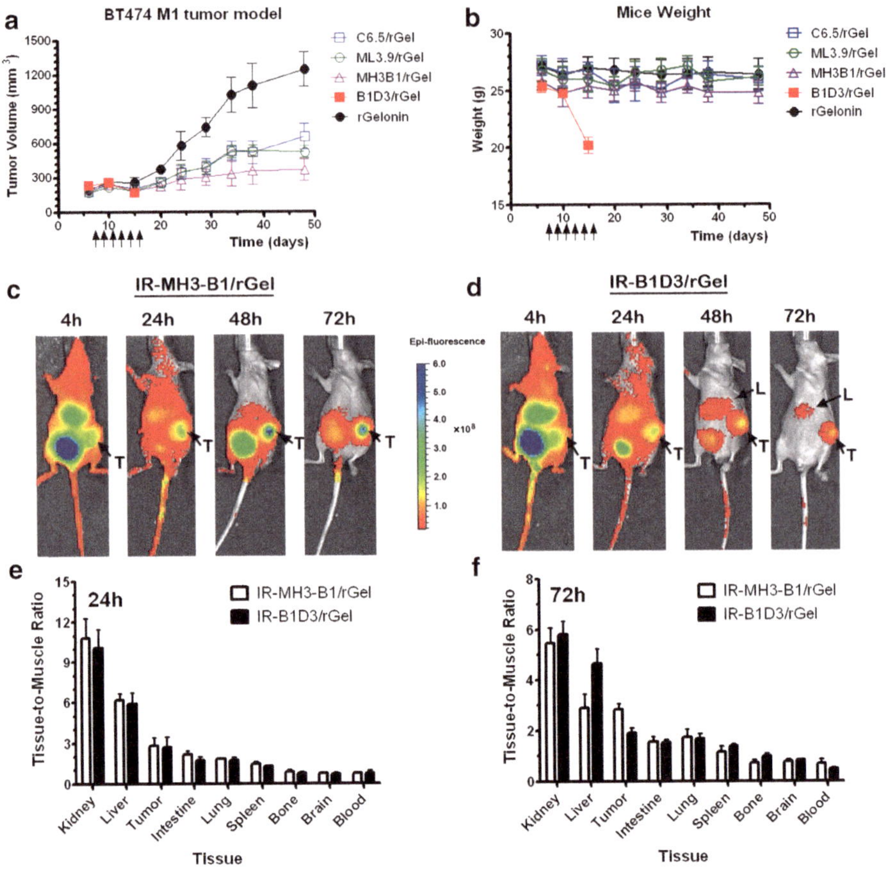

Fig. 18.6 *In vivo* study of the immunotoxins against BT474 M1 tumor xenografts in nude mice. (**a**) Treatment of BT474 M1 tumors with scFv/rGel fusions at the dose of 24 mg/kg. Mean tumor volume was calculated by W×L×H as measured by digital calipers. (**b**) Average body weight of the mice during the immunotoxin treatment. (**c**, **d**) Whole-body imaging results of the mice i.v. injected with either IR-MH3-B1/rGel or IR-B1D3/rGel at 4, 24, 48, and 72 h. *Arrows* pointed at tumor (*T*) and liver (*L*). (**e**, **f**) The comparison of tissue-to-muscle ratio (*TMR*) of IR–MH3–B1/rGel and IR–B1D3/rGel at 24 h and 72 h after injection into xenograft mice ($n = 5$)

of paramount importance to design immunotoxins with minimal toxicity to normal tissues. Previous concepts focused on employing the highest-affinity antibodies available for use in immunotoxin constructs, and the current study suggests that high-affinity constructs are the most vulnerable to the presence of shed antigen. Intermediate-affinity antibodies appear to be preferable for this application since their targeting ability is high enough to show reliable specificity and targeted toxicity but low enough to avoid interference by shed antigen.

Shedding of cell surface antigens is an important biological process used to modulate cellular response to signals in the extracellular environment [130, 131]. Measurement of shed HER2/neu antigen levels in the blood of mice bearing BT474

M1 tumor showed that HER2/neu levels increase in parallel with tumor size. Levels of HER2/neu in serum increased from 2 to 12 nM for mice with 200 mm^3 tumors up to 1,800 mm^3, respectively. The correlation between shed HER2/neu levels and tumor volume was found to be significant with a correlation coefficient of 0.797 ($p<0.01$). At sufficiently high HER2/neu levels, the efficacy of high-affinity targeted therapeutics could be impacted.

Our in vitro studies demonstrated that the activity of B1D3/rGel could be impaired by the presence of added ECD, and this is likely because B1D3 displays a higher association constant rate and a lower dissociation rate than the other scFv tested. As a result, immune complex formation with B1D3/rGel was shown to reduce in vitro cytotoxicity and with a corresponding significant increase in in vivo toxicity. Biodistribution studies in BT474 M1 tumor-bearing mice indicated that there was little difference in the liver and tumor uptake of MH3-B1/rGel and B1D3/rGel at 24 h, but there was a significant difference between the two at 72 h (Fig. 18.6c–f). There was a statistically significant decrease in tumor localization for the high-affinity B1D3/rGel compared to intermediate-affinity MH3-B1/rGel 72 h after i.v. injection with a corresponding increase in liver accumulation (Fig. 18.7a, b). This accumulation paralleled liver toxicity as assessed by increasing serum levels of alanine aminotransferase (ALT), aspartate aminotransferase (AST), and LDH (Fig. 18.7c–e). In addition, toxicity was confirmed by postmortem histopathologic examination of liver tissue from B1D3/rGel-treated mice (Fig. 18.7f). This data is consistent with the finding that the high-affinity B1D3/rGel construct formed immune complexes with soluble, tumor-derived antigen leading to clearance by the hepatic RES and a reduction in ability to distribute to the tumor. The intermediate-affinity MH3-B1/rGel construct showed a comparatively better distribution to tumor and a reduced hepatotoxicity profile compared to the high-affinity construct. It is important to note that murine studies of species-specific anti-human HER2/neu antibody constructs may underrepresent the eventual clinical toxicity of these agents against normal tissues expressing low levels of HER2/neu antigen. Nevertheless, our study clearly demonstrated that when high-affinity immunotoxins form complexes in vivo with tumor-derived HER2/neu antigen, this additionally results in significantly increased hepatic toxicity.

The hepatotoxicity of immunotoxins as a result of normal tissue expression of the antigen is a common problem observed in clinical trials [14, 125, 132, 133]. Immunotoxins containing toxins such as ricin toxin A (RTA), PE, or DT appear to bind to hepatocytes or vascular endothelial cells and have demonstrated dose-limiting toxicities which include renal and liver toxicity as well as vascular leak syndrome (VLS) [134–136]. However, clinical studies with rGel-based immunotoxins have not demonstrated such nontarget effects. In addition, distinct from PE-based anti-HER2/neu immunotoxins, which appear to effectively target cells bearing low levels of antigen [40, 41], the use of rGel-based constructs may be particularly important to consider in cases of low level expression of antigen on normal tissues since previous studies have demonstrated that there appears to be a relatively high minimal threshold of HER2/neu antigen sites (~1.5×10^5 sites per cell) present on a target cell before specific toxicity is enabled [30]. This appears to be unique compared to studies with other toxins.

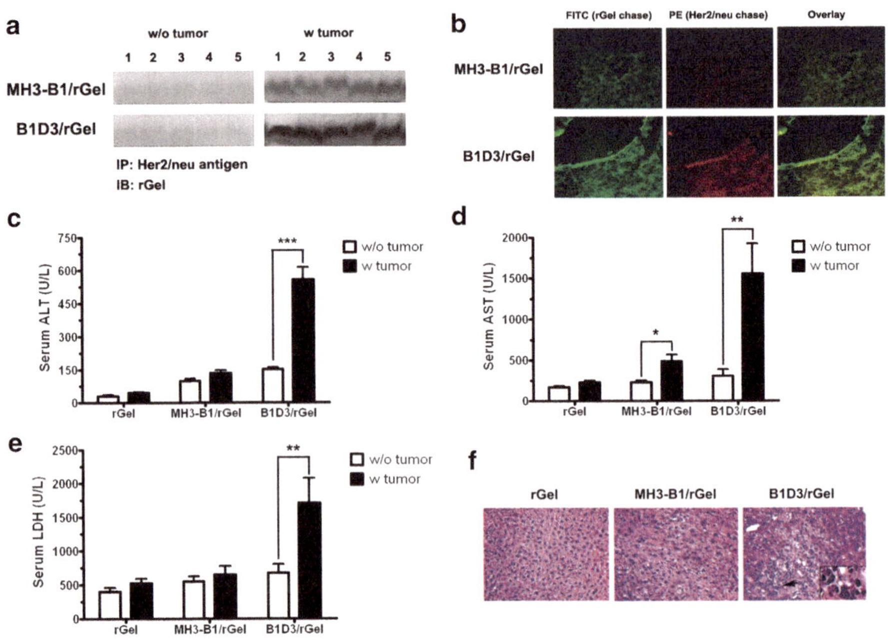

Fig. 18.7 Analysis of the accumulation of HER2/neu antigen and scFv/rGel (MH3-B1/rGel or B1D3/rGel) complex-driven liver toxicity after 72 h injection. (**a**) Coimmunoprecipitation of HER2/neu antigen and scFv/rGel in the liver from the mice with or without BT474 M1 tumors. Liver homogenates were subjected to HER2/neu immunoprecipitation, followed by western blot for rGel. (**b**) Immunofluorescence colocalization of scFv/rGel (*green*) and HER2/neu antigen (*red*) in the liver of the BT474 M1 burden mice. (**c**–**e**) Enzymatic activities of ALT, AST, and LDH in the serum of mice with or without tumors, treated with rGel, MH3-B1/rGel, or B1D3/rGel. Values are expressed as mean ± SD ($n=5$). *, ** and ***, statistically different from own control mice at $p<0.05$, $p<0.01$, and $p<0.002$, respectively. (**f**) Histologic findings of the livers from tumor burden mice after immunotoxin application. All the sections were stained with hematoxylin and eosin (primary magnification: 100×). *Inset* showed multiple necrosis of hepatocytes (primary magnification: 400×)

From Preclinical Development to Therapeutic Application

There has been remarkable progress in the development of immunotoxins to fulfill an unmet medical need for novel agents with unique spectra of action. Preclinical testing of these anti-HER2/neu immunotherapeutics has generated impressive results. There is a potential to improve the therapeutic window of these new agents by making immunotoxins either more potent, thereby lowering the efficacious dose or less nonspecifically toxic and thereby increasing the maximal tolerated dose.

Several clinical trials are currently addressing the efficiency of anti-HER2/neu immunotoxins for the treatment of the patients with solid or metastatic carcinoma known to express HER2/neu [63, 125, 127, 137]. Clinical manifestations of toxicity regularly included VLS and hepatotoxicity [79, 125, 138]. VLS is characterized by hypoalbuminemia, peripheral edema with resultant weight gain, and pulmonary edema in the most severe cases. These conditions were the results of increased vascular permeability from endothelial cell damage likely due to direct binding of the toxin component to endothelial cells. All anti-HER2/neu immunotoxins tested to date appear to cause VLS, but it was most severe in patients treated with RTA-containing immunotoxins [78, 134]. Hepatotoxicity has limited the clinical dose escalation of some immunotoxins, including erb-38 [125] and (FRP5)-ETA [14]; as mentioned above, likely due to binding of the constructs to HER2/neu on hepatocytes ($\sim 5 \times 10^4$ sites per cell) [139, 140]. The binding affinity of these immunotoxins was 27×10^{-9} M for erb-38 [41] and 6.5×10^{-9} M for (FRP5)-ETA [122]. Both constructs demonstrated cytotoxicity to human A431 epidermoid carcinoma cells expressing low levels of HER2/neu (2×10^4 sites per cell) [40]. This suggests that HER2/neu-targeted immunotoxins with affinities in the nanomolar range may effectively target both tumor and normal cells expressing low antigen levels. The development of anti-HER2/neu immunotoxins containing human antibodies or fragments with intermediate affinities of 10^{-10} M can be generated with relative ease using standard mutagenesis techniques including error-prone PCR and DNA shuffling [90, 141–144], and this may provide a novel source of agents for further development.

The use of anti-HER2/neu immunotoxins is further hampered by the relatively strong immunogenicity of some toxins. Humoral immune responses to toxins can be observed after just one treatment course. This immunological response does not only reduce serum half-life but also significantly inhibits cytotoxic activity, especially in cases in which repeated treatment courses are required. Several approaches were therefore pursued to decrease the immunogenicity of toxins, specifically the modification of the toxins or coadministration of immunosuppressive agents [137, 145, 146]. Pastan et al. identified 7 major epitope groups and 9 of 13 epitope subgroups, associated with the PE38 toxin. Epitope modification produced an immunotoxin in a fully active but significantly less immunogenic molecule using site-directed mutagenesis [147, 148]. For the plant toxin rGel, clinical studies thus far have not demonstrated that patients mount a robust immune response to administered immunoconjugates. Nevertheless, we have engineered a number of rGel analogs by deleting known antigenic regions, replacing defined immunogenic regions with human homologous sequences, or modest sequence changes to modify B or T cell epitopes. Conjugation of the toxin component with polyethylene glycol (PEGylation) of the toxin to cover potential immunogenic regions or genetic engineering to generate humanized toxins is a promising approach for overcoming the problem of immunogenicity [149, 150]. Guo et al. [35, 39, 151] developed novel liposomes loaded with PE toxin and conjugated with an anti-HER2/neu Fab. This approach was designed to improve the pharmacological and therapeutic properties of drugs administered parenterally, providing a unique practical means of reducing toxicity and immunogenicity [34, 38, 150]. Another promising strategy is to deliver immunotoxin therapy through gene therapy vectors. Huang et al. [152] evaluated a gene therapy approach designed to express intratumoral therapeutic levels of the e23/PE40 fusion protein to target HER2/neu-expressing tumors. The advantages of gene therapy vectors are that they can mediate continuous and prolonged immunotoxin production and may provide reduced host immune response [140, 153].

Evidence from a number of laboratory studies suggests that immunotoxins targeting HER2/neu can display synergistic effects in combination with other antitumor agents. Combinations of external radiation and anti-HER2/neu immunotoxins can demonstrate synergistic inhibition of clonogenic growth of ovarian and breast cancer cells [20, 36]. Antibody binding and activation of HER2/neu cellular signaling and cross talk with other receptors may lead to signaling events which could protect the cells from toxin-mediated killing. Therefore, a bispecific immunotoxin approach to simultaneously target HER2/neu and EGFR [37, 46], or HER2/neu and EpCAM [33], may offer advantages for tumor therapy with superior in vitro and in vivo activity over monospecific immunotoxins.

New Approaches

Although the biological activity in vitro and in vivo of bacterial and plant toxin-based anti-HER2/neu immunotoxins has demonstrated remarkable potency, there are a number of obstacles that limit their clinical application [145]. The toxin component of these fusion proteins can elicit a high degree of humoral response in humans, and patients in developed countries are generally immunized against some bacterial toxins such as DT, which could result in neutralization of the related immunotoxins [79, 154, 155]. In addition, both bacterial and plant toxins are large molecules which are difficult to humanize completely. In order to overcome these problems, several groups have focused on the construction of anti-HER2/neu immunotoxins composed of novel, highly cytotoxic human proteins as replacements for bacterial or plant toxins. Anti-HER2/neu constructs containing human GrB, human ribonucleases (RNase), or other proapoptotic proteins are described below.

GrB is a serine protease generated by cytotoxic lymphocytes to induce apoptotic cell death in target cells. GrB is released after the target cell membrane has been permeabilized by the prior exposure to the transmembrane, pore-forming molecule perforin [156, 157] allowing GrB entry to the cytosol. Since GrB is present in plasma in both normal and pathological states, it is unlikely that this molecule would engender an immune response. Studies by Liu et al. first demonstrated that fusion constructs containing a cell-targeting scFv or growth factor fused to human GrB displayed highly cytotoxic targeted effects [158–160]. In addition, these constructs could be composed of completely human proteins, and the resulting proteins had a unique, proapoptotic mechanism of biological action. Subsequent studies by Wels et al. described the GrB-scFv (FRP5) fusion construct targeting HER2/neu and displayed selective and rapid tumor cell killing, accompanied by clear signs of apoptosis such as chromatin condensation, membrane blebbing, formation of apoptotic bodies, and activation of endogenous initiator and effector caspases [161, 162]. Yang et al. demonstrated that injection of Jurkat cells producing and secreting

GrB fused to anti-HER2/neu scFv was capable of selectively targeting HER2/neu-overexpressing tumor cells [74, 95, 163].

RNases once internalized into cells efficiently degrade RNA causing cell death via inhibition of protein synthesis [164, 165]. RNases constitute a large superfamily spread across several species. Human RNases are encoded by at least eight different genes out of which five (RNase 1–5) have been identified at the protein level. De Lorenzo et al. demonstrated the availability of an anti-HER2/neu scFv fused to human pancreatic RNase (RNase I or HP-RNase) [166–169]. The resulting construct was found to induce a remarkable reduction (86%) in tumor volume in xenograft models. Further, introduction of a dimeric mutant RNase construct (ERB-HH2-RNase) or anti-HER2/neu human compact antibody-RNase (Erb-hcAb-RNase) demonstrated improved biologic properties compared to the original monomeric version [170–174].

Insights gained from studies of the early anti-HER2/neu immunotoxins with respect to antibody affinity, valency, linker construction, and composition have improved our understanding of immunotoxin design approaches and have led to a promising new generation of humanized protein therapeutics. Incorporation of novel human proteins to replace plant and bacterial toxins has expanded our abilities to generate fusion proteins with unique mechanisms of action and which are demonstrating pronounced antitumor effects against HER2/neu-positive tumor xenografts. Additionally, there are a wide range of other cytotoxic human proteins which might be considered excellent candidates for incorporation into fusion constructs such as caspase 3 [175, 176], caspase 6 [177, 178], and BH3-interacting domain death agonist (BID) [179–182]. Finally, proteases, kinases, or other enzyme classes or proteins may be effective when used as payloads for therapeutics targeting HER2/neu.

Since the discovery of its pivotal roles in tumorigenesis and metastatic spread, HER2/neu has attracted enormous attention as a focal point for the development of novel therapeutics. Anti-HER2/neu immunotoxins are tumor-directed biological constructs containing highly cytotoxic protein payloads with the potential to effectively target and suppress the growth of a number of malignancies overexpressing HER2/neu. Although currently no anti-HER2/neu immunotoxins have been approved by the FDA, a variety of potent agents are under development or undergoing clinical trials. New discoveries and further understanding of co-targeting strategies, reduction of toxicity, and immunogenicity can only serve to speed the development of anti-HER2/neu immunotoxins. A new generation of immunotoxins containing novel, cytotoxic proteins of human origin will continue to drive innovation in this arena.

References

1. Coussens L, Yang-Feng TL, Liao YC, Chen E, Gray A, McGrath J et al (1985) Tyrosine kinase receptor with extensive homology to EGF receptor shares chromosomal location with neu oncogene. Science 230:1132–1139
2. King CR, Kraus MH, Aaronson SA (1985) Amplification of a novel v-erbB-related gene in a human mammary carcinoma. Science 229:974–976

3. Yamamoto T, Ikawa S, Akiyama T, Semba K, Nomura N, Miyajima N et al (1986) Similarity of protein encoded by the human c-erb-B-2 gene to epidermal growth factor receptor. Nature 319:230–234
4. Bargmann CI, Hung MC, Weinberg RA (1986) The neu oncogene encodes an epidermal growth factor receptor-related protein. Nature 319:226–230
5. Barros FF, Powe DG, Ellis IO, Green AR (2010) Understanding the HER family in breast cancer: interaction with ligands, dimerization and treatments. Histopathology 56:560–572
6. Scholl S, Beuzeboc P, Pouillart P (2001) Targeting HER2 in other tumor types. Ann Oncol 12(Suppl 1):S81–S87
7. Tamborini E, Perrone F, Frattini M, Negri T, Aiello A, Gloghini A et al (2008) Genetic markers in sporadic tumors. In: Bronchud MH, Foote M, Giaccone G, Olopade OI, Workman P (eds) Principles of molecular oncology, 3rd edn., pp 43–84
8. Press MF, Pike MC, Hung G, Zhou JY, Ma Y, George J et al (1994) Amplification and overexpression of HER-2/neu in carcinomas of the salivary gland: correlation with poor prognosis. Cancer Res 54:5675–5682
9. Daniele L, Sapino A (2009) Anti-HER2 treatment and breast cancer: state of the art, recent patents, and new strategies. Recent Pat Anticancer Drug Discov 4:9–18
10. Pohlmann PR, Mayer IA, Mernaugh R (2009) Resistance to trastuzumab in breast cancer. Clin Cancer Res 15:7479–7491
11. Murphy CG, Fornier M (2010) HER2-positive breast cancer: beyond trastuzumab. Oncology (Williston Park) 24:410–415
12. Moulder SL, Arteaga CL (2003) A Phase I/II Trial of trastuzumab and gefitinib in patients with Metastatic Breast Cancer that overexpresses HER2/neu (ErbB-2). Clin Breast Cancer 4:142–145
13. Jones KL, Buzdar AU (2009) Evolving novel anti-HER2 strategies. Lancet Oncol 10:1179–1187
14. Wels W, Biburger M, Muller T, Dalken B, Giesubel U, Tonn T et al (2004) Recombinant immunotoxins and retargeted killer cells: employing engineered antibody fragments for tumor-specific targeting of cytotoxic effectors. Cancer Immunol Immunother 53:217–226
15. Milenic DE (2002) Monoclonal antibody-based therapy strategies: providing options for the cancer patient. Curr Pharm Des 8:1749–1764
16. Bast RC Jr, Boyer CM, Jacobs I, Xu FJ, Wu S, Wiener J et al (1993) Cell growth regulation in epithelial ovarian cancer. Cancer 71:1597–1601
17. Boyer CM, Pusztai L, Wiener JR, Xu FJ, Dean GS, Bast BS et al (1999) Relative cytotoxic activity of immunotoxins reactive with different epitopes on the extracellular domain of the c-erbB-2 (HER-2/neu) gene product p185. Int J Cancer 82:525–531
18. Dean GS, Pusztai L, Xu FJ, O'Briant K, DeSombre K, Conaway M et al (1998) Cell surface density of p185(c-erbB-2) determines susceptibility to anti-p185(c-erbB-2)-ricin A chain (RTA) immunotoxin therapy alone and in combination with anti-p170(EGFR)-RTA in ovarian cancer cells. Clin Cancer Res 4:2545–2550
19. Rodriguez GC, Boente MP, Berchuck A, Whitaker RS, O'Briant KC, Xu F et al (1993) The effect of antibodies and immunotoxins reactive with HER-2/neu on growth of ovarian and breast cancer cell lines. Am J Obstet Gynecol 168:228–232
20. Xu F, Leadon SA, Yu Y, Boyer CM, O'Briant K, Ward K et al (2000) Synergistic interaction between anti-p185HER-2 ricin A chain immunotoxins and radionuclide conjugates for inhibiting growth of ovarian and breast cancer cells that overexpress HER-2. Clin Cancer Res 6:3334–3341
21. Xu FJ, Boyer CM, Bae DS, Wu S, Greenwald M, O'Briant K et al (1994) The tyrosine kinase activity of the C-erbB-2 gene product (p185) is required for growth inhibition by anti-p185 antibodies but not for the cytotoxicity of an anti-p185-ricin-A chain immunotoxin. Int J Cancer 59:242–247
22. Zhou XX, Ji F, Zhao JL, Cheng LF, Xu CF (2010) Anti-cancer activity of anti-p185HER-2 ricin A chain immunotoxin on gastric cancer cells. J Gastroenterol Hepatol 25:1266–1275
23. Maier LA, Xu FJ, Hester S, Boyer CM, McKenzie S, Bruskin AM et al (1991) Requirements for the internalization of a murine monoclonal antibody directed against the HER-2/neu gene product c-erbB-2. Cancer Res 51:5361–5369

24. Crews JR, Maier LA, Yu YH, Hester S, O'Briant K, Leslie DS et al (1992) A combination of two immunotoxins exerts synergistic cytotoxic activity against human breast-cancer cell lines. Int J Cancer 51:772–779
25. Casalini P, Caldera M, Canevari S, Menard S, Mezzanzanica D, Tosi E et al (1993) A critical comparison of three internalization assays applied to the evaluation of a given mAb as a toxin-carrier candidate. Cancer Immunol Immunother 37:54–60
26. Di LC, Digiesi G, Tecce R, Lotti LV, Torrisi MR, Natali PG (1994) Immunotoxins to the HER-2 oncogene product: functional and ultrastructural analysis of their cytotoxic activity. Cancer Immunol Immunother 39:318–324
27. Natali PG, Nicotra MR, Digiesi G, Cavaliere R, Bigotti A, Trizio D et al (1994) Expression of gp185HER-2 in human cutaneous melanoma: implications for experimental immunotherapeutics. Int J Cancer 56:341–346
28. Ricci C, Polito L, Nanni P, Landuzzi L, Astolfi A, Nicoletti G et al (2002) HER/erbB receptors as therapeutic targets of immunotoxins in human rhabdomyosarcoma cells. J Immunother 25:314–323
29. Tecce R, Digiesi G, Savarese A, Trizio D, Natali PG (1993) Characterization of cytotoxic activity of saporin anti-gp185/HER-2 immunotoxins. Int J Cancer 55:122–127
30. Rosenblum MG, Shawver LK, Marks JW, Brink J, Cheung L, Langton-Webster B (1999) Recombinant immunotoxins directed against the c-erb-2/HER2/neu oncogene product: in vitro cytotoxicity, pharmacokinetics, and in vivo efficacy studies in xenograft models. Clin Cancer Res 5:865–874
31. Cao Y, Marks JD, Marks JW, Cheung LH, Kim S, Rosenblum MG (2009) Construction and characterization of novel, recombinant immunotoxins targeting the HER2/neu oncogene product: in vitro and in vivo studies. Cancer Res 69:8987–8995
32. Cao Y, Marks JD, Huang Q, Rudnick SI, Xiong C, Hittelman WN et al (2012) Single-chain antibody-based immunotoxins targeting HER2/neu: design optimization and impact of affinity on antitumor efficacy and off-target toxicity. Mol Cancer Ther 11:143–153
33. Stish BJ, Chen H, Shu Y, Panoskaltsis-Mortari A, Vallera DA (2007) Increasing anticarcinoma activity of an anti-erbB2 recombinant immunotoxin by the addition of an anti-EpCAM sFv. Clin Cancer Res 13:3058–3067
34. Skrepnik N, Zieske AW, Bravo JC, Gillespie AT, Hunt JD (1999) Recombinant oncotoxin AR209 (anti-P185erbB-2) diminishes human prostate carcinoma xenografts. J Urol 161:984–989
35. Gao J, Kou G, Wang H, Chen H, Li B, Lu Y et al (2009) PE38KDEL-loaded anti-HER2 nanoparticles inhibit breast tumor progression with reduced toxicity and immunogenicity. Breast Cancer Res Treat 115:29–41
36. Schmidt M, McWatters A, White RA, Groner B, Wels W, Fan Z et al (2001) Synergistic interaction between an anti-p185HER-2 pseudomonas exotoxin fusion protein [scFv(FRP5)-ETA] and ionizing radiation for inhibiting growth of ovarian cancer cells that overexpress HER-2. Gynecol Oncol 80:145–155
37. Schmidt M, Hynes NE, Groner B, Wels W (1996) A bivalent single-chain antibody-toxin specific for ErbB-2 and the EGF receptor. Int J Cancer 65:538–546
38. Kuan CT, Pastan I (1996) Recombinant immunotoxin containing a disulfide-stabilized Fv directed at erbB2 that does not require proteolytic activation. Biochemistry 35:2872–2877
39. Chen H, Gao J, Lu Y, Kou G, Zhang H, Fan L et al (2008) Preparation and characterization of PE38KDEL-loaded anti-HER2 nanoparticles for targeted cancer therapy. J Control Release 128:209–216
40. Mazor Y, Noy R, Wels WS, Benhar I (2007) chFRP5-ZZ-PE38, a large IgG-toxin immunoconjugate outperforms the corresponding smaller FRP5(Fv)-ETA immunotoxin in eradicating ErbB2-expressing tumor xenografts. Cancer Lett 257:124–135
41. Bera TK, Onda M, Brinkmann U, Pastan I (1998) A bivalent disulfide-stabilized Fv with improved antigen binding to erbB2. J Mol Biol 281:475–483
42. Spyridonidis A, Schmidt M, Bernhardt W, Papadimitriou A, Azemar M, Wels W et al (1998) Purging of mammary carcinoma cells during ex vivo culture of CD34+ hematopoietic progenitor cells with recombinant immunotoxins. Blood 91:1820–1827

43. Shinohara H, Morita S, Kawai M, Miyamoto A, Sonoda T, Pastan I et al (2002) Expression of HER2 in human gastric cancer cells directly correlates with antitumor activity of a recombinant disulfide-stabilized anti-HER2 immunotoxin. J Surg Res 102:169–177
44. Kuge S, Miura Y, Nakamura Y, Mitomi T, Habu S, Nishimura T (1995) Superantigen-induced human CD4+ helper/killer T cell phenomenon. Selective induction of Th1 helper/killer T cells and application to tumor immunotherapy. J Immunol 154:1777–1785
45. Gurkan C, Ellar DJ (2003) Expression in Pichia pastoris and purification of a membrane-acting immunotoxin based on a synthetic gene coding for the Bacillus thuringiensis Cyt2Aa1 toxin. Protein Expr Purif 29:103–116
46. Schmidt M, Wels W (1996) Targeted inhibition of tumour cell growth by a bispecific single-chain toxin containing an antibody domain and TGF alpha. Br J Cancer 74:853–862
47. Ming-Kai X, Cheng-Gang Z (2006) Gene expression and function study of fusion immunotoxin anti-Her-2-scFv-SEC2 in Escherichia coli. Appl Microbiol Biotechnol 70:78–84
48. Reiter Y, Brinkmann U, Kreitman RJ, Jung SH, Lee B, Pastan I (1994) Stabilization of the Fv fragments in recombinant immunotoxins by disulfide bonds engineered into conserved framework regions. Biochemistry 33:5451–5459
49. Reiter Y, Brinkmann U, Jung SH, Lee B, Kasprzyk PG, King CR et al (1994) Improved binding and antitumor activity of a recombinant anti-erbB2 immunotoxin by disulfide stabilization of the Fv fragment. J Biol Chem 269:18327–18331
50. Jeschke M, Wels W, Dengler W, Imber R, Stocklin E, Groner B (1995) Targeted inhibition of tumor-cell growth by recombinant heregulin-toxin fusion proteins. Int J Cancer 60:730–739
51. Bera TK, Viner J, Brinkmann E, Pastan I (1999) Pharmacokinetics and antitumor activity of a bivalent disulfide-stabilized Fv immunotoxin with improved antigen binding to erbB2. Cancer Res 59:4018–4022
52. Barok M, Tanner M, Koninki K, Isola J (2011) Trastuzumab-DM1 causes tumour growth inhibition by mitotic catastrophe in trastuzumab-resistant breast cancer cells in vivo. Breast Cancer Res 13:R46
53. Barok M, Tanner M, Koninki K, Isola J (2011) Trastuzumab-DM1 is highly effective in preclinical models of HER2-positive gastric cancer. Cancer Lett 306:171–179
54. Junttila TT, Li G, Parsons K, Phillips GL, Sliwkowski MX (2011) Trastuzumab-DM1 (T-DM1) retains all the mechanisms of action of trastuzumab and efficiently inhibits growth of lapatinib insensitive breast cancer. Breast Cancer Res Treat 128:347–356
55. Lewis Phillips GD, Li G, Dugger DL, Crocker LM, Parsons KL, Mai E et al (2008) Targeting HER2-positive breast cancer with trastuzumab-DM1, an antibody-cytotoxic drug conjugate. Cancer Res 68:9280–9290
56. Junutula JR, Flagella KM, Graham RA, Parsons KL, Ha E, Raab H et al (2010) Engineered thio-trastuzumab-DM1 conjugate with an improved therapeutic index to target human epidermal growth factor receptor 2-positive breast cancer. Clin Cancer Res 16:4769–4778
57. Krop IE, Beeram M, Modi S, Jones SF, Holden SN, Yu W et al (2010) Phase I study of trastuzumab-DM1, an HER2 antibody-drug conjugate, given every 3 weeks to patients with HER2-positive metastatic breast cancer. J Clin Oncol 28:2698–2704
58. Burris HA III, Rugo HS, Vukelja SJ, Vogel CL, Borson RA, Limentani S et al (2011) Phase II study of the antibody drug conjugate trastuzumab-DM1 for the treatment of human epidermal growth factor receptor 2 (HER2)-positive breast cancer after prior HER2-directed therapy. J Clin Oncol 29:398–405
59. Mandler R, Kobayashi H, Hinson ER, Brechbiel MW, Waldmann TA (2004) Herceptin-geldanamycin immunoconjugates: pharmacokinetics, biodistribution, and enhanced antitumor activity. Cancer Res 64:1460–1467
60. Mehta RR, Bratescu L, Graves JM, Green A, Mehta RG (2000) Differentiation of human breast carcinoma cells by a novel vitamin D analog: 1alpha-hydroxyvitamin D5. Int J Oncol 16:65–73
61. Eigenbrot C, Ultsch M, Dubnovitsky A, Abrahmsen L, Hard T (2010) Structural basis for high-affinity HER2 receptor binding by an engineered protein. Proc Natl Acad Sci USA 107:15039–15044

62. Gundla R, Kazemi R, Sanam R, Muttineni R, Sarma JA, Dayam R et al (2008) Discovery of novel small-molecule inhibitors of human epidermal growth factor receptor-2: combined ligand and target-based approach. J Med Chem 51:3367–3377
63. Frankel AE, Kreitman RJ, Sausville EA (2000) Targeted toxins. Clin Cancer Res 6:326–334
64. Pennell CA, Erickson HA (2002) Designing immunotoxins for cancer therapy. Immunol Res 25:177–191
65. Brinkmann U (2000) Recombinant antibody fragments and immunotoxin fusions for cancer therapy. In Vivo 14:21–27
66. Ramakrishnan S, Fryxell D, Mohanraj D, Olson M, Li BY (1992) Cytotoxic conjugates containing translational inhibitory proteins. Annu Rev Pharmacol Toxicol 32:579–621
67. Johannes L, Decaudin D (2005) Protein toxins: intracellular trafficking for targeted therapy. Gene Ther 12:1360–1368
68. Kawakami K, Nakajima O, Morishita R, Nagai R (2006) Targeted anticancer immunotoxins and cytotoxic agents with direct killing moieties. ScientificWorldJournal 6:781–790
69. Senter PD (2009) Potent antibody drug conjugates for cancer therapy. Curr Opin Chem Biol 13:235–244
70. Govindan SV, Griffiths GL, Hansen HJ, Horak ID, Goldenberg DM (2005) Cancer therapy with radiolabeled and drug/toxin-conjugated antibodies. Technol Cancer Res Treat 4:375–391
71. Chen J, Jaracz S, Zhao X, Chen S, Ojima I (2005) Antibody-cytotoxic agent conjugates for cancer therapy. Expert Opin Drug Deliv 2:873–890
72. Chari RV (1998) Targeted delivery of chemotherapeutics: tumor-activated prodrug therapy. Adv Drug Deliv Rev 31:89–104
73. Goyal A, Batra JK (2000) Inclusion of a furin-sensitive spacer enhances the cytotoxicity of ribotoxin restrictocin containing recombinant single-chain immunotoxins. Biochem J 345(Pt 2):247–254
74. Wang T, Zhao J, Ren JL, Zhang L, Wen WH, Zhang R et al (2007) Recombinant immunoproapoptotic proteins with furin site can translocate and kill HER2-positive cancer cells. Cancer Res 67:11830–11839
75. Izidoro MA, Gouvea IE, Santos JA, Assis DM, Oliveira V, Judice WA et al (2009) A study of human furin specificity using synthetic peptides derived from natural substrates, and effects of potassium ions. Arch Biochem Biophys 487:105–114
76. Kibirev VK, Osadchuk TV (2007) Radavskii I [Furin and its biological role]. Ukr Biokhim Zh 79:5–18
77. Baluna R, Coleman E, Jones C, Ghetie V, Vitetta ES (2000) The effect of a monoclonal antibody coupled to ricin A chain-derived peptides on endothelial cells in vitro: insights into toxin-mediated vascular damage. Exp Cell Res 258:417–424
78. Vitetta ES (2000) Immunotoxins and vascular leak syndrome. Cancer J 6(Suppl 3):S218–S224
79. Mathew M, Verma RS (2009) Humanized immunotoxins: a new generation of immunotoxins for targeted cancer therapy. Cancer Sci 100:1359–1365
80. Huhn M, Sasse S, Tur MK, Matthey B, Schinkothe T, Rybak SM et al (2001) Human angiogenin fused to human CD30 ligand (Ang-CD30L) exhibits specific cytotoxicity against CD30-positive lymphoma. Cancer Res 61:8737–8742
81. Jain M, Chauhan SC, Singh AP, Venkatraman G, Colcher D, Batra SK (2005) Penetratin improves tumor retention of single-chain antibodies: a novel step toward optimization of radioimmunotherapy of solid tumors. Cancer Res 65:7840–7846
82. Batra SK, Jain M, Wittel UA, Chauhan SC, Colcher D (2002) Pharmacokinetics and biodistribution of genetically engineered antibodies. Curr Opin Biotechnol 13:603–608
83. Jain RK (2001) Delivery of molecular and cellular medicine to solid tumors. Adv Drug Deliv Rev 46:149–168
84. Batra JK, Kasprzyk PG, Bird RE, Pastan I, King CR (1992) Recombinant anti-erbB2 immunotoxins containing Pseudomonas exotoxin. Proc Natl Acad Sci USA 89:5867–5871
85. Carter P, Presta L, Gorman CM, Ridgway JB, Henner D, Wong WL et al (1992) Humanization of an anti-p185HER2 antibody for human cancer therapy. Proc Natl Acad Sci USA 89: 4285–4289

86. Adams GP, Schier R, Marshall K, Wolf EJ, McCall AM, Marks JD et al (1998) Increased affinity leads to improved selective tumor delivery of single-chain Fv antibodies. Cancer Res 58:485–490
87. Harwerth IM, Wels W, Schlegel J, Muller M, Hynes NE (1993) Monoclonal antibodies directed to the erbB-2 receptor inhibit in vivo tumour cell growth. Br J Cancer 68:1140–1145
88. De LC, Cozzolino R, Carpentieri A, Pucci P, Laccetti P, D'Alessio G (2005) Biological properties of a human compact anti-ErbB2 antibody. Carcinogenesis 26:1890–1895
89. Gelardi T, Damiano V, Rosa R, Bianco R, Cozzolino R, Tortora G et al (2010) Two novel human anti-ErbB2 immunoagents are active on trastuzumab-resistant tumours. Br J Cancer 102:513–519
90. Schier R, McCall A, Adams GP, Marshall KW, Merritt H, Yim M et al (1996) Isolation of picomolar affinity anti-c-erbB-2 single-chain Fv by molecular evolution of the complementarity determining regions in the center of the antibody binding site. J Mol Biol 263:551–567
91. Schier R, Marks JD, Wolf EJ, Apell G, Wong C, McCartney JE et al (1995) In vitro and in vivo characterization of a human anti-c-erbB-2 single-chain Fv isolated from a filamentous phage antibody library. Immunotechnology 1:73–81
92. Rudnick SI, Adams GP (2009) Affinity and avidity in antibody-based tumor targeting. Cancer Biother Radiopharm 24:155–161
93. Adams GP, Schier R, McCall AM, Simmons HH, Horak EM, Alpaugh RK et al (2001) High affinity restricts the localization and tumor penetration of single-chain fv antibody molecules. Cancer Res 61:4750–4755
94. Zhang Y, Pastan I (2008) High shed antigen levels within tumors: an additional barrier to immunoconjugate therapy. Clin Cancer Res 14:7981–7986
95. Zhang L, Zhao J, Wang T, Yu CJ, Jia LT, Duan YY et al (2008) HER2-targeting recombinant protein with truncated pseudomonas exotoxin A translocation domain efficiently kills breast cancer cells. Cancer Biol Ther 7:1226–1231
96. Clemente R, de la Torre JC (2007) Cell-to-cell spread of Borna disease virus proceeds in the absence of the virus primary receptor and furin-mediated processing of the virus surface glycoprotein. J Virol 81:5968–5977
97. Ackerman ME, Pawlowski D, Wittrup KD (2008) Effect of antigen turnover rate and expression level on antibody penetration into tumor spheroids. Mol Cancer Ther 7:2233–2240
98. Austin CD, De Maziere AM, Pisacane PI, van Dijk SM, Eigenbrot C, Sliwkowski MX et al (2004) Endocytosis and sorting of ErbB2 and the site of action of cancer therapeutics trastuzumab and geldanamycin. Mol Biol Cell 15:5268–5282
99. Pirie CM, Hackel BJ, Rosenblum MG, Wittrup KD (2011) Convergent potency of internalized gelonin immunotoxins across varied cell lines, antigens, and targeting moieties. J Biol Chem 286:4165–4172
100. Sandvig K (2002) van DB. Membrane traffic exploited by protein toxins. Annu Rev Cell Dev Biol 18:1–24
101. Sandvig K, van DB (2005) Delivery into cells: lessons learned from plant and bacterial toxins. Gene Ther 12:865–872
102. Potala S, Sahoo SK, Verma RS (2008) Targeted therapy of cancer using diphtheria toxin-derived immunotoxins. Drug Discov Today 13:807–815
103. Lambert JM, Blattler WA, McIntyre GD, Goldmacher VS, Scott CF Jr (1988) Immunotoxins containing single-chain ribosome-inactivating proteins. Cancer Treat Res 37:175–209
104. Olsnes S (2004) The history of ricin, abrin and related toxins. Toxicon 44:361–370
105. Nielsen K, Boston RS (2001) Ribosome-inactivating proteins: a plant perspective. Annu Rev Plant Physiol Plant Mol Biol 52:785–816
106. Stirpe F, Battelli MG (2006) Ribosome-inactivating proteins: progress and problems. Cell Mol Life Sci 63:1850–1866
107. Rosenblum MG, Cheung LH, Liu Y, Marks JW III (2003) Design, expression, purification, and characterization, in vitro and in vivo, of an antimelanoma single-chain Fv antibody fused to the toxin gelonin. Cancer Res 63:3995–4002

108. Zhou H, Marks JW, Hittelman WN, Yagita H, Cheung LH, Rosenblum MG et al (2011) Development and characterization of a potent immunoconjugate targeting the Fn14 receptor on solid tumor cells. Mol Cancer Ther 10:1276–1288
109. Lyu MA, Cheung LH, Hittelman WN, Marks JW, Aguiar RC, Rosenblum MG (2007) The rGel/BLyS fusion toxin specifically targets malignant B cells expressing the BLyS receptors BAFF-R, TACI, and BCMA. Mol Cancer Ther 6:460–470
110. Thorburn J, Horita H, Redzic J, Hansen K, Frankel AE, Thorburn A (2009) Autophagy regulates selective HMGB1 release in tumor cells that are destined to die. Cell Death Differ 16: 175–183
111. Maiuri MC, Zalckvar E, Kimchi A, Kroemer G (2007) Self-eating and self-killing: crosstalk between autophagy and apoptosis. Nat Rev Mol Cell Biol 8:741–752
112. Thorburn A (2008) Apoptosis and autophagy: regulatory connections between two supposedly different processes. Apoptosis 13:1–9
113. Carter PJ, Senter PD (2008) Antibody-drug conjugates for cancer therapy. Cancer J 14: 154–169
114. Pegram MD, Lipton A, Hayes DF, Weber BL, Baselga JM, Tripathy D et al (1998) Phase II study of receptor-enhanced chemosensitivity using recombinant humanized anti-p185HER2/ neu monoclonal antibody plus cisplatin in patients with HER2/neu-overexpressing metastatic breast cancer refractory to chemotherapy treatment. J Clin Oncol 16:2659–2671
115. Pegram M, Hsu S, Lewis G, Pietras R, Beryt M, Sliwkowski M et al (1999) Inhibitory effects of combinations of HER-2/neu antibody and chemotherapeutic agents used for treatment of human breast cancers. Oncogene 18:2241–2251
116. Baselga J, Tripathy D, Mendelsohn J, Baughman S, Benz CC, Dantis L et al (1996) Phase II study of weekly intravenous recombinant humanized anti-p185HER2 monoclonal antibody in patients with HER2/neu-overexpressing metastatic breast cancer. J Clin Oncol 14:737–744
117. Leary AF, Hanna WM, van de Vijver MJ, Penault-Llorca F, Ruschoff J, Osamura RY et al (2009) Value and limitations of measuring HER-2 extracellular domain in the serum of breast cancer patients. J Clin Oncol 27:1694–1705
118. Kreitman RJ, Pastan I (2006) Immunotoxins in the treatment of hematologic malignancies. Curr Drug Targets 7:1301–1311
119. Frankel AE, Kreitman RJ (2005) CLL immunotoxins. Leuk Res 29:985–986
120. Jain M, Venkatraman G, Batra SK (2007) Optimization of radioimmunotherapy of solid tumors: biological impediments and their modulation. Clin Cancer Res 13:1374–1382
121. Beckman RA, Weiner LM, Davis HM (2007) Antibody constructs in cancer therapy: protein engineering strategies to improve exposure in solid tumors. Cancer 109:170–179
122. Wels W, Harwerth IM, Mueller M, Groner B, Hynes NE (1992) Selective inhibition of tumor cell growth by a recombinant single-chain antibody-toxin specific for the erbB-2 receptor. Cancer Res 52:6310–6317
123. King CR, Fischer PH, Rando RF, Pastan I (1996) The performance of e23(Fv)PEs, recombinant toxins targeting the erbB-2 protein. Semin Cancer Biol 7:79–86
124. Kihara A, Pastan I (1995) Cytotoxic activity of chimeric toxins containing the epidermal growth factor-like domain of heregulins fused to PE38KDEL, a truncated recombinant form of Pseudomonas exotoxin. Cancer Res 55:71–77
125. Pai-Scherf LH, Villa J, Pearson D, Watson T, Liu E, Willingham MC et al (1999) Hepatotoxicity in cancer patients receiving erb-38, a recombinant immunotoxin that targets the erbB2 receptor. Clin Cancer Res 5:2311–2315
126. Maurer-Gebhard M, Schmidt M, Azemar M, Altenschmidt U, Stocklin E, Wels W et al (1998) Systemic treatment with a recombinant erbB-2 receptor-specific tumor toxin efficiently reduces pulmonary metastases in mice injected with genetically modified carcinoma cells. Cancer Res 58:2661–2666
127. Azemar M, Djahansouzi S, Jager E, Solbach C, Schmidt M, Maurer AB et al (2003) Regression of cutaneous tumor lesions in patients intratumorally injected with a recombinant single-chain antibody-toxin targeted to ErbB2/HER2. Breast Cancer Res Treat 82:155–164

128. Ghetie MA, Ghetie V, Vitetta ES (1997) Immunotoxins for the treatment of B-cell lymphomas. Mol Med 3:420–427
129. Bang S, Nagata S, Onda M, Kreitman RJ, Pastan I (2005) HA22 (R490A) is a recombinant immunotoxin with increased antitumor activity without an increase in animal toxicity. Clin Cancer Res 11:1545–1550
130. Arribas J, Borroto A (2002) Protein ectodomain shedding. Chem Rev 102:4627–4638
131. Dello SP, Rovida E (2002) Transmodulation of cell surface regulatory molecules via ectodomain shedding. Biol Chem 383:69–83
132. Wolf P, Alt K, Wetterauer D, Buhler P, Gierschner D, Katzenwadel A et al (2010) Preclinical evaluation of a recombinant anti-prostate specific membrane antigen single-chain immunotoxin against prostate cancer. J Immunother 33:262–271
133. Morgan AC Jr, Manger R, Pearson JW, Longo D, Abrams P, Sivam G et al (1991) Immunoconjugates of Pseudomonas exotoxin A: evaluation in mice, monkeys, and man. Cancer Detect Prev 15:137–143
134. Baluna R, Vitetta ES (1997) Vascular leak syndrome: a side effect of immunotherapy. Immunopharmacology 37:117–132
135. Vallera DA, Panoskaltsis-Mortari A, Blazar BR (1997) Renal dysfunction accounts for the dose limiting toxicity of DT390anti-CD3sFv, a potential new recombinant anti-GVHD immunotoxin. Protein Eng 10:1071–1076
136. Brown J, Rasamoelisolo M, Spearman M, Bosc D, Cizeau J, Entwistle J et al (2009) Preclinical assessment of an anti-EpCAM immunotoxin: locoregional delivery provides a safer alternative to systemic administration. Cancer Biother Radiopharm 24:477–487
137. Schrama D, Reisfeld RA, Becker JC (2006) Antibody targeted drugs as cancer therapeutics. Nat Rev Drug Discov 5:147–159
138. Frankel AE, Tagge EP, Willingham MC (1995) Clinical trials of targeted toxins. Semin Cancer Biol 6:307–317
139. Brand FX, Ravanel N, Gauchez AS, Pasquier D, Payan R, Fagret D et al (2006) Prospect for anti-HER2 receptor therapy in breast cancer. Anticancer Res 26:715–722
140. Krauss WC, Park JW, Kirpotin DB, Hong K, Benz CC (2000) Emerging antibody-based HER2 (ErbB-2/neu) therapeutics. Breast Dis 11:113–124
141. Schaffitzel C, Hanes J, Jermutus L, Pluckthun A (1999) Ribosome display: an in vitro method for selection and evolution of antibodies from libraries. J Immunol Methods 231:119–135
142. Hanes J, Pluckthun A (1997) In vitro selection and evolution of functional proteins by using ribosome display. Proc Natl Acad Sci USA 94:4937–4942
143. Hanes J, Schaffitzel C, Knappik A, Pluckthun A (2000) Picomolar affinity antibodies from a fully synthetic naive library selected and evolved by ribosome display. Nat Biotechnol 18:1287–1292
144. Jermutus L, Honegger A, Schwesinger F, Hanes J, Pluckthun A (2001) Tailoring in vitro evolution for protein affinity or stability. Proc Natl Acad Sci USA 98:75–80
145. Frankel AE (2004) Reducing the immune response to immunotoxin. Clin Cancer Res 10:13–15
146. De Groot AS, Scott DW (2007) Immunogenicity of protein therapeutics. Trends Immunol 28: 482–490
147. Benhar I, Brinkmann U, Webber KO, Pastan I (1994) Mutations of two lysine residues in the CDR loops of a recombinant immunotoxin that reduce its sensitivity to chemical derivatization. Bioconjug Chem 5:321–326
148. Onda M, Beers R, Xiang L, Nagata S, Wang QC, Pastan I (2008) An immunotoxin with greatly reduced immunogenicity by identification and removal of B cell epitopes. Proc Natl Acad Sci USA 105:11311–11316
149. Benhar I, Wang QC, FitzGerald D, Pastan I (1994) Pseudomonas exotoxin A mutants. Replacement of surface-exposed residues in domain III with cysteine residues that can be modified with polyethylene glycol in a site-specific manner. J Biol Chem 269:13398–13404
150. Pasquetto MV, Vecchia L, Covini D, Digilio R, Scotti C (2011) Targeted drug delivery using immunoconjugates: principles and applications. J Immunother 34:611–628
151. Gao J, Zhong W, He J, Li H, Zhang H, Zhou G et al (2009) Tumor-targeted PE38KDEL delivery via PEGylated anti-HER2 immunoliposomes. Int J Pharm 374:145–152

152. Liu X, Wu J, Zhang S, Li C, Huang Q (2009) Novel strategies to augment genetically delivered immunotoxin molecular therapy for cancer therapy. Cancer Gene Ther 16:861–872
153. Vasir JK, Labhasetwar V (2005) Targeted drug delivery in cancer therapy. Technol Cancer Res Treat 4:363–374
154. Hall PD, Virella G, Willoughby T, Atchley DH, Kreitman RJ, Frankel AE (2001) Antibody response to DT-GM, a novel fusion toxin consisting of a truncated diphtheria toxin (DT) linked to human granulocyte-macrophage colony stimulating factor (GM), during a phase I trial of patients with relapsed or refractory acute myeloid leukemia. Clin Immunol 100:191–197
155. Hertler AA, Spitler LE, Frankel AE (1987) Humoral immune response to a ricin A chain immunotoxin in patients with metastatic melanoma. Cancer Drug Deliv 4:245–253
156. Rousalova I, Krepela E (2010) Granzyme B-induced apoptosis in cancer cells and its regulation (review). Int J Oncol 37:1361–1378
157. Kurschus FC, Jenne DE (2010) Delivery and therapeutic potential of human granzyme B. Immunol Rev 235:159–171
158. Liu Y, Zhang W, Niu T, Cheung LH, Munshi A, Meyn RE Jr et al (2006) Targeted apoptosis activation with GrB/scFvMEL modulates melanoma growth, metastatic spread, chemosensitivity, and radiosensitivity. Neoplasia 8:125–135
159. Liu Y, Cheung LH, Hittelman WN, Rosenblum MG (2003) Targeted delivery of human proapoptotic enzymes to tumor cells: In vitro studies describing a novel class of recombinant highly cytotoxic agents. Mol Cancer Ther 2:1341–1350
160. Liu Y, Cheung LH, Thorpe P, Rosenblum MG (2003) Mechanistic studies of a novel human fusion toxin composed of vascular endothelial growth factor (VEGF)121 and the serine protease granzyme B: directed apoptotic events in vascular endothelial cells. Mol Cancer Ther 2:949–959
161. Dalken B, Giesubel U, Knauer SK, Wels WS (2006) Targeted induction of apoptosis by chimeric granzyme B fusion proteins carrying antibody and growth factor domains for cell recognition. Cell Death Differ 13:576–585
162. Giesubel U, Dalken B, Mahmud H, Wels WS (2006) Cell binding, internalization and cytotoxic activity of human granzyme B expressed in the yeast Pichia pastoris. Biochem J 394:563–573
163. Zhao J, Zhang LH, Jia LT, Zhang L, Xu YM, Wang Z et al (2004) Secreted antibody/granzyme B fusion protein stimulates selective killing of HER2-overexpressing tumor cells. J Biol Chem 279:21343–21348
164. Chang CH, Gupta P, Michel R, Loo M, Wang Y, Cardillo TM et al (2010) Ranpirnase (frog RNase) targeted with a humanized, internalizing, anti-Trop-2 antibody has potent cytotoxicity against diverse epithelial cancer cells. Mol Cancer Ther 9:2276–2286
165. De LC, D'Alessio G (2008) From immunotoxins to immunoRNases. Curr Pharm Biotechnol 9:210–214
166. De LC, Arciello A, Cozzolino R, Palmer DB, Laccetti P, Piccoli R et al (2004) A fully human antitumor immunoRNase selective for ErbB-2-positive carcinomas. Cancer Res 64:4870–4874
167. De LC, D'Alessio G (2009) Human anti-ErbB2 immunoagents—immunoRNases and compact antibodies. FEBS J 276:1527–1535
168. De LC, Nigro A, Piccoli R, D'Alessio G (2002) A new RNase-based immunoconjugate selectively cytotoxic for ErbB2-overexpressing cells. FEBS Lett 516:208–212
169. De LC, Di MC, Cali G, Troise F, Nitsch L, D'Alessio G (2007) Intracellular route and mechanism of action of ERB-hRNase, a human anti-ErbB2 anticancer immunoagent. FEBS Lett 581:296–300
170. Di DA, Cafaro V, D'Alessio G (1994) Ribonuclease A can be transformed into a dimeric ribonuclease with antitumor activity. J Biol Chem 269:17394–17396
171. Riccio G, Borriello M, D'Alessio G, De LC (2008) A novel human antitumor dimeric immunoRNase. J Immunother 31:440–445
172. Piccoli R, Di GS, De LC, Grauso M, Monaco C, Spalletti-Cernia D et al (1999) A dimeric mutant of human pancreatic ribonuclease with selective cytotoxicity toward malignant cells. Proc Natl Acad Sci USA 96:7768–7773
173. Di GS, D'alessio G, Piccoli R (2001) Second generation antitumour human RNase: significance of its structural and functional features for the mechanism of antitumour action. Biochem J 358:241–247

174. Borriello M, Laccetti P, Terrazzano G, D'Alessio G, De LC (2011) A novel fully human antitumour immunoRNase targeting ErbB2-positive tumours. Br J Cancer 104:1716–1723
175. Jia LT, Zhang LH, Yu CJ, Zhao J, Xu YM, Gui JH et al (2003) Specific tumoricidal activity of a secreted proapoptotic protein consisting of HER2 antibody and constitutively active caspase-3. Cancer Res 63:3257–3262
176. Zhang DX, Zhao PT, Xia L, Liu LL, Liang J, Zhai HH et al (2010) Potent inhibition of human gastric cancer by HER2-directed induction of apoptosis with anti-HER2 antibody and caspase-3 fusion protein. Gut 59:292–299
177. Xu YM, Wang LF, Jia LT, Qiu XC, Zhao J, Yu CJ et al (2004) A caspase-6 and anti-human epidermal growth factor receptor-2 (HER2) antibody chimeric molecule suppresses the growth of HER2-overexpressing tumors. J Immunol 173:61–67
178. Wang LF, Zhou Y, Xu YM, Qiu XC, Zhou BG, Wang F et al (2009) A caspase-6 and anti-HER2 antibody chimeric tumor-targeted proapoptotic molecule decreased metastasis of human osteosarcoma. Cancer Invest 27:774–780
179. Qiu XC. Single-chain antibody/activated BID chimeric protein effectively suppresses HER2-positive tumor growth. 2008.
180. Shan LQ, Qiu XC, Xu YM, Ji ZG, Yang TT, Chen X et al (2008) scFv-mediated delivery of truncated BID suppresses HER2-positive osteosarcoma growth and metastasis. Cancer Biol Ther 7:1717–1722
181. Shan LQ, Ma S, Qiu XC, Wang T, Yu SB, Ma BA et al (2011) A novel recombinant immuno-tBid with a furin site effectively suppresses the growth of HER2-positive osteosarcoma cells in vitro. Oncol Rep 25:325–331
182. Wang F, Ren J, Qiu XC, Wang LF, Zhu Q, Zhang YQ et al (2010) Selective cytotoxicity to HER2-positive tumor cells by a recombinant e23sFv-TD-tBID protein containing a furin cleavage sequence. Clin Cancer Res 16:2284–2294
183. Wels W, Beerli R, Hellmann P, Schmidt M, Marte BM, Kornilova ES et al (1995) EGF receptor and p185erbB-2-specific single-chain antibody toxins differ in their cell-killing activity on tumor cells expressing both receptor proteins. Int J Cancer 60:137–144
184. Wang L, Liu B, Schmidt M, Lu Y, Wels W, Fan Z (2001) Antitumor effect of an HER2-specific antibody-toxin fusion protein on human prostate cancer cells. Prostate 47:21–28
185. Skrepnik N, Araya JC, Qian Z, Xu H, Hamide J, Mera R et al (1996) Effects of anti-erbB-2 (HER-2/neu) recombinant oncotoxin AR209 on human non-small cell lung carcinoma grown orthotopically in athymic nude mice. Clin Cancer Res 2:1851–1857
186. Skrepnik N, Zieske AW, Robert E, Bravo JC, Mera R, Hunt JD (1998) Aggressive administration of recombinant oncotoxin AR209 (anti-ErbB-2) in athymic nude mice implanted with orthotopic human non-small cell lung tumours. Eur J Cancer 34:1628–1633
187. Kasprzyk PG, Sullivan TL, Hunt JD, Gubish CT, Scoppa CA, Oelkuct M et al (1996) Activity of anti-erbB-2 recombinant toxin OLX-209 on lung cancer cell lines in the absence of erbB-2 gene amplification. Clin Cancer Res 2:75–80
188. Fischer PH, Bird RE, Kasprzyk PG, King CR, Turner NA, Pastan I et al (1994) In vitro and in vivo activity of a recombinant toxin, OLX-209, which targets the erbB-2 oncoprotein. Adv Enzyme Regul 34:119–128
189. Yang D, Kuan CT, Payne J, Kihara A, Murray A, Wang LM et al (1998) Recombinant heregulin-Pseudomonas exotoxin fusion proteins: interactions with the heregulin receptors and antitumor activity in vivo. Clin Cancer Res 4:993–1004
190. King CR, Kasprzyk PG, Fischer PH, Bird RE, Turner NA (1996) Preclinical testing of an anti-erbB-2 recombinant toxin. Breast Cancer Res Treat 38:19–25
191. Altenschmidt U, Schmidt M, Groner B, Wels W (1997) Targeted therapy of schwannoma cells in immunocompetent rats with an erbB2-specific antibody-toxin. Int J Cancer 73:117–124
192. Chen SY, Yang AG, Chen JD, Kute T, King CR, Collier J et al (1997) Potent antitumour activity of a new class of tumour-specific killer cells. Nature 385:78–80
193. Mazor Y, Barnea I, Keydar I, Benhar I (2007) Antibody internalization studied using a novel IgG binding toxin fusion. J Immunol Methods 321:41–59

Chapter 19
The Preclinical and Clinical Evaluation of VB6-845: An Immunotoxin with a De-Immunized Payload for the Systemic Treatment of Solid Tumors

Joycelyn Entwistle, Mark Kowalski, Jennifer Brown, Jeannick Cizeau, and Glen C. MacDonald

Introduction

One of the challenges in cancer therapy is to eradicate tumor cells while minimizing the toxic side effects to normal tissue that can rapidly become dose-limiting. In this regard, the unique specificity of antibodies enables the targeting of antigens that are differentially or aberrantly expressed on tumor cells while ignoring their normal counterparts [1]. To date, six IgG antibodies have received FDA approval for the treatment of cancer, Herceptin™ (Trastuzumab), Rituxan™ (Rituximab), Avastin™ (Bevacizumab), Campath™ (Alemtuzumab), Erbitux™ (Cetuximab), and Vectibix™ (Panitumumab), and all have shown varying degrees of clinical and commercial success [2]. While designed to target tumor cells with nanomolar affinity, clinical evidence would suggest that the anticancer mechanisms mediated by these antibodies are not on their own sufficient to provide a prolonged clinical benefit [3].To that end, other strategies have been explored to enhance antibody potency while still exploiting their targeting function. One such approach has been to attach a cytotoxic payload to an antibody that when delivered to a cancer cell induces a highly potent cell death signal [4]. The most common payloads attached to antibodies or antibody fragments are small molecule drugs, radionucleotides, and toxins [1, 5–8]. Two radionucleotide-conjugated antibodies Zevalin (Ibritumomab tiuxetan) and Bexxar (Tositumomab-/I131) and one antibiotic-conjugated antibody Mylotarg (Gemtuzumab ozogamicin) have been approved, although Mylotarg was subsequently withdrawn [9]. In addition, Ontak a diptheria toxin (DT) conjugated to an IL2 cytokine received approval for the treatment of cutaneous T cell lymphoma [10]. A variety of antibody–drug conjugates (ADCs) such as the anti-HER2 trastuzumab-DM1 are currently being evaluated in the clinic as antibody conjugates have proven themselves superior to the naked antibody in xenograft tumor models [11].

J. Entwistle • M. Kowalski • J. Brown • J. Cizeau • G.C. MacDonald (✉)
Viventia Biotechnologies Inc., 147 Hamelin Street, Winnipeg, MB R3T 3Z1, Canada
e-mail: gmacdonald@viventia.com

G.L. Phillips (ed.), *Antibody-Drug Conjugates and Immunotoxins: From Pre-Clinical Development to Therapeutic Applications*, Cancer Drug Discovery and Development,
DOI 10.1007/978-1-4614-5456-4_19, © Springer Science+Business Media New York 2013

Similarly, a variety of immunotoxins have been evaluated in the clinic, but as yet none have received FDA approval; however, those targeting leukemic cancers such as BL22, an anti-CD22 dsFv linked to truncated *Pseudomonas* exotoxin A (ETA), have been particularly successful [12, 13].

Despite the potency of immunotoxins, their inherent immunogenicity has limited their clinical use [14, 15]. In most cases the targeting antibodies are human or humanized scFv or Fab fragments which minimize the likelihood of a patient immune response; however, toxins are entirely foreign proteins and therefore highly immunogenic [16–18]. As a consequence, the humoral response in patients elicits the formation of antidrug antibodies (ADAs), resulting in rapid drug clearance, and hence, limited therapeutic effectiveness. Historically, cancers of hematological origin have responded better to immunotoxin-based therapies due to both the accessibility of the malignant cells as well as the immunocompromised state of these patients, thereby permitting multiple cycles of treatment [8]. For solid tumors, ADAs rapidly become dose-limiting after only a few weeks of treatment [19]. One strategy for circumventing immunogenicity is to use loco-regional administration, an approach that is only applicable in a limited number of indications. The immunotoxin, VB4-845, an anti-EpCAM scFv (4D5MOCB) linked to a truncated form of *Pseudomonas* ETA, has been evaluated in early clinical trials for squamous cell carcinomas of the head and neck (SCCHN) as well as transitional cell carcinomas of the bladder; drug administration was intratumoral for SCCHN and intravesical for bladder cancer [20–22]. In both indications, the drug was efficacious, well tolerated, and unaffected by a humoral response. However, most solid cancers cannot be treated effectively using loco-regional delivery strategies and thus require a systemically administered drug given in multiple cycles. Several approaches have been used to reduce the immunogenicity of the toxin moiety including the co-administration of immunosuppressant drugs, PEGylation, as well as the identification and removal of putative B and T cell epitopes from the protein [23–28]. Each approach has demonstrated some success in preclinical studies, but a final assessment of a de-immunization strategy can only be obtained by analyzing patient samples following repeat administration. The approach we have taken is to create a toxin, de-bouganin, in which the T cell epitopes were removed to create a cytotoxic payload with negligible immunogenic potential. In this chapter, we describe the 'bench to clinic' development of an anti-EpCAM immunotoxin carrying the de-immunized payload, de-bouganin, designed for the systemic treatment of solid tumors.

De-Bouganin for Use in Immunotoxins

Bouganin is a plant-derived toxin isolated as a 29 kDa single polypeptide chain (Type 1) ribosome inactivating protein with RNA N-glycosidase activity that directly inhibits translation [29–31]. The selection of bouganin was based upon its proven cytotoxic potential when conjugated to a targeting antibody as well as its favorable toxicity profile in animal models when compared to other type I RIPs [32, 33].

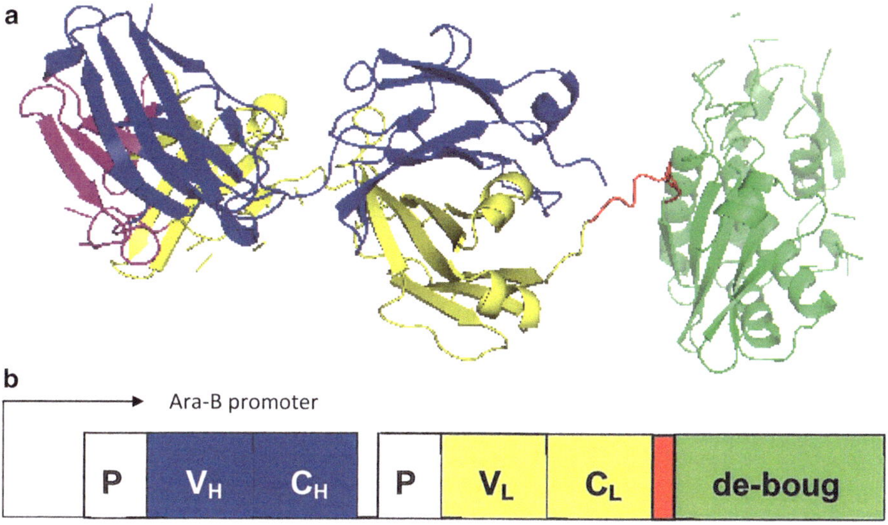

Fig. 19.1 (**a**) Ribbon representation of VB6-845. The de-bouganin moiety (*green*) is fused to the light chain (*yellow*) of the Fab fragment via a peptidic linker containing the furin proteolytic site (*red*). The heavy chain is shown in *blue* and CDRs loop in *magenta*. (**b**) Schematic representation of the VB6-845-C_L dicistronic unit under the control of the Arabinose (Ara-B) promoter of pING3302 expression vector. V_H, V_L, C_H, and C_L abbreviations correspond to the variable heavy and light chain and heavy and kappa chain conserved domain, respectively, P to the *Pel*B leader sequence and de-boug to de-bouganin. The furin linker is indicated in *red*

The absence of a cell binding domain, often associated with other toxins, contributes to its favorable toxicity profile. In order to address the potential immunogenicity of bouganin, overlapping peptides covering the entire sequence were tested in a T cell proliferation assay. Subsequently, reactive peptides corresponding to potential T cell epitopes were identified and removed [34]. This T cell epitope-depleted form of Bouganin (de-bouganin) was shown to have minimal immunogenic potential in vitro while preserving the potency of the parent molecule [34].

In order to clinically evaluate de-bouganin, the 77 kDa VB6-845 immunotoxin was constructed as a recombinant fusion protein comprised of an anti-EpCAM humanized Fab fragment, derived from 4D5MOCB scFv [34, 35] (Fig. 19.1a). There are several compelling reasons that make EpCAM a clinically relevant target for immunotherapy. First, although expressed on normal epithelia, EpCAM is generally overexpressed on carcinomas and increased expression is often associated with disease progression and poor patient prognosis [36–38]. Second, the cell surface distribution differs between normal and tumor epithelia such that EpCAM is more readily accessible on tumor cells [39–41]. Third, the pivotal role of EpCAM in proliferation, mitogenic signal transduction, and transformation underscores its importance as a therapeutic target [42]. To create VB6-845, de-bouganin was attached to a humanized EpCAM targeting Fab fragment using a furin-cleavable linker (Fig. 19.1b). The choice of a Fab-toxin format for VB6-845 was based upon

Table 19.1 VB6-845 reactivity and potency

Cell line	Indication	Reactivity[a]	IC_{50} (nM)
NIH:OVCAR-3	Ovarian	59	0.4
Caov-3	Ovarian	107	0.4
MCF 7	Breast	113	0.4
NCI-H69	Lung	31	1.5
HT-29	Colon	58	1.7
CAL 27	Head and neck	87	1.8
LNCaP	Prostate	43	11
HT-3	Cervical	29	23
HEC-1-A	Endometrial	42	43
RL95-2	Endometrial	4.9	100
SK-OV-3	Ovarian	4.3	>100
A-375	Melanoma	1.1	>100

[a]Values are representative of three independent experiments. Reactivity is defined as the mean fluorescence fold increase over the PBS control

the consideration of an optimal molecular size that would permit extravasation from the vasculature and subsequent penetration into the tumor bed while remaining stable in serum. The Fab-toxin format was manufactured as a fusion protein using a scalable, cost-effective microbial expression system.

Preclinical Evaluation of VB6-845

A preclinical evaluation of VB6-845 was performed to support clinical development in accordance with the ICH S6 (ICH S6 Preclinical Safety Evaluation of Biotechnology-derived Pharmaceuticals) guidelines. The preliminary investigation of VB6-845 examined its specificity, cytotoxicity, and reactivity with normal human tissue and identified appropriate clinical indications for the drug. This was followed by a comprehensive series of pharmacology and toxicology studies to determine the safety profile of VB6-845 for human use as well as establish a safe starting clinical dose.

In Vitro Specificity and Cytotoxicity of VB6-845

To illustrate the specificity and potency of VB6-845, a panel of epithelial tumor cell lines was tested for binding reactivity and cytotoxicity (Table 19.1). The tumor cell line selection was based, in part, upon the availability of established mouse xenograft models for follow-up efficacy studies as well as areas of perceived clinical need. As expected, VB6-845 potency varied according to EpCAM expression with no measurable cytotoxicity in EpCAM-negative cell lines. High EpCAM expression was associated with a sub-nanomolar IC_{50}. To further demonstrate the targeted

Table 19.2 Cytotoxic activity of common chemotherapeutic drugs

	IC_{50} (nM)			
Drug	NIH:OVCAR-3	A-375	Daudi	HMEC
Paclitaxel	$<10^{-6}$	4.9×10^{-6}	$<10^{-6}$	$<10^{-6}$
Docetaxel	$<10^{-6}$	$<10^{-6}$	$<10^{-6}$	$<10^{-6}$
Vincristine	4.4×10^{-6}	$<10^{-6}$	$<10^{-6}$	$<10^{-6}$
Topotecan	0.071	1.5	0.009	4.1
VB6-845	**1.0**	**>1,000**	**>1,000**	**220**
Doxorubicin	3.0	2.8	16×10^{-6}	16
Mitomycin C	28	14	2.8	50
Bleomycin Sulfate	30	170	22	600
Bleomycin A5	150	290	130	1,000
Irinotecan	180	900	190	1,000
Etoposide	210	280	1.7	600
Methotrexate	>1,000	6.0	3.6	41
Fluorouracil	>1,000	>1,000	>1,000	>1,000
Cyclophosphamide	>1,000	>1,000	>1,000	>1,000
Cisplatin	>1,000	>1,000	>1,000	>1,000

Representative IC_{50} of two independent experiments. Adapted with permission from Cizeau et al. [34]

specificity of VB6-845, the potency of VB6-845 was compared against a panel of chemotherapeutics on representative EpCAM-positive and EpCAM-negative tumor cell lines as well as a normal cell line (Table 19.2). In direct contrast to chemotherapeutics that showed no specificity, VB6-845 exhibited potent killing only against the EpCAM-positive tumor cell line (NIH:OVCAR-3) with minimal to no potency against the EpCAM-negative melanoma cell line (A-375), the lymphoid-derived tumor B cell line (Daudi), or the normal human mammary epithelial cell line (HMEC).

Immunohistochemical Staining with VB6-845

In accordance with FDA regulations, the reactivity of VB6-845 with normal human tissues was investigated using immunohistochemical analysis [43]. The GLP study tested a panel of 35 normal frozen human tissues for immune reactivity using an optimized concentration for staining. Of the 35 tissues examined, some degree of binding was noted in 20 tissue types with no binding being detected in the adrenal, bone marrow, brain, cerebellum, cervix, esophagus, eye, heart, liver, lymph node, muscle, placenta, skin, spinal cord, spleen, tonsil tissues, or white blood cells. The binding of VB6-845 in epithelia was membrane associated and consistent with the expression of EpCAM in normal tissues reported for other antibodies [44–46]. VB6-845 bound strongly to carcinomas of various origins including colon, rectum, head and neck, breast, prostate, esophagus, lung, endometrial, and ovarian, all of which are known to express higher levels of EpCAM relative to their normal counterparts [46].

In Vivo Efficacy

Since VB6-845 was highly potent against ovarian cell lines, SCID mice bearing established subcutaneous NIH:OVCAR-3 human tumor xenografts were used to evaluate the in vivo efficacy and tolerability of VB6-845 using 10 and 20 mg/kg doses. No significant weight loss was observed over the course of the treatment, indicating that both dose levels were well tolerated. The maximum tumor volume in the 10 mg/kg treated group was on average 40 mm^3 at the end of the study with 3/15 mice being tumor free. However, tumor growth was negligible in the 20 mg/kg treated group with a significantly higher number of tumor free mice (12/15) than observed in the control group [34] (Fig. 19.2a). Of the 15 mice in the untreated group, 11 reached the 750 mm^3 endpoint tumor volume. In contrast, treatment with 10 and 20 mg/kg of VB6-845 resulted in 100% survival by the end of the study with none of the treated mice reaching the 750 mm^3 endpoint tumor volume (Fig. 19.2b).

Given the promising in vitro and in vivo efficacy data, a comprehensive pharmacokinetic and toxicokinetic program was undertaken to determine the safety profile of this drug and to establish a safe starting dose in humans.

Selection of an Animal Model

In order to establish a pharmacologically relevant model for use in toxicology studies, several animal species (mouse, rat, and dog) including non-human primates (cynomolgus monkey, Rhesus monkey, and chimpanzee) were screened for binding cross-reactivity with VB6-845 through immunohistochemical analysis. With the exception of chimpanzees, no tissue cross-reactivity was observed. Given the ethical concerns surrounding the use of chimpanzees, this species was not considered suitable for toxicological testing. Therefore, it was determined that VB6-845 would not be pharmacologically active in terms of EpCAM binding in species typically used to conduct toxicology studies. This outcome was expected and observed in a previous preclinical evaluation of an EpCAM targeting scFv linked to *Pseudomonas* ETA [47, 48]. Consequently, the Sprague–Dawley rat was chosen for single-dose toxicological testing as it represented a well-characterized model for immunotoxin testing and in the case of some ETA-based immunotoxins has shown symptoms closely resembling VLS in humans [49, 50]. Given the lack of a cross-reactive species, it was decided that a second repeat-dose toxicity study would be performed in a non-human primate model (cynomolgus monkey) to provide another level of safety that would mimic the treatment regimen and route of administration to be used in the clinic. This same approach was used in the repeated-dose toxicology testing of the ADC Mylotarg, where its target antigen was only expressed in humans and larger primates [51]. It is important to note that subsequent to this study, IHC S6 regulations were amended to stipulate that tissue cross-reactivity is not an appropriate criterion for selecting a relevant species for the safety evaluation of immunotherapeutics.

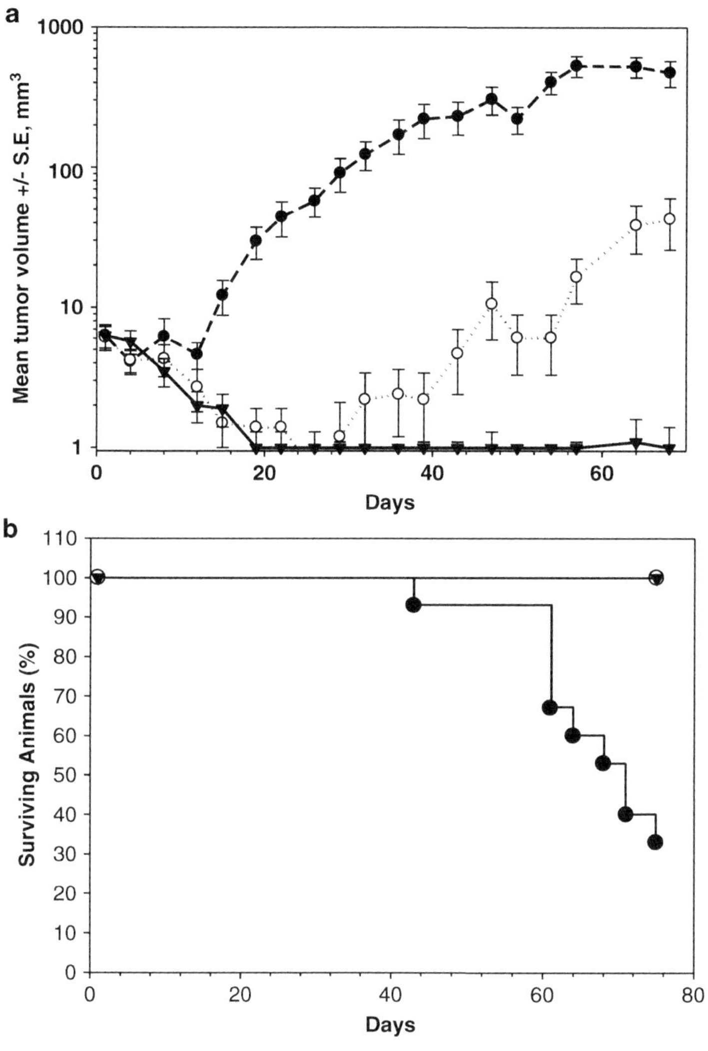

Fig. 19.2 Median tumor growth curves and survival plots. (**a**) NIH:OVCAR-3 human ovarian xenografts were generated from tumor fragments implanted subcutaneously into the flank of each mouse. On Day 1 of the study (8 days post-implantation), mice were randomly sorted into three groups ($n=15$). Group 1, untreated mice (*filled circles*), served as tumor growth controls. Mice in Groups 2 (*open circles*) and 3 (*inverted filled triangle*) received 10 and 20 mg/kg doses, respectively, administered on a 5-days-on, 2-days-off cycle for 3 weeks, followed by twice weekly for 4 weeks. The route of administration was a bolus intravenous (*IV*) injection into the tail vein until Day 26, followed by intraperitoneal (*IP*) injection for the remaining doses due to tail swelling. Animals were monitored for tumor size and were euthanized when their tumors reached the endpoint volume (750 mm^3) or on the last day of the study, Day 75. Animals dosed at 20 mg/kg showed no increase in median tumor volume, $p<0.001$. Reprinted with permission from Cizeau et al. [34]. (**B**) Kaplan–Meier survival plots. Animals from both treatment groups survived beyond the end of the study

Transgenic animals were also considered; however, their pattern of EpCAM expression was different when compared to humans and they were therefore unsuitable as pharmacologically relevant models [52–54].

Animal Toxicology Studies

Single-Dose Toxicology in Sprague–Dawley Rats

Sprague–Dawley rats (three/sex/dose) were administered a single IV bolus of VB6-845 via the lateral tail vein at doses of 6.25, 25, 50, 100, or 200 mg/kg, followed by a 2-week observation period. No overt adverse clinical signs were observed in animals administered up to and including 100 mg/kg of VB6-845. However, rats administered 200 mg/kg demonstrated clinical signs that included excessive licking of forepaws, reddened skin on fore and hind paws, edema of the forepaws, and a slight decrease in activity level. Rats in both the 100 and 200 mg/kg dose groups showed less body weight gain when compared to the control group.

Dose-dependent increases in alanine aminotransferase (ALT) and aspartate aminotransferase (AST) levels were detected following the administration of VB6-845 at 100 and 200 mg/kg. In both treatment groups, the changes in hepatic function were transient as AST returned to control levels by Day 8, and ALT returned to control levels by Day 15. On the basis of the elevated AST and ALT levels, as well as the paw oedema, the MTD was determined to be 200 mg/kg. The no-observable-adverse-effect level (NOAEL) for VB6-845 was determined to be 100 mg/kg. From these results, a repeated-dose toxicology study was undertaken in a non-human primate model mimicking the proposed clinical strategy for drug delivery.

Repeated-Dose Toxicology in Cynomolgus Monkeys

A GLP study was conducted to evaluate the systemic effects of repeated doses of VB6-845 administered via IV infusion in cynomolgus monkeys. In all, four treatment groups of Two/sex/group were administered VB6-845 at 10, 30, 60, or 90 mg/kg on Days 1 and 8 with additional recovery groups of one/sex/group (administered 60 or 90 mg/kg) maintained for a 20-day recovery period. The test article was administered to all groups via a 3 h infusion on Days 1 and 8, at a dose volume of 10 mL/kg/h, to mimic the route and infusion time intended for the clinic. Given the foreign nature of VB6-845 in this species and the expected immune response, repeat dosing was limited to two treatments. Parameters monitored included mortality, clinical signs, and body weight and food consumption. Blood samples were collected for hematology and clinical chemistry evaluations as well as for the determination of the pharmacokinetic profile and immunogenicity of VB6-845. At the end of the study, complete necropsy examinations were performed and a standard panel of tissues was microscopically examined.

There were no mortalities or changes in body weight. Treatment-related clinical signs were limited to decreased activity and hunched posture following the second treatment at all dose levels, with no indication of a dose relationship. These clinical signs generally resolved by the next day. Red cell parameters (erythrocytes, hemoglobin, and hematocrit) were comparably decreased in all treatment groups on Day 7, and continued to decrease through Day 14 in the Recovery Group, suggestive of a test article-related effect. Increased reticulocytes on Day 14 were compatible with a delayed bone marrow regenerative response. Transient and reversible increases in liver enzymes (AST, ALT, and SDH) were observed throughout the treatment; however, the changes did not appear to be dose-dependent and resolved by Day 20 in the Recovery Group.

Histopathological changes related to the administration of VB6-845 were dose-dependent and were limited to the kidneys, liver, spleen (female only), and lymph nodes (female only). All treatment-related effects, with the exception of tubular degeneration at 60 and 90 mg/kg that was still ongoing, were resolved by the end of the observation period. Due to the lack of tissue cross-reactivity in this model, these findings would not be unexpected as these organs represent the primary routes of metabolic elimination for a protein of this size.

Based on the results, the NOAEL was determined to be 30 mg/kg and therefore used as the basis for calculating a safe starting dose in the clinic [55, 56]. A dose level of 30 mg/kg in cynomolgus monkeys approximates a 10 mg/kg dose in humans [55] and applying the generally accepted 1 log lower safety margin resulted in the starting dose for humans being set at 1 mg/kg.

Pharmacokinetics in Cynomolgus Monkeys

The toxicokinetic profile of VB6-845 was evaluated as part of the repeated-dose toxicology study in cynomolgus monkeys, using an ELISA. Plasma samples were taken from two males and two females in the main study group at 0, 0.5, 1, 2, 4, and 24 h following a 3 h infusion of 10, 30, 60, and 90 mg/kg of VB6-845. Analysis indicated a proportional relationship between dose level and pharmacokinetic parameters in samples collected on both Day 1 and Day 8 (Table 19.3). Dose escalation was directly proportional to the mean peak (C_{max}) as well as the extent of the exposure ($AUC_{(last)}$). Although C_{max} values increased in a dose proportional manner on both Day 1 and Day 8, peak exposure levels were lower on Day 8 at all dose levels. The lower C_{max} on Day 8 at all dose levels had an effect on clearance (CL) and volume distribution (V_d) that was most likely due to an immune response in the animals. The mean half-life ($t_{1/2}$) values of VB6-845 on Days 1 and 8 were 2.5 ± 0.1 and 2.4 ± 0.5 h, respectively. The half-life was in the expected range for a 77 kDa drug and was similar to that obtained in a previous study with VB4-845 an anti-EpCAM scFv-ETA immunotoxin [48]. Some variability was observed between males and females; however, a statistical difference could not be calculated due to the limited sample size in each dosing group. The approximate 2.5 h half-life of VB6-845 indicated that full clearance of the drug would be expected between doses when patients are administered a once-weekly dose.

Table 19.3 Pharmacokinetic parameters in Cynomolgus monkeys

Dose level (mg/kg)	Day	C_{max} (μg/mL)	$AUC_{(last)}$ (h μg/mL)	$t_{1/2}$ (h)	CL (mL/h/kg)	V_d (mL/kg)
10	1	139±30.8	801±348	2.4±0.1	14.5±6.4	50.9±24.4
	8	74.6±22.5	291±124	2.7±0.4	39.6±17.1	158±84.0
30	1	335±47.3	1,784±107	2.5±0.1	16.9±1.0	59.5±4.4
	8	245±49.6	792±160	2.7±0.6	39.1±8.3	147±14.9
60	1	716±134	3,682±415	2.6±0.1	16.4±1.9	62.0±6.5
	8	433.5±179	1,354±496	2.3±0.3	48.7±16.4	165±70.9
90	1	1,255±270	6,770±2214	2.5±0.1	14.2±3.7	51.1±15.3
	8	648±230	2,585±902	1.9±0.2	38.2±13.3	108±45.3

Data for males and females are combined. Values are means ± SD, $n=4$. C_{max} maximum observed drug concentration in plasma; $AUC_{(last)}$ area under the drug concentration–time curve from time 0 to time t, where t is the time of the last measurable plasma concentration; $t_{1/2}$ elimination; *CL* apparent plasma clearance; V_d apparent volume of distribution

Immunogenicity in Cynomolgus Monkeys

As both the antibody and toxin moieties of VB6-845 were foreign proteins to the cynomolgus monkeys, an immune response was expected and not considered predictive for humans. However, determining the immunogenic potential of protein therapeutics in animal models, particularly non-human primates, is important for identifying potential safety concerns that may arise in patients [57].

The immunogenicity of VB6-845 was evaluated in cynomolgus monkeys as part of the repeated-dose toxicology study with plasma samples taken from Main Study Group animals on Days 0 and 7 (Two/sex/dose) and from Recovery Group animals on Days 0, 7, 14, 21, and 28 (one male and one female per dose cohort) following IV administration of VB6-845. Samples were analyzed by ELISA to determine the presence of antibodies against the Fab fragment (4D5MOCB) and de-bouganin. Antibodies were detected 14 days after the first infusion with the majority of the response being directed towards the Fab portion of the molecule and to a lesser extent against the de-immunized bouganin moiety (Fig. 19.3). While this result demonstrated that de-bouganin was minimally immunogenic, a final assessment of the effectiveness of the de-immunization strategy can only be determined following repeat dosing in patients.

Summary of Preclinical Evaluation

The in vitro and in vivo preclinical data demonstrated the specificity and nanomolar potency of VB6-845 against EpCAM-positive cell lines and human tumor xenografts, respectively. A comprehensive toxicological program showed the safety and tolerability profile of VB6-845 and determined a safe starting dose of 1 mg/kg in the clinic.

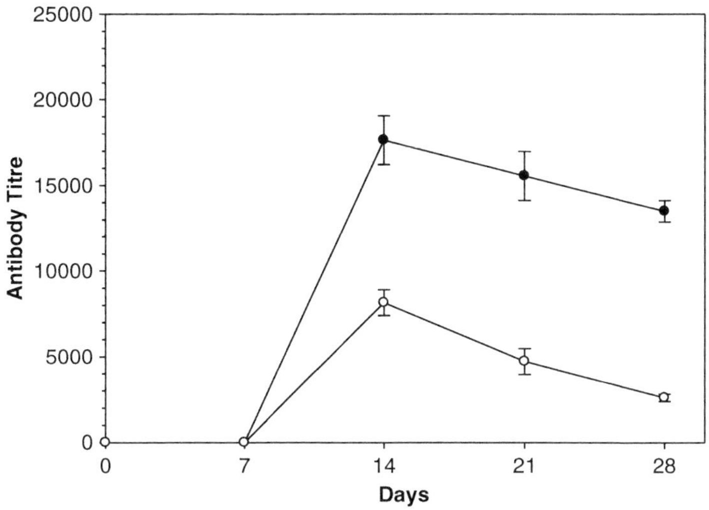

Fig. 19.3 Immunogenicity in Cynomolgous monkeys dosed at 90 mg/kg against the Fab fragment (*filled circles*) and de-bouganin (*open circles*). Mean antibody titers ± SE, $n=2$.

Clinical Experience with VB6-845

Study Design and Dose Escalation

The primary study objective of the Phase I trial was to determine the maximum tolerated dose (MTD) and evaluate the safety and tolerability of VB6-845 when administered as an IV monotherapy infusion, once weekly, in 4-week cycles. Secondary objectives included evaluating the pharmacokinetic profile, assessing exploratory efficacy, and in particular examining the immunogenicity of VB6-845.

Dose cohorts of a minimum of 3 subjects with EpCAM-positive, advanced refractory solid tumors of epithelial origin as detected by immunohistochemistry were entered into the study which was carried out at a total of six investigative sites. The occurrence of a dose-limiting toxicity (DLT) in a cohort required the expansion of that dose cohort to six subjects and subjects who discontinued from the study prior to having received a minimum of four doses of VB6-845 were replaced. The starting dose was defined as 1 mg/kg and doses were escalated, according to a modified Fibonacci design, until an MTD was reached. The MTD was defined as the highest dose at which <2 out of six patients experienced a DLT. Subjects continued to receive treatment until an unacceptable toxicity occurred, all lesions completely disappeared, disease progression was determined, or the study was terminated. Patients were assessed for safety by monitoring of adverse events (AEs), clinical laboratory tests, standard 12-lead ECGs, vital signs, and physical examinations. AEs were graded according to the National Cancer Institute Common Terminology Criteria for Adverse Events, version 3.0 (NCI CTC AE v3.0).

A total of 15 subjects were enrolled into the study with solid tumors that included renal, ovary, breast, gastric, pancreas, non-small cell lung, and colorectal cancers. Three subjects were enrolled at the first cohort dose level of 1 mg/kg, ten subjects at the second cohort dose level of 2 mg/kg, and two subjects at the third cohort dose level of 3.34 mg/kg. The study was terminated when sufficient data had been collected to assess the immunogenicity of VB6-845 (see below). The maximum treatment duration was 16 weeks.

Safety Evaluation

Only one DLT was reported. This event was a grade 4 acute infusion reaction which occurred in a subject (cohort 2 at 2.0 mg/kg) with metastatic renal cell carcinoma. The subject developed hypotension and weakness during the third infusion, which was assessed as probably related to VB6-845. The event responded well to medicated therapy and was considered to be resolved 1 day after onset, without any sequelae. The MTD of VB6-845 was not reached at the time of study termination.

Of the 15 subjects who received treatment, 5 subjects reported a total of 5 serious adverse events (SAEs). Two of the reported SAEs were reported as related to study treatment. Both treatment-related SAEs were infusion reactions and consisted of a symptom complex characterized in both cases by hypotension, fever, and nausea, and on an individual basis included dizziness, weakness, drowsiness, chills, and hyperemia of the face and neck. The first infusion reaction event was grade 3 and resolved with standard therapy. The subject continued subsequent VB6-845 infusions with corticosteroid and H1 and H2-receptor antagonist pre-medication; the second event was grade 4 and assessed as the single reported DLT, as described above. The subject was discontinued from the study in accordance with the protocol treatment stopping criteria.

Due to the early closure of the trial, adverse event results are based on data available in the clinical database at the time of study termination. At least one treatment-related AE (defined as possibly, probably, or definitely related) was experienced by ten subjects. The majority of the treatment-related AEs reported were assessed as mild or moderate in severity and resolved within 1–2 days. The most frequently reported treatment-related AEs were associated with general disorders and administration site conditions. Within this group, pyrexia was reported most frequently.

Exploratory Efficacy Evaluation

A secondary endpoint of the study was to make an exploratory assessment of efficacy. Patients had full imaging performed (including, but not limited to, the chest, abdomen, pelvis, and bone architecture) at baseline in order to establish all existing lesions using standard imaging techniques (CT/MRI for chest, abdomen, and pelvis; and a bone scan for bone architecture with following CT/MRI if bone scan is positive for any lesions). Post-baseline assessments of all sites of disease were made every 4 weeks using the same techniques as used at baseline. Up to ten sites of measurable disease were identified as "target" lesions for the assessment of tumor response. Non-radiographically measurable tumors were assessed for a clinical response by the Investigator.

Exploratory efficacy data reported on seven subjects enrolled in cohorts 1 and 2 who completed one full cycle (4 weeks) of treatment revealed encouraging preliminary results. Five of the seven subjects showed stable disease on CT scans 1 week after the completion of the fourth dose. Of the three subjects who continued to receive study treatment past the first cycle, one subject continued to have stable disease at the completion of their second (8 weeks) and third (12 weeks) cycles. In addition, objective tumor responses, based on data reported by the investigative sites at the time of study termination, demonstrated a decrease in measurable target tumor size in two patients in the second dose cohort; one with renal cell carcinoma and another with breast carcinoma. At baseline, the subject with renal cell carcinoma had six measurable target lesions in the lungs, as well as a measurable target lesion in a pulmonary lymph node and the pelvic mesentery. At the final visit (following the week 3 infusion), reported CT scan results showed decreases in all measurable target lesions, with decreases in individual lesions ranging from 11 to 29%. Other nontarget, nonmeasurable lesions appeared unchanged and the appearance of a potentially new brain lesion (inaccessible to VB6-845 therapy) was noted. At baseline, the subject with breast carcinoma had five measurable target lesions in the liver as well as three additional measurable target lymph nodes in the mediastinal, pre-tracheal, and bifurcational areas. CT scan results reported following the completion of 4 weekly infusions of VB6-845 revealed decreases in four of the five measurable target lesions in the liver, with decreases in individual lesions ranging from 4 to 15%. Nontarget, nonmeasurable lesions in lungs, liver, and bones were reported as stable.

Pharmacokinetics

Patient blood samples were taken for pharmacokinetic analysis on weeks 1 and 3 before, during, and after the 3 h infusion; analysis was completed only for the 1 and 2 mg/kg cohorts. The slow infusion rate was chosen to avoid a cytokine response and to maintain an elevated drug plasma concentration for a longer period of time than would have been achieved with a bolus injection. Sampling was performed according to the following schedule: pre-infusion, midpoint infusion (1.5 h), end of infusion, post-infusion 10 and 30 min; and 1, 2, 4, 6, 8, 12, and 24 h post-dose. The level of VB6-845 was measured using a GLP-validated, MTS-based potency assay. The assay detected VB6-845-mediated killing of CAL-27 cells, an EpCAM-positive cell line, and the IC_{50} values obtained are directly proportional to the concentration of intact drug; the lower detection limit of the assay was 14 pg/mL.

Table 19.4a Pharmacokinetic parameters in patients

Dose level (mg/kg)	Week	C_{max} (μg/mL)	$t_{1/2}$ (h)	$AUC_{(last)}$ (h μg/mL)	Cl (mL/h/kg)	V_d (mL/kg)
1	1	9.6±2.3	3.8±1.3	35.2±13.3	30.8±9.5	183±99.6
	3	1.4±1.8	2.2±1.6	4.6±6.1	859±936	4,020±5970
2	1	16.3±5.8	4.9±1.5	60.3±24.8	40.5±22.8	309±245
	3	10.9±9.6	2.6±2.2	41.7±46.5	299±399	552±503

Data for males and females are combined. Values are means±SD. C_{max}, maximum observed drug concentration in plasma; $t_{1/2}$ elimination half-life; $AUC_{(last)}$ area under the drug concentration–time curve from time 0 to time *t*, where *t* is the time of the last measurable plasma concentration; *CL* apparent plasma clearance; V_d apparent volume of distribution

Table 19.4b Kinetics of VB6-845 plasma clearance in patients

	Mean VB6-845 plasma concentration (nM)							
Dose level (mg/kg)	Infusion time interval		Post-infusion time intervals (h)					
	Pre-dose	Infusion-3 h	1	2	4	8	12	24
1	N/A	123.95 (206.6)	63.53 (105.9)	39.07 (65.1)	15.50 (25.8)	2.68 (4.5)	1.02 (1.7)	0.2 (0.3)
2	N/A	196.93 (328.2)	108.98 (181.6)	52.15 (86.9)	21.98 (36.6)	3.80 (6.3)	1.46 (2.43)	0.41 (0.68)

Values in parentheses represent the fold increase in nM concentration of VB6-845 expressed as a function of the VB6-845 IC_{50} concentration versus ovarian carcinoma cell line NIH:OVCAR-3

Standard pharmacokinetic parameters were determined for both dose levels (Table 19.4a). The maximum concentration (C_{max}) measured for patients dosed at 1 mg/kg ranged from 8.08–12.26 μg/mL in week 1 to 0.07–3.50 μg/mL at week 3. For patients dosed at the 2 mg/kg level, the C_{max} values ranged from 4.76–23.2 μg/mL in week 1 to 1.15–21.6 μg/mL at week 3. The mean maximal plasma concentration for both dose cohorts was at the end of the 3 h infusion. A comparison of the two dose cohorts indicated a dose proportionality that was concentration dependent similar to that observed in the non-human primate study. The mean elimination time ($t_{1/2}$) for patients dosed at 1 mg/kg was 3.8 h on week 1 and 2.2 h on week 3 and for the 2 mg/kg group was 4.9 h on week 1 and subsequently 2.6 h on week 3. The peak exposure levels and half-life of VB6-845 were lower in all patients by week 3; however, the reduction was considerably less in the 2 mg/kg group. VB6-845 was cleared fairly rapidly within the first 24 h following infusion consistent with its molecular size. The highest concentration of drug detected for each dose cohort was >2 logs over the IC_{50} value of VB6-845 (0.6 nM) versus the ovarian carcinoma cell line NIH:OVCAR-3, whereas the lowest drug concentration at the 24 h time point approximated the IC_{50} concentration (Table 19.4b).

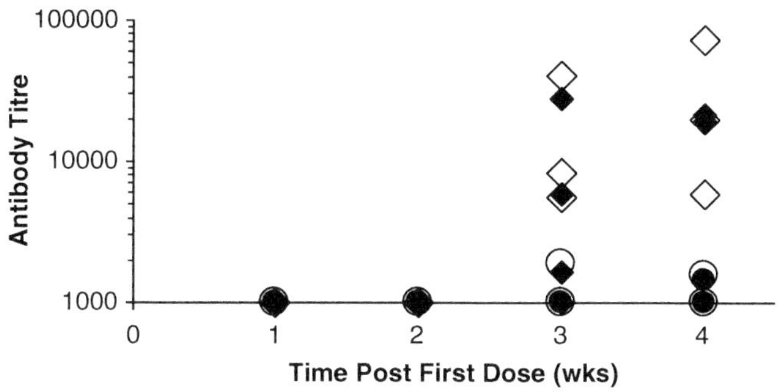

Fig. 19.4 Antibody titers measured against de-bouganin (1 mg cohort (*filled circles*); 2 mg cohort (*open circles*) and the Fab moiety (1 mg cohort (*open diamonds*); 2 mg cohort (*filled diamonds*)) of VB6-845. For 1 mg cohort n=3 for all weeks. For 2 mg cohort, n=9 for weeks 1 and 2, n=4 for week 3, and n=2 for week 4

Immunogenicity

To assess the effectiveness of the bouganin de-immunization strategy, patient plasma samples were tested for immune responsiveness to the humanized Fab and de-bouganin portions of VB6-845 (Fig. 19.4). No measurable antibody titers were directed against either molecule in any of the patients after 2 weeks. A relatively weak anti-de-bouganin titer was measured in only one of the patients after the first 3 weeks of treatment, as compared to six of seven patients who showed anti-Fab titers at the same time point. By week 4, all patients from both dose cohorts had measurable anti-Fab titers (mean titer=27,858±25,744, n=5). In contrast, only two of these patients had berely detectable anti-de-bouganin titers (mean titer 1,513±65.1). The lack of immune responsiveness towards de-bouganin, a totally foreign protein, in these patients illustrates the validity of the T cell epitope-depletion approach to dampen the immune response and strongly supports the utility of de-bouganin as a cytotoxic payload for systemic delivery. Even though the CDR loops of the mouse anti-EpCAM antibody were grafted onto a humanized framework, immune reactivity is not necessarily unexpected as humanized and even fully human antibodies can exhibit some degree of immunogenicity in the clinic [58]. The strength and degree of this antibody response on efficacy and/or safety will often depend upon the antibody itself and the indication being treated. In order to reintroduce VB6-845 to the clinic, the T cell epitopes of the Fab fragment have been identified and removed while preserving specificity and potency.

Summary

The potency and efficacy of immunotoxins as cancer therapeutics, particularly for treating cancers of hematologic origin, have been well demonstrated over the last two decades. However, the clinical effectiveness of immunotoxins for solid cancer therapy has been limited by their immunogenicity directed primarily at the toxin moiety. VB6-845 was well tolerated and showed preliminary efficacy in the exploratory Phase I trial. The clinical data supported the continued development of VB6-845 as a promising new therapy for advanced solid tumors of epithelial origin. An important endpoint of this study was to assess the immunogenicity of VB6-845 as the appearance of ADAs would reduce the number of treatment cycles and limit clinical benefit. The study showed the de-bouganin payload to be of low immunogenic potential with a minimal de-bouganin response and therefore represents a first-in-man demonstration of a successfully de-immunized protein toxin. On the strength of the clinical experience with VB6-845, Viventia is currently evaluating several Fab-de-bouganin molecules specific to solid tumors. These antibodies were characterized using an immune driven antibody platform which comprises a novel screening method to generate fully human antibody fragments, thus circumventing the need to de-immunize the targeting moiety [59]. Reducing or completely ablating the appearance of anti-toxin antibodies with de-immunization strategies will permit a true assessment of the clinical benefit of immunotoxins in targeted cancer therapy.

References

1. Carter PJ, Senter PD (2008) Antibody-drug conjugates for cancer therapy. Cancer J 14(3):154–69
2. Boyiadzis M, Foon KA (2008) Approved monoclonal antibodies for cancer therapy. Expert Opin Biol Ther 8(8):1151–58
3. Ross JS, Gray K, Gray GS, Worland PJ, Rolfe M (2003) Anticancer antibodies. Am J Clin Pathol 119:472–85
4. Teicher BA (2009) Antibody-drug conjugate targets. Curr Cancer Drug Targets 9:982–1004
5. Hellström I, Hellström KE, Siegall CB, Trail PA (1995) Immunoconjugates and immunotoxins for therapy of carcinomas. Adv Pharmacol 33:349–88
6. Reiter Y (2001) Recombinant immunotoxins in targeted cancer cell therapy. Adv Cancer Res 81:93–124
7. Stirpe F, Battelli MG (2006) Ribosome-inactivating proteins: progress and problems. Cell Mol Life Sci 63:1850–66
8. Kreitman RJ (2006) Immunotoxins for targeted cancer therapy. AAPS J 8(3):E532–51
9. Van Arnum P (2008) Antibody drug conjugates: a marriage of biologics and small molecules. Pharm Technol. http://pharmtech.findpharma.com/pharmtech/Ingredients+Insider/Antibody-Drug-Conjugates-A-Marriage-of-Biologics-a/ArticleStandard/Article/detail/522139. Accessed 5 Nov 2010
10. Turturro F (2007) Denileukin diftitox: a biotherapeutic paradigm shift in the treatment of lymphoid-derived disorders. Expert Rev Anticancer Ther 7(1):11–17
11. Phillips GD, Li G, Duggar DL, Crocker LM, Parsons KL, Mai E, Blattler WA, Lambert JM, Chari RV, Lutz RJ, Wong WL, Jacobson FS, Koeppen H, Schwall RH, Kenkare-Mitra SR, Spencer SD, Sliwkowski MX (2008) Targeting HER2-positive breast cancer with Trastuzumab-DM1 an antibody-cytotoxic drug conjugate. Cancer Res 68(22):9280–9290
12. Kreitman RJ, Pastan I (2006) Immunotoxins in the treatment of hematologic malignancies. Curr Drug Targets 7(10):1301–11
13. Wayne AS, Kreitman RJ, Findley HW, Lew G, Delbrook C, Steinberg SM, Stetler-Stevenson M, FitzGerald DJ, Pastan I (2010) Anti-CD22 immunotoxin RFB4(dsFv)-PE38 (BL22) for

CD22-positive hematologic malignancies of childhood: preclinical studies and Phase I clinical trial. Clin Cancer Res 16(6):1894–1903
14. Frankel AE (2004) Reducing the immune response to immuntotoxin. Commentary re R. Hassan et al., Pretreatment with Rituximab does not inhibit the human immune response against the immunogenic protein LMB-1. Clin Cancer Res 10:13–15
15. MacDonald GC, Glover N (2005) Effective tumor targeting: strategies for the delivery of armed antibodies. Curr Opin Drug Discov Devel 8(2):177–83
16. Niv R, Cohen CJ, Denkberg G, Segal D, Reiter Y (2001) Antibody engineering for targeted therapy of cancer: recombinant Fv-immunotoxins. Curr Pharm Biotechnol 2:19–46
17. Brinkmann U, Keppler-Hafkemeyer A, Hafkemeyer P (2001) Recombinant immunotoxins for cancer therapy. Expert Opin Biol Ther 1(4):693–702
18. Li Z, Yu T, Zhao P, Ma J (2005) Immunotoxins and cancer therapy. Cell Mol Immunol 2(2):106–12
19. Pastan I, Hassan R, FitzGerald DJ, Kreitman RJ (2007) Immunotoxin treatment of cancer. Annu Rev Med 58:221–37
20. MacDonald GC, Rasamoelisolo M, Entwistle J, Cizeau J, Bosc D, Cuthbert W, Kowalski M, Spearman M, Glover N (2008) A Phase I clinical study of VB4-845: weekly intratumoral administration of an anti-EpCAM recombinant fusion protein in patients with sqamous cell carcinoma of the head and neck. Drug Des Dev Ther 2:105–14
21. MacDonald GC, Rasamoelisolo M, Entwistle J, Cuthbert W, Kowalski M, Spearman MA, Glover N (2009) A Phase I clinical study of intratumorally administered VB4-845, an anti-epithelial cell adhesion molecule recombinant fusion protein, in patients with squamous cell carcinoma of the head and neck. Med Oncol 26(3):257–64
22. Kowalski M, Entwistle J, Cizeau J, Niforos D, Loewen S, Chapman W, MacDonald GC (2010) A phase I study of an intravesically administered immunotoxin targeting EpCAM for the treatment of non muscle-invasive bladder cancer in BCG-refractory and BCG-intolerant patients. Drug Des Devel Ther 4:313–20
23. Tsutsumi Y, Onda M, Nagata S, Lee B, Kreitman RJ, Pastan I (2000) Site-specific chemical modification with polyethylene glycol of recombinant immunotoxin anti-Tac(Fv)-PE38 (LMB-2) improves antitumor activity and reduces animal toxicity and immunogenicity. Proc Natl Acad Sci USA 97(15):8548–53
24. Onda M, Beers R, Xiang L, Nagata S, Wang Q, Pastan I (2008) An immunotoxin with greatly reduced immunogenicity by identification and removal of B cell epitopes. Proc Natl Acad Sci USA 105(32):11311–16
25. Nagata S, Pastan I (2009) Removal of B cell epitopes as a practical approach for reducing the immunogenicity of foreign protein-based therapeutics. Adv Drug Deliv Rev 61(11):977–85
26. De Groot AS, Scott DW (2007) Immunogenicity of protein therapeutics. Trends Immunol 28(11):482–90
27. Stas P, Lasters I (2009) Strategies for preclinical immunogenicity assessment of protein therapeutics. IDrugs 12(3):169–73
28. Baker MP, Reynolds HM, Lumicisi B, Bryson CJ (2010) Immunogenicity of protein therapeutics the key causes, consequences and challenges. Self/Nonself 1(4):314–22
29. Bolognesi A, Barbieri L, Carnicelli D, Abbondanza A, Cenini P, Falasca AI, Dinota A, Stirpe F (1989) Purification and properties of a new ribosome-inactivating protein with RNA *N*-glycosidase activity suitable for immunotoxin preparation from the seeds of *Momordica cochinchinensis*. Biochim Biophys Acta 993:287–92
30. Bolognesi A, Barbieri L, Abbondanza A, Falasca AI, Carnicelli D, Battelli MG, Stirpe F (1990) Purification and properties of new ribosome-inactivating proteins with RNA *N*-glycosidase activity. Biochim Biophys Acta 1087:293–302
31. Barbieri L, Battelli MG, Stirpe F (1993) Ribosome-inactivating proteins from plants. Biochim Biophys Acta 1154:237–82
32. Bolognesi A, Polito L, Tazzari PL, Lemoli RM, Lubelli C, Fogli M, Boon L, De Boer M, Stirpe F (2000) *In vitro* anti-tumour activity of anti-CD80 and anti-CD86 immunotoxins containing type 1 ribosome-inactivating proteins. Br J Haematol 110:351–61

33. den Hartog MT, Lubelli C, Boon L, Heerkens S (2002) Ortiz Buijsse AP, de Boer M, Stirpe F. Cloning and expression of cDNA coding for bouganin. A type-I ribosome-inactivating protein from *Bougainvillea spectabilis* Willd. Eur J Biochem 269:1772–79
34. Cizeau J, Grenkow DM, Brown JG, Entwistle J, MacDonald GC (2009) Engineering and biological characterization of VB6-845, an anti-EpCAM immunotoxin containing a T-cell epitope-depleted variant of the plant toxin bouganin. J Immunother 32(6):574–84
35. Willuda J, Honegger A, Waibel R, Schubiger A, Stahel R, Zangemeister-Wittke U, Pluckthun A (1999) High thermal stability is essential for tumor targeting of antibody fragments: engineering of a humanized anti-epithelial glycoprotein-2 (epithelial cell adhesion molecule) single-chain Fv fragment. Cancer Res 59:5758–67
36. Litvinov SV, van Driel W, van Rhijn CM, Bakker HAM, van Krieken H, Fleuren GJ, Warnaar SO (1996) Expression of Ep-CAM in cervical squamous epithelia correlates with an increased proliferation and the disappearance of markers for terminal differentiation. Am J Pathol 148(3):865–75
37. Went P, Dirnhofer S, Schöpf D, Moch H, Spizzo G (2008) Expression and prognostic significance of EpCAM. J Cancer Mol 3(6):169–74
38. Ralhan R, Cao J, Lim T, MacMillan C, Freeman JL, Walfish PG (2010) EpCAM nuclear localization identifies aggressive thyroid cancer and is a marker for poor prognosis. BMC Cancer 10:331–41
39. Momburg F, Moldenhauer G, Hämmerling GJ, Möller P (1987) Immunohistochemical study of the expression of a M_r 34,000 human epithelium-specific surface glycoprotein in normal and malignant tissues. Cancer Res 47:2883–91
40. Ogura E, Senzaki H, Yoshizawa K, Hioki K, Tsubura A (1998) Immunohistochemical localization of epithelial glycoprotein EGP-2 and carcinoembryonic antigen in normal colonic mucosa and colorectal tumors. Anticancer Res 18:3669–75
41. Xie X, Wang C, Cao Y, Wang W, Zhuang R, Chen L, Dang N, Fang L, Jin B (2005) Expression pattern of epithelial cell adhesion molecule on normal and malignant colon tissues. World J Gastroenterol 11(3):344–47
42. Münz M, Kieu C, Mack B, Schmitt B, Zeidler R, Gires O (2004) The carcinoma-associated antigen EpCAM upregulates c-*myc* and induces cell proliferation. Oncogene 23:5748–58
43. Food and Drug Administration (FDA) (1997) Points to consider in the manufacture and testing of monoclonal antibody products for human use
44. Balzar M, Winter MJ, de Boer CJ, Litvinov SV (1999) The biology of the 17-1A antigen (Ep-CAM). J Mol Med 77:699–712
45. Winter MJ, Nagtegaal ID, Han J, van Krieken JM, Litvinov SV (2003) The epithelial cell adhesion molecule (Ep-CAM) as a morphoregulatory molecule is a tool in surgical pathology. Am J Pathol 163(6):2139–48
46. Went PTH, Lugli A, Meier S, Bundi M, Mirlacher M, Sauter G, Dirnhofer S (2004) Frequent EpCam protein expression in human carcinomas. Hum Pathol 35(1):122–28
47. Brown JG, Entwistle J, Glover N, MacDonald GC (2008) Preclinical safety evaluation of immunotoxins. In: Cavagnaro JA (ed) Preclinical safety evaluation of biopharmaceuticals. A science-based approach to facilitating clinical trials. John Wiley & Sons, Hoboken, NJ, pp 649–68
48. Brown J, Rasamoelisolo M, Spearman M, Bosc D, Cizeau J, Entwistle J, MacDonald GC (2009) Preclinical assessment of an anti-EpCAM immunotoxin: locoregional delivery provides a safer alternative to systemic administration. Cancer Biother Radiopharm 24(4):477–87
49. Siegall CB, Liggitt D, Chace D, Tepper MA, Fell HP (1994) Prevention of immunotoxin-mediated vascular leak syndrome in rats with retention of antitumor activity. Proc Natl Acad Sci USA 91(20):9514–18
50. Frankel AE, Kreitman RJ, Sausville EA (2000) Targeted toxins. Clin Cancer Res 6:326–34
51. Bross PF, Beitz J, Chen G, Chen XH, Duffy E, Kieffer L, Roy S, Sridhara R, Rahman A, Williams G, Pazdur R (2001) Approval summary: gemtuzumab ozogamicin in relapsed acute myeloid leukemia. Clin Cancer Res 7:1490–96
52. McLaughlin PMJ, Kroesen B, Dokter WHA, van der Molen H, de Groot M, Brinker MGL, Kok K, Ruiters MHJ, Buys CHCM, de Leij LFMH (1999) An EGP-2/Ep-CAM-expressing

transgenic rat model to evaluate antibody-mediated immunotherapy. Cancer Immunol Immunother 48:303–11
53. McLaughlin PMJ, Harmsen MC, Dokter WH, Kroesen B, van der Molen H, Brinker MGL, Hollema H, Ruiters MHJ, Buys CHCM, de Leij LFMH (2001) The epithelial glycoprotein 2 (EGP-2) promoter-driven epithelial-specific expression of EGP-2 in transgenic mice: a new model to study carcinoma-directed immunotherapy. Cancer Res 61(10):4105–11
54. Mosolits S, Campbell F, Litvinov SV, Fagerberg J, Crowe JS, Mellstedt H, Ellis JH (2004) Targeting human Ep-CAM in transgenic mice by anti-idiotype and antigen based vaccines. Int J Cancer 112:669–77
55. Food and Drug Administration (FDA) (2005) Estimating the safe starting dose in clinical trial for therapeutics in adult healthy volunteers
56. Food and Drug Administration (FDA) (2006) General guide for starting dose selection for a cytotoxic agent in cancer patients. Available from http://www.fda.gov/cder/cancer/docs/doseflow.pdf. Accessed on 3 Nov 2010
57. Wierda D, Smith HW, Zwickl CM (2001) Immunogenicity of biopharmaceuticals in laboratory animals. Toxicology 158:71–74
58. Harding FA, Stickler MM, Razo J, DuBridge RB (2010) The immunogenicity of humanized and fully human antibodies. Residual immunogenicity resides in the CDR regions. mAbs 2(3):256–65
59. Cizeau J, Torres MGP, Cowling SG, Stibbard S, Premsukh A, Entwistle J, MacDonald GC (2011) Fusogenics: a recombinant immunotoxin-based screening platform to select internalizing tumor-specific antibody fragments. J Biomol Screen 16(1):90–100

Index

G.L. Phillips (ed.), *Antibody-Drug Conjugates and Immunotoxins: From Pre-Clinical Development to Therapeutic Applications*, Cancer Drug Discovery and Development,
DOI 10.1007/978-1-4614-5456-4,

GPSR Compliance

The European Union's (EU) General Product Safety Regulation (GPSR) is a set of rules that requires consumer products to be safe and our obligations to ensure this.

If you have any concerns about our products, you can contact us on ProductSafety@springernature.com

In case Publisher is established outside the EU, the EU authorized representative is:

Springer Nature Customer Service Center GmbH
Europaplatz 3
69115 Heidelberg, Germany

Batch number: 10755329

Printed by Printforce, the Netherlands